INDUSTRIAL PHARMACY
A Textbook

INDUSTRIAL PHARMACY
A Textbook

Marina Koland
Professor & Head
Anoop Narayanan V
D.S. Sandeep
Assistant Professor
Department of Pharmaceutics
NGSM Institute of Pharmaceutical Sciences
'Nitte (Deemed to be University)', Mangalore, Karnataka

R. Harshitha
Assistant Professor
Department of Pharmaceutics
Vivekananda College of Pharmacy
Bengaluru, Karnataka

M.P. Gowrav
Assistant Professor
Department of Pharmaceutics
JSS College of Pharmacy
Mysuru, Karnataka

I.K. International Pvt. Ltd.
NEW DELHI

Published by
I.K. International Pvt. Ltd.
4435-36/7, Ansari Road, Daryaganj
New Delhi-110 002 (India)
E-mail: info@ikinternational.com
Website: www.ikbooks.com

ISBN 978-93-90620-65-4

Published by Krishan Makhijani for I.K. International Pvt. Ltd., 4435-36/7, Ansari Road, Daryaganj, New Delhi-110 002 and Printed by Rekha Printers Pvt. Ltd., Okhla Industrial Area, Phase II, New Delhi–110 020.

PREFACE

Industrial Pharmacy is meant for the B.Pharm students. It gives a simplified narrative of the formulation, processing and evaluation of various pharmaceutical dosage forms manufactured by the pharmaceutical industry. The pharmaceutical industry is also involved in drug discovery, and drug development followed by quality control and quality assurance aspects of pharmaceuticals and other drug products. These activities must be in conformity with standard regulations. This book covers all the topics prescribed in the syllabus for the Bachelor of Pharmacy (B.Pharm) program (Semester Scheme) by the Pharmacy Council of India (PCI) of course regulations 2014.

The first half of the book describes the formulation, manufacture, and quality control of tablets, capsules, parenteral dosage forms, liquid orals, ophthalmic dosage forms and aerosols. The additives and vehicles used in the formulation have been described with adequate examples. Labelled figures of equipment used in the manufacture with descriptions are also included. In addition, topics such as 'Pre-formulation', 'Cosmetics' and 'Packaging Material Science' have also been briefly discussed.

The second half of the book has been designed with the objective of imparting knowledge of the pilot plant scale-up considerations of different dosage forms. The student will be able to understand the technology transfer process from R & D to production with the necessary documentation. This subject also provides brief information about drug regulations, roles and responsibilities of drug regulatory professionals, and different regulatory requirements such as ANDA, and NDA that are required for the approval of clinical trials on new drugs for their registration. Quality management systems (QMSs) and the organizational structure, responsibilities of Indian drug regulatory authority (CDSCO) along with its regulatory requirements and approval procedures for new drugs in India can also be well understood from the subject. There are 12 chapters as per the course content of the syllabus for Industrial Pharmacy-I and 5 chapters as per Industrial Pharmacy-II. Each chapter is provided with 5 to 6 learning objectives and a set of review questions at the end.

We, the contributing authors, do hope that this book would provide to the B.Pharm student, all the information necessary to study for the examinations.

Authors

CONTENTS

Preface *v*

1. PREFORMULATION STUDIES **1**

1.1 Introduction 1
1.2 Objectives and Goals of Preformulation Studies 1
1.3 Physical Properties 2
1.3.1 Physical Forms 2
1.3.2 Particle Size and Surface Area 3
1.3.3 Determination of Particle Size 4
1.3.4 Particle Shape 4
1.3.5 Shape Factor to Determine the Shape of a Particle 4
1.3.6 Powder Flow Property 5
1.3.7 Solubility **8**
1.4 Chemical Properties 11
1.4.1 Hydrolysis 11
1.4.2 Ester Hydrolysis 12
1.4.3 Oxidation 12
1.4.4 Racemisation Reaction or Optical Isomerisation 13
1.4.5 Polymerisation 13
1.5 Biopharmaceutical Classification System (BCS) 14
1.5.1 Significance of BCS Classification 15
1.5.2 Application of Preformulation Considerations in the Development of Solid, Liquid Oral and Parenteral Dosage Form and Its Impact on Stability of Dosage Forms 15
Review Questions *16*

2. TABLETS **17**

2.1 Introduction 17
2.2 Ideal Characteristics of Tablets 17
2.3 Classification of Tablets 18
2.3.1 Tablets Ingested Orally 18
2.3.2 Tablets Used in Oral Cavity 19
2.3.3 Tablets Administered by Other Routes 19
2.3.4 Tablets Used to Prepare Solutions 19
2.4 Tablet Excipients and Formulation 20
2.5 Manufacturing of Tablets 22
2.5.1 Direct Compression 22
2.5.2 Compression Granulation 23

2.6 Wet or Moist Granulation 26
2.6.1 Weighing and Blending 26
2.6.2 Preparing the Damp Mass 27
2.6.3 Screening the Damp Mass into Pellets or Granules 28
2.6.4 Sizing the Granulation by Dry Screening 28
2.6.5 Adding Lubrication and Blending 28
2.7 Equipment and Tablet Tooling 28
2.8 Tablet Compression Machines 30
2.8.1 Single Punch Tablet Press 31
2.8.2 Components/Functional Parts of a Single Punch Tablet Press 31
2.8.3 Advantages of the Single Punch Tablet Press 32
2.9 Multi-Station Press or Rotary Tablet Machine 32
2.9.1 Features of the Rotary Press 32
2.10 Working of the Rotary Press and the Tablet Compression Cycle 33
2.10.1 Advantages of the Rotary Press 34
2.11 Compression and Processing Problems in Tablet Manufacturing (Tablet Defects) 34
2.11.1 Processing Problems 35
2.12 Quality Control Tests for Tablets: In-Process and Finished Product Tests 37
2.12.1 General Appearance 38
2.12.2 Organoleptic Properties 38
2.12.3 Strength Tests 39
2.12.4 Friability 40
2.12.5 Drug Content Tests 41
2.12.6 Uniformity of Drug Content 41
2.12.7 Drug Release Tests 42
2.13 Features of the USP Dissolution Test Apparatus 44
2.14 Dissolution Parameters 45
Review Questions *46*

3. TABLET COATING **47**

3.1 Introduction 47
3.2 Sugar Coating 47
3.2.1 Sugar Coating Process 49
3.3 Film Coating 50
3.3.1 Types of Film Coating Methods 50
3.4 Coating Equipment 52
3.4.1 Materials Used for Film Coating 55
3.5 General Formulation of Coating Solution 56
3.5.1 Film Formers: Synthetic Polymers 56
3.5.2 Solvents 58
3.5.3 Plasticizers 59
3.5.4 Colourants 59
3.5.5 Opaquant Extenders 60
3.6 Quality Control Test for Coated Tablet 60
3.6.1 Film Defects 60
3.7 Specialized Coating 61
Review Questions *62*

4. LIQUID ORALS 63

4.1 Introduction 63
4.2 Additives and Components 68
4.3 Formulation Components of Suspension 72
4.4 Manufacturing Considerations 73
4.4.1 Raw Materials 73
4.4.2 Equipment 74
4.4.3 Manufacturing Procedure 74
4.5 Filling and Packing of Liquid Orals 75
Review Questions *76*

5. HARD GELATIN CAPSULES 77

5.1 Introduction 77
5.2 Hard Gelatin Capsules 77
5.2.1 Production of Hard Gelatin Capsule Shells 78
5.2.2 Other Capsule Shell Components 79
5.2.3 Production of Capsule Shells 79
5.2.4 Sizes of Capsules 80
5.2.5 Formulation of Hard Gelatin Capsules 81
5.2.6 Filling of Hard Gelatin Capsules 81
5.2.7 Special Techniques in Capsules 83
5.2.8 Quality Control Tests for Capsules 84
Review Questions *84*

6. SOFT GELATIN CAPSULES 85

6.1 Introduction 85
6.1.1 Advantages 85
6.1.2 Disadvantages 85
6.1.3 Composition of Soft Gelatin Capsules 86
6.1.4 Formulation of Soft Gelatin Capsules 86
6.1.5 Manufacturing of Soft Gelatin Capsule 87
6.1.6 Quality Control Test for Capsules 88
6.1.7 Packaging and Storage Stability for Capsules 89
Review Questions *89*

7. PELLETS 90

7.1 Introduction 90
7.1.1 Advantages of Pellets 90
7.1.2 Technological Advantages 90
7.1.3 Therapeutic Advantages 91
7.1.4 Limitations of Pellets 91
7.2 Pelletization Techniques 91
7.2.1 Extrusion/Spheronization 91
7.2.2 Hot Melt Extrusion 93
7.2.3 Layering Techniques 94

7.2.4 Dry Powder Layering 94
7.2.5 Balling 94
7.2.6 Compression 94
7.2.7 Globulation 94
7.2.8 Spray Drying 95
7.3 Desirable Properties of Pellets 95
Review Questions *95*

8. PARENTERAL DOSAGE FORMS 96

8.1 Introduction 96
8.2 Routes of Injection 97
8.2.1 Intradermal Route 98
8.2.2 Subcutaneous (SC) or Hypodermic Route 98
8.2.3 Intramuscular Injection (IM) 98
8.2.4 Intravenous (IV) Route 98
8.3 Preformulation 99
8.4 Types of Parenterals 99
8.5 Formulation 100
8.5.1 Vehicles 100
8.5.2 Added Solutes 106
8.6 Containers and Closures 110
8.6.1 Glass 110
8.6.2 Plastic 113
8.6.3 Rubber Closures 115
8.7 Parenteral Dosage Forms 116
8.7.1 Solutions 116
8.7.2 Suspensions 117
8.7.3 Emulsions 119
8.7.4 Dry Powders (Sterile Solids) 120
8.7.5 Subdermal Implants 124
8.8 Pyrogens and Their Significance in Parenteral Dosage Forms 125
8.8.1 Source of Pyrogens and Their Control 125
8.9 Production Facilities 127
8.9.1 Design of Production Area 127
8.9.2 Flow Plan 127
8.10 Production 135
8.10.1 Cleaning Containers, Closures and Equipment 136
8.10.2 Compounding 138
8.10.3 Filtration 139
8.10.4 Filling 139
8.10.5 Sealing 141
8.10.6 Sterilization 143
8.10.7 Quality Assurance and Control 144
8.10.8 Packaging and Labelling 144
8.10.9 Quality Control 145
Review Questions *152*

9. OPHTHALMIC DOSAGE FORMS **154**

9.1 Introduction 154
9.2 Anatomy and Physiology of the Human Eye 154
9.3 Site of Application for Topical Ophthalmic Dosage Forms 156
9.4 Optimum Volumes of Administration for Topical Preparations 156
9.5 Types of Ophthalmic Dosage Forms 157
9.5.1 Ophthalmic Solutions 157
9.5.2 Ophthalmic Gel Forming Solutions 157
9.5.3 Ophthalmic Suspensions 157
9.5.4 Ophthalmic Emulsions 158
9.5.5 Ophthalmic Ointments and Gels 159
9.5.6 Ocular Inserts 160
9.5.7 Intraocular Dosage Forms 161
9.6 Requirements of Ophthalmic Dosage Forms 161
9.6.1 Sterility 162
9.6.2 Use of Preservatives or Antimicrobial Agents (AMA) 163
9.6.3 Clarity 164
9.6.4 Viscosity 164
9.6.5 Stability 165
9.6.6 Tonicity 167
9.6.7 Particle Size 167
9.6.8 Use of Surfactants 167
9.7 Formulation and Preparation of Eye Drops 168
9.7.1 Formulation 168
9.7.2 Manufacture of Ophthalmic Solutions and Suspensions (Eye Drops, Eye Lotions and Intaocular Solutions) 169
9.8 Formulation and Preparation of Eye Ointments 170
9.8.1 Formulation 170
9.8.2 Manufacture of Ophthalmic Ointments 171
9.9 Packaging and Labelling of Ophthalmic Dosage Forms 171
9.9.1 Containers for Eye Drops 172
9.9.2 Containers for Eye Lotions and Intraocular Solutions 175
9.9.3 Containers for Eye Ointments/Gels 175
9.9.4 Tamper Proof Feature 176
9.10 Quality Control 176
Review Questions *177*

10. PHARMACEUTICAL AEROSOLS **178**

10.1 Introduction 178
10.1.1 Advantages of Aerosols over Other Dosage Forms 179
10.2 Components of Aerosol Package 179
10.2.1 Propellants 180
10.2.2 Containers 182
10.2.3 Valves 183
10.2.4 Actuators 185

10.3 Formulation of Pharmaceutical Aerosols 186
10.4 Types of Systems 187
10.4.1 Solution System/Two-phase System 187
10.4.2 Water Based System/Three-phase System 187
10.4.3 Two-layer System/Aquasol System 188
10.4.4 Suspension or Dispersion System 188
10.4.5 Foam System 189
10.5 Manufacture of Pharmaceutical Aerosols 190
10.5.1 Pressure Filling Apparatus 191
10.5.2 Cold Filling Apparatus 191
10.6 Compressed Gas Filling Apparatus 192
10.7 Stability Testing of Pharmaceutical Aerosols 192
10.8 Quality Control for Pharmaceutical Aerosols 193
10.9 Testing of Pharmaceutical Aerosols 195
Review Questions *199*

11. COSMETICS **200**

11.1 Introduction 200
11.2 Lipstick 200
11.2.1 Characteristics of a Good Lipstick 201
11.2.2 Formulation 201
11.2.3 Manufacture 204
11.3 Shampoos 205
11.3.1 Characteristics of a Good Shampoo 205
11.3.2 Formulation 205
11.3.3 Manufacture of Liquid Shampoo 210
11.4 Cold Cream 211
11.4.1 Characteristics 211
11.4.2 Formulation 211
11.4.3 Method of Preparation 211
11.5 Vanishing Cream 212
11.5.1 Characteristics 212
11.5.2 Formulation 212
11.5.3 Method of Preparation 213
11.6 Toothpaste 213
11.6.1 Basic Requirements of a Toothpaste 213
11.6.2 Formulation 214
11.6.3 Manufacture of Toothpaste 216
11.7 Hair Dyes 216
11.7.1 Requirements of a Good Hair Dye 216
11.7.2 Hair Colouring Formulations 216
11.7.3 Formulation 219
11.7.4 Method of Preparation 220

11.8 Sunscreens 220
11.8.1 Effects of UV Radiation 220
11.8.2 Sun Protection Factor (SPF) 221
11.8.3 Formulation of Sunscreen Products 221
11.8.4 Types of Sunscreen Products 223
Review Questions *224*

12. PACKAGING MATERIALS SCIENCE **225**

12.1 Introduction 225
12.1.1 Levels of Packaging 225
12.1.2 Materials used for Packaging of Pharmaceutical Products 226
12.1.3 Glass Containers 226
12.1.4 Plastic Containers 227
12.1.5 Disadvantages 229
12.1.6 Metal and Metal Containers 229
12.1.7 Rubber Based Components 230
12.2 Factors Influencing Choice of Containers 231
12.2.1 The Product 231
12.2.2 The Market 231
12.2.3 The Distribution System 231
12.2.4 Manufacturing Facilities 231
12.2.5 Drug-Plastic Considerations 232
12.2.6 Permeation 232
12.2.7 Leaching 232
12.2.8 Sorption 232
12.2.9 Chemical Reactivity 232
12.2.10 Polymer Modification 233
12.3 Legal and Official Requirements for Containers 233
12.3.1 FDA Regulations 233
12.3.2 Stability Aspects of Packaging Materials 233
12.4 Quality Control of Packaging Materials 234
12.5 Quality Control of Glass Containers 235
12.5.1 Evaluation Parameters 235
12.6 Quality Control of Plastic Containers 237
12.7 Quality Control of Rubber Closures 237
Review Questions *238*

13. PILOT PLANT SCALE-UP TECHNIQUES **239**

13.1 Introduction 239
13.2 Pilot Plant Design 240
13.3 Pilot Plant Operation 241
13.4 General Considerations 243
13.5 GMP Considerations 245

13.6 Steps in Scale Up 246
13.6.1 Pilot Plant Design for Tablets 246
13.6.2 Critical Aspects of Liquid Manufacturing 252
13.6.3 Pilot Plant Scale-up for Semi-solid Products 253
13.6.4 Scale-up of Liquid and Semi-solid Manufacturing Processes 254
13.6.5 Scale-up and Post-approval Changes (SUPAC) 255
13.6.6 Current Requirements for Post-approval Changes 256
Review Questions *262*

14. TECHNOLOGY DEVELOPMENT AND TRANSFER 263

14.1 Introduction 263
14.2 Scope 268
14.3 Organization & Management 269
14.4 Project Team 270
14.5 Production: Transfer 270
14.5.1 Processing, Packaging and Cleaning 270
14.5.2 Starting Materials 271
14.6 Active Pharmaceutical Ingredient (API) 271
14.7 Excipients 272
14.8 Packaging 275
14.9 Cleaning 275
14.10 Quality Control: Analytical Method Transfer 276
14.11 Premises and Equipment 278
14.11.1 Premises 278
14.11.2 Equipment 278
14.12 Documentation 279
14.13 Qualification and Validation 279
14.14 Approved Regulatory Bodies and Agencies 280
14.14.1 TIFAC (Technology Information Forecasting and Assessment Council) 280
14.14.2 National Research Development Corporation (NRDC) 280
14.14.3 BCIL (Biotech Consortium India Limited) 281
14.14.4 SIDBI (Small Industries Development Bank of India) 281
14.14.5 APCTT (Asian and Pacific Centre for Transfer of Technology) 281
14.14.6 TBSE (Technology Bureau for Small Enterprises) 282
14.15 Technology of Transfer (ToT) 283
14.15.1 Introduction - Why Licence? 283
14.15.2 Is Licensing the Right Strategy? 283
14.15.3 Patent Information 284
14.15.4 What is Patent Information? 284
14.15.5 Content of Patent Documents 284
14.15.6 Memorandum of Understanding (MoU) or Letter of Intent 285
14.15.7 Subject Matter 285
Review Questions *286*

15. REGULATORY AFFAIRS 287

15.1 Introduction 287
15.2 Basic Need of RA Department 287
15.3 Objectives of RA Department 288
15.4 Historical Overview of Regulatory Affairs 288
15.4.1 Sulphanilamide Tragedy 289
15.4.2 Thalidomide Disaster 289
15.4.3 Tuskegee Syphilis Study (1932-1972) 289
15.4.4 Nazi Experiments 290
15.5 Regulatory Authorities 290
15.5.1 World Health Organization (WHO) 290
15.5.2 United States Food and Drug Administration (USFDA) 291
15.5.3 Central Drugs Standards Control Organization (CDSCO) 291
15.5.4 European Medicines Agency (EMA) 292
15.5.5 Medicines and Healthcare Products Regulatory Agency (MHRA) 292
15.5.6 Health Canada 293
15.5.7 Therapeutic Goods Administration (TGA) 293
15.6 Role of Regulatory Affairs Department 295
15.7 Job Responsibilities of RA Department 295
15.8 Job Profile of RA Professionals in Drug Product/Finished Product Manufacturing Company 295
15.9 Regulatory Requirements for Drug Approval 296
15.9.1 Drug Development Teams 296
15.10 Non-clinical Drug Development 298
15.10.1 Types of Non-clinical Studies 299
15.11 Pharmacology 300
15.12 Drug Metabolism 300
15.13 Toxicology 300
15.13.1 Types of Toxicity 301
15.14 Investigational New Drug Application (INDA) 301
15.14.1 Types of IND 302
15.14.2 INDA Content and Format 302
15.15 FDA Review Process of IND 304
15.16 Investigator's Brochure 305
15.17 New Drug Application (NDA) 308
15.17.1 Goals of NDA 308
15.17.2 NDA Document Contents 309
15.18 Review and Approval of NDA 311
15.19 Bioequivalence Studies 311
15.20 Types of BE Studies 312
15.20.1 Pharmacokinetic Studies 312
15.20.2 Pharmacodynamic Studies 312
15.20.3 Comparative Clinical Studies 313
15.20.4 *In vitro* Dissolution Studies 313

15.21 Clinical Research Protocol (CRP) 313
15.21.1 Components of Clinical Research Protocols 313
15.22 Biostatistics in Pharmaceutical Product Development 315
15.22.1 Basic Biostatistics Approach 316
15.22.2 Commonly used Terms in Biostatistics 316
15.22.3 Types of Measurement Scales 316
15.23 Data Presentation for FDA Submissions 317
15.23.1 Format of Text 317
15.23.2 Tabular Presentation 318
15.24 Management of Clinical Trials 319
Review Questions *320*

16. QUALITY MANAGEMENT SYSTEMS (QMSS) 322

16.1 Introduction 322
16.2 Important Elements in QMS 322
16.3 Concept of Quality 323
16.4 Need of Quality 323
16.5 Quality Aspects 323
16.6 Concept of Quality Management Triology 324
16.6.1 Quality Planning 324
16.6.2 Quality Control 324
16.6.3 Quality Improvement 324
16.7 Total Quality Management (TQM) 324
16.7.1 Key Elements of TQM 325
16.7.2 TQM Tools for Quality Problem Solving 325
16.8 Quality by Design (QbD) 327
16.8.1 The Key Elements of QbD 328
16.9 Six Sigma Concept 329
16.9.1 Six Sigma Methods 329
16.9.2 Out of Specifications (OoS) 330
16.10 Change Control 333
16.10.1 Scope of Change Control 333
16.10.2 Change Control Principles 333
16.10.3 Steps of Change Control 334
16.10.4 Classification of Changes 334
16.10.5 Minor Changes 334
16.10.6 Major Changes 335
16.11 ISO 9000 335
16.11.1 Objectives of ISO 9000 Standards 335
16.11.2 ISO 9000 Series 336
16.11.3 Benefits of ISO 9000 Series Standards 336
16.11.4 ISO 9000 Series Clauses 336
16.11.5 ISO 14000 336
16.11.6 ISO 14000 Policy 337
16.11.7 ISO 14000 Series Standards 337
16.11.8 Benefits of ISO 14000 Standards 338

16.12 National Accreditation Board for Testing and Calibration Laboratories (NABL) 338
16.12.1 Benefits of NABL Accreditation 339
16.12.2 NABL Accreditation/Certification Process 339
16.13 Good Laboratory Practices (GLP) 342
16.13.1 Objectives of GLP 342
16.13.2 Basic Elements of GLP 342
Review Questions *344*

17. INDIAN REGULATORY REQUIREMENTS **346**
17.1 Introduction 346
17.2 Organizational Structure of CDSCO 346
17.2.1 Drugs Controller General of India (DCGI) 346
17.2.2 Responsibilities of CDSCO 347
17.3 State Licensing Authority 348
17.3.1 Responsibilities of State Licensing Authority 348
17.4 Certificate of Pharmaceutical Product (COPP) 349
17.4.1 Definition 349
17.4.2 Purpose 349
17.4.3 Aim and Scope 349
17.4.4 Types of COPP 350
17.4.5 Content of the COPP 351
17.5 Certificate of a Pharmaceutical Product 352
17.6 Types of Drugs for Which COPP May be Issued 354
17.7 Approval of New Drug in India 356
17.7.1 Purpose 357
17.7.2 New Drug Application (NDA) 357
Review Questions *361*

INDEX **362**

1

PREFORMULATION STUDIES

Learning Objectives

After going through this chapter, you would be able to:

1. Know the objectives of preformulation.
2. List out the physicochemical characteristics of drug substances.
3. Explain the physical properties and chemical properties of drug substances.
4. Describe the biopharmaceutical classification system.

1.1 INTRODUCTION

For design of the dosage forms, preformulation is an important step used to characterize the properties of drug substance and also to understand the challenges that a particular compound may possess during the formulation.

Preformulation is the initial stage of the conversion of a molecule to a drug where various important physical, chemical, and biopharmaceutical properties of drug molecules are assessed. With the knowledge of a new molecule's physical, chemical and biopharmaceutical properties, a suitable dosage form can be designed which improves patient compliance and also ease of administration.

Initial learning phase related to drug is known as prefornulation. All the studies performed on a newly identified drug substance and all the activities carried out at and before formulation stage of dosage form, are called preformulation studies. This information provides an outline for the drug combination with additives in the manufacturing of safe, therapeutically effective and robust dosage form.

Once an optimized molecule is selected for formulation development, it is important to understand the biopharmaceutical properties of drug entity with respect to its *in vivo* absorption and disposition. This information is helpful in making appropriate formulation choice to maximize the drug's bioavailability.

The overall objective of preformulation testing is to generate information useful to the formulator in developing stable and bioavailable dosage forms that can be produced in mass.

1.2 OBJECTIVES AND GOALS OF PREFORMULATION STUDIES

GOAL: To convert active drug moiety into suitable dosage form.

Objectives

- Choosing the suitable drug based on the type of dosage form developed.
- Physical and chemical properties of the drug substance are evaluated.

- To understand biopharmaceutical properties of drug.
- To determine kinetic rate profile.
- To determine stability of drug.
- To establish drug compatibility with common excipients.
- To decrease the time and expenses of product development.
- To produce robust, safe and effective drug delivery system.

Study of Physicochemical Characteristics of Drug Substances

Physicochemical studies of a new drug substance would include:

- Appearance, colour, particle size, surface area, particle shape, crystalline structure, polymorphism, melting point, bulk density, tap density, and compressibility.
- Solubility in water and other solvents
- pH profile
- pKa
- Vapour pressure
- Hygroscopicity

1.3 PHYSICAL PROPERTIES

1.3.1 Physical Forms

Amorphous form: Defined as substance that are not crystalline in nature and therefore have no defined long range molecular structure. Because of this:

- They are "energetic" solid (higher thermodynamic energy than crystalline form).
- They have higher dissolution rates.
- They have higher solubility.
- Have better compression properties.
- They tend to be less stable. This thermodynamic instability can occur during bulk processing or within dosage form and become a major disadvantage.

***Crystalline form*:** Crystals are repetitious spacing of constituent atoms or molecules in a three-dimensional array.

Crystal habit and the internal structure of a drug can affect physicochemical properties which range from flowability to chemical stability.

Crystal habit: It is the outer appearance of a crystal.

Internal structure: It is the molecular arrangement within the solid.

A single internal structure for a compound can have several different habits, depending on the environment for growing crystals.

***Polymorphism*:** When a substance exists in more than one crystalline form, the different forms are designated as polymorphs and the phenomenon as polymorphism.

Polymorphism can be classified as two types:

1. **Enantiotropic**: One form of polymorph can be reversibly changed into another by varying temperature and pressure.
   Ex: sulphur
2. **Monotropic**: One polymorphic form is unstable at all temperatures and pressures.
   Ex: glyceryl stearates
   - Since polymorphism varies with the internal structure of the solid drug rather than chemical difference, it influences the drug's pharmaceutical properties like solubility, melting point, hardness, density, and compression characteristics.
   - They are made by crystallizing the drug in a variety of solvents under diverse conditions.
   - The polymorph can be determined by using methods such as differential scanning calorimetry [DSC], X-ray powder diffraction, and optical crystallography. They are also used to distinguish between different polymorphs.
   - If a compound exhibits polymorphism, one of the forms will be more physically stable and another is in meta stable form.
   - Important aspects of stable form are lowest energy state, highest melting point, least aqueous solubility.
   - Important aspects of metastable form are higher energy state, low melting points, higher aqueous solubility, dissolution rate will also be higher.

Due to their higher energy state metastable forms have a tendency to convert to the stable form. If the metastable polymorph is kept dry, it may be stable for years and it is therefore not referred to as an unstable but, rather a metastable polymorph.

- A crystalline compound may contain crystallization solvent.
- When solvent molecules are entrapped within the crystal lattice of the solid, they are referred to as *solvate.*
- When the incorporated solvent is water within the crystal lattice of the solid, the complex is called *hydrate.*
- A compound not containing any water within its crystal structure is termed *anhydrous.*

The anhydrous form of a drug has greater aqueous solubility than the hydrates because the hydrates are already in interaction with water and therefore have less energy for crystal breakup and for further interaction with water in comparison to the anhydrates. The organic (non-aqueous) solvates have greater aqueous solubility than the non-solvates.

1.3.2 Particle Size and Surface Area

Particle size is a basic physical feature of a solid, the size of particle is of greater importance. Particle size and surface area are inversely related to each other, as the particle size of the material decreases, the surface area increases.

The size gives an idea about the size distribution and therefore the total surface area of the particle not only depends on size but shape too influences the flow and mixing efficiency of the powders and granules.

For spherical particle the size is measured in terms of diameter but if the shape is other than spherical then particle size is expressed as the diameter which is an equivalent diameter.

1.3.3 Determination of Particle Size

Particle size can be determined by:

- Optical microscopy
- Sedimentation method
- Sieve analysis
- Coulter counter method/volume method

De-mixing effects can occur when the active components and excipients have large size differences. If materials become too fine, then undesirable properties such as electrostatic effects and other surface-active properties lead to aggregation, increase in hydrophobicity and lowers dissolution rate.

Fine materials are relatively more open to attack from atmospheric oxygen, heat, light, humidity and interacting excipients than coarse materials. It is important to decide the desired size range and to maintain it.

It is safest to grind drugs having particles that are above approximately 100 μm in diameter, particles of 30 μm or less, then grinding is unnecessary. Grinding should reduce coarse material to the 10-40 μm range.

1.3.4 Particle Shape

- Particle shape is related to geometric shape and surface irregularity.
- Particle shape will influence the surface area, flow properties, packing and compaction properties of the particles.
- Surface area per unit weight or volume is an important characteristic which determines surface adsorption and dissolution rate of the particle.
- A sphere has a minimum surface area per unit volume. The surface area per unit volume of a particle increases as it becomes more asymmetric. It may be necessary to determine the extent of asymmetry in a particle.
- Spherical particle exhibits better flow than irregularly shaped particles.
- Irregular particles because of surface roughness interlock with each other, resulting in poor flow and bridging with hopper.
- Irregular shaped particles have higher interparticle contacts. During compression, the corners and edges can undergo greater deformation and promote higher bond strength.

1.3.5 Shape Factor to Determine the Shape of a Particle

Shape factor is a numerical value expressed to describe quantitatively the shape of an irregular particle.

- Shape factor cannot be described for a irregularly shaped particle.
- It is possible to determine whether the shape of a particle is spherical or asymmetric.

A sphere has minimum surface area per unit volume. These properties can be compared for spheres and asymmetric particles (consider projected diameter, d_p), in order to decide the shape.

Surface area of a sphere is given by:

$$S = \pi d^2$$

While its volume is given by:

$$V = \pi d^3/6$$

where d is the diameter of the particles.

where α_s and α_v are the surface area factor and volume factor, for the asymmetric particle.

Solving for α_s and α_v by equation the appropriate properties (surface area and volume) provide:

$$\alpha_s = \frac{\pi d^2 s}{d^2 p}$$

$$\alpha_v = \frac{\pi d^3}{6d^3 p}$$

When d_s are made equal to d_p, the relationship may be written as

$$\alpha_s = \pi = 3.124$$

$$\alpha_v = \frac{\pi}{6} = 5.24$$

The shape factor of particle can be expressed as the ratio of surface to volume.

$$\text{Shape factor} = \frac{\alpha_s}{\alpha_v} = \frac{3.124}{0.524} = 6$$

The minimum possible value for shape factor is 6, which represents a sphere. If the ratio exceeds this factor 6, the particle is considered asymmetric.

1.3.6 Powder Flow Property

Flowability is the ability of a powder to flow through reliably.

The flow properties of powder are an important parameter to be considered in the production of pharmaceutical dosage forms since most of the processes such as uniform filling of dies during tabletting and proper filling of capsules during capsule filling directly depends on the flow properties of the powder mass. The poor flow in powders is generally due to one or more of the following reasons.

Flow properties of a powder are affected by:

- Small variation on particle size, shape, density, electrostatic charge and moisture level.
- Cohesiveness or stickiness between particles.
- Adhesion between the particle and the container wall due to the presence of vander Waal's force, electrostatic forces, moisture.
- Physical interlocking of particles due to their irregular shape.
- Friction between particles due to surface roughness.

A powder flow investigation helps to assess an improvement in various stages of the formulation developments. Angle of repose, bulk density, tapped density, Carr's compressibility index, and Hausner's ratio are the methods available for measuring powder flow.

1. ***Angle of repose:*** The flow characteristics are measured by angle of repose. Improper flow of powder is due to frictional force between the particles. These frictional forces are quantified by angle of repose.

"Angle of repose is defined as the maximum angle possible between the surface of a pile of the powder and the horizontal plane."

The angle of repose (θ) was calculated as follows:

$$\tan\theta = \frac{h}{r}$$

$$\theta = \tan^{-1}\frac{h}{r}$$

where, h = height of pile in cm

r = radius of the base of the pile in cm

θ = angle of repose

Procedure:

- A glass funnel is held in place with a clamp on the ring support.
- Approximately 100 gm of granules are poured into the funnel while the orifice of the funnel is blocked by the thumb.
- As the thumb is removed, a cone shaped pile is formed on the glass plate.
- Repeat the process until the distance is adjusted appropriately.
- Pour the granules back into the funnel and allow powder or granules to flow through an orifice of funnel from a certain height.
- The granules form a conical heap on the horizontal surface.
- Measure the height of the pile with a ruler.
- The angle which the heap forms with the horizontal surface is the angle of repose and it is determined by the above formula.

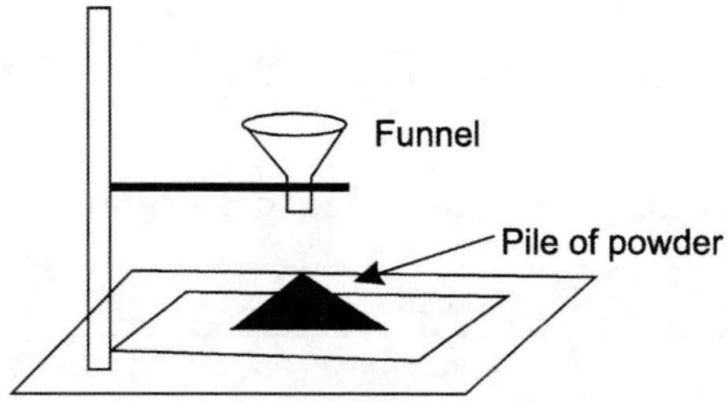

Fig. 1.1: Determination of angle of repose

Table 1.1: Relationship between angle of repose (θ) ànd flow properties of powder

Angle of repose (θ)	Flow properties
<25	Excellent
25–30	Good
30–40	Satisfactory
40–50	Poor
>50	Very poor

2. ***Bulk density:*** It is defined as mass of powder divided by the bulk volume. Bulk density is used to check the uniformity of the bulk chemicals and to determine the proper size of packing materials or containers, mixing apparatus and the size of empty gelatin capsules for given mass of powder.

   Procedure: Weighed amount of powder is transferred into a dry 100 mL graduated cylinder. Carefully level the powder without compacting, if necessary, and read the unsettled apparent volume. The density is calculated by using the formula.

$$\text{Bulk density} = \frac{\text{wt. of power}}{\text{Bulk volume}}$$

3. ***Tapped density***: It is determined by mechanically tapping a graduated cylinder containing the sample until further volume change is observed.

$$\text{Tapped density} = \frac{\text{wt. of power}}{\text{Tapped volume}}$$

4. ***Carr's compressibility index and Hausner ratio***: Carr's compressibility index (CI) and Hausner ratio (HR) are determined by calculating bulk and tapped densities to provide a measure of the flow properties and compressibility of powder.

$$\text{Carr's compressibility index} = \frac{\text{Tapped density- Bulk density}}{\text{Tapped density}} \times 100$$

$$\text{Hausner's ratio} = \frac{\text{Tapped density}}{\text{Bulk density}}$$

Table 1.2: Relationship of Carr's index and Hausner's ratio with poweder flowability

Carr's index	Hausner's ratio	Flowability
5–15	1.05–1.18	Excellent
12–16	1.14–1.20	Good
18–21	1.22–1.26	Fair-passable
23–35	1.30–1.54	Poor
33–38	1.50–1.61	Very poor
>40	>1.67	Very, very poor

1.3.7 Solubility

Solubility is the ability of a solute to dissolve in a solvent to form a saturated solution under a specific condition of temperature and pressure."

The solubility of a solid substance is defined as the concentration at which the solution phase is in equilibrium with a given solid phase at a stated temperature and pressure.

Solid drugs administered orally for systemic activity must dissolve in the gastrointestinal fluid prior to their absorption. Thus, the solubility is an important physicochemical property as it affects the dissolution parameters, rate of drug release, bioavailability of the drug and ultimately therapeutic efficiency.

The solubility of the molecules in various solvents is determined as a first step. The solubility is usually determined in a variety of commonly used solvents. Since aqueous solubility indicates the amount of compound dissolved and therefore the amount available for absorption, bioavailability depends on solubility.

In order to be transported across biological membrane, drug molecules are required to be present in a dissolved form. Therefore, low aqueous solubility can delay or decrease drug absorption.

The solubility of every new drug must be determined as a function of pH over the physiological pH range of 1 to 8. If the solubility is considered too low or too high, efforts to alter it may be undertaken.

1. ***pKa Ionisation constant:*** When a weakly acidic or basic drug is administered, it will undergo ionisation in GI fluids. Determination of the dissociation constant for a drug capable of ionisation within a pH range of 1 to 10 is important since solubility and absorption can be altered by changing pH. The concentration of ionised and unionised drug can be estimated by **Henderson- Hasselbalch equation.**

   For basic compounds

$$pH = pKa + \log [\text{unionised drug}]/[\text{ionised drug}]$$

For acidic compounds

pH = pKa +log [ionised drug]/[unionised drug]

It is customary to express the dissociation constants of both acidic and basic drugs by pKa value. The lower the pKa of an acidic drug, stronger the acid (greater the proportion of ionised form at a particular pH). The higher the pKa of a basic drug, stronger the base.

The unionised form of drugs is more lipid-soluble and hence more rapidly absorbed than ionised form. Of the ionic forms, the anionic solute is absorbed faster than the cationic form.

The factors that are important in the absorption of weakly acidic or basic compounds are:

- The pH at the absorption site
- The ionisation constant
- The lipid solubility

Methods to determine pKa

1. Potentiometric method
2. Spectrophotometric method
3. HPLC technique
4. Solubility measurement
5. Capillary zone electrophoresis.

2. pH: Since most drugs are weak acids or weak bases, their degree of ionisation depends on the pH of the biological fluid.

Depending on the pH, the drug undergoes dissociation at dissociation equilibrium. The drug is present in unionised as well as ionised forms in the solution. If pH of the medium favours the formation of unionised species, the drug can be rapidly diffused across the lipoidal bio-membrane.

Example: Acidic drugs such as aspirin will be present in unionised form at gastric pH.

Acidic drugs are largely in ionised form in the intestinal pH. Hence, intestine is unfavourable for the absorption of weakly acidic drugs.

Weakly basic drugs are largely in ionised form in the gastric pH. Hence, gastric pH is unfavourable for the absorption of basic drugs.

pH is defined as a negative logarithm of hydrogen ion concentration.

$$pH = -\log [H_3O^+]$$

or

$$pH = \log 1 [H_3O^+]$$

Most of the drugs are either weak acids or weak bases and are poorly soluble in water.

The solubility of such drug is markedly affected by change in pH. If the pH of a solution is reduced, the solubility of weak acidic drug or its salts decreases and the solubility of weak basic drug or their salts increases.

The relationship between the pH, solubility and pka value of an acidic drug is given by

$$pH_p = pK_a + \log S - S_0 / S_0$$

$$pH_p = pK_a + \log S_0 / S - S_0$$

where; pHp = pH below which the drug precipitates from solution.

S = overall solubility of the drug.

S_0 = solubility of its unionised form.

3. **Partition coefficient:** "The partition coefficient, log P is defined as the ratio of unionised drug distributed between the organic phase and aqueous phase at equilibrium".

It is an important physicochemical property that is used to predict the diffusion of drugs. The higher the partition coefficient, the better is its lipid solubility. When a solute is added to two immiscible liquids that are in contact with each other, it will distribute itself between the two phases in a fixed ratio. This ratio is known as the *partition coefficient* or the *distribution coefficient.*

$$\text{Partition coefficient (pc)} = \frac{\text{Conc. of drug in oil phase}}{\text{Conc. of drug in water phase}}$$

The lipid solubility of a drug is an important factor in the assessment of its absorption potential. An indication of the relative lipid solubility can be obtained by determining how a drug substance distributes itself between water and an immiscible organic solvent.

GI fluids represent the aqueous phases and GI membrane represents the lipid phase. The administered drug will undergo partition between these two phases. Thus, partition coefficient is useful in predicting the drug absorption. The unionised form is more lipid soluble and therefore, better diffused through lipoidal membrane.

Various organic solvents such as chloroform, ether, amyl acetate, isopropyl myristate, carbon tetrachloride and n-octanol can be used in the determination of the partition coefficient.

Method for determining partition or distribution coefficient is *"shake flask method"*.

Procedure: The drug is dissolved in either the aqueous or the organic phase, and the known volume of the two phases is equilibrated by shaking. The phases are separated by standing. Aliquot is taken and analysed for the drug content.

1.4 CHEMICAL PROPERTIES

Preformulation stability studies are the quantitative assessment of chemical stability of a new drug.

All medicinal agents are to be investigated for their degradation. Most drugs contain one or more functional groups and therefore may undergo different chemical reactions. Environmental factors such as moisture, heat, light, and radiation affect the physical and chemical stability of drugs.

The major objectives of the preformulation stability studies are to identify conditions to which the compound is sensitive and interpret degradation profiles under these conditions.

A few degradation reactions are enumerated here.

- Hydrolysis
- Oxidation
- Reduction
- Racemization
- Polymerisation

1.4.1 Hydrolysis

Hydrolysis is the reaction of a molecule with water resulting in the cleavage of chemical bond within that molecule, resulting in two compounds. At the same time water molecule splits into two, with a hydrogen transferring to one of the compounds and a hydroxide to the other compound. Hydrolysis occurs via nucleophilic attack of the water molecule on bonds.

Drugs are either weak acids or bases. These may be available as ionised or unionised form. Hydrolysis reaction between ionic species proceeds faster than with unionised form. Therefore, hydrolysis of a drug depends on the pH condition. Hydrolysis reactions are catalysed by H^+ and OH^- ions.

Drugs that tend to degrade by hydrolytic cleavage of an ester or amide linkage are anaesthetics, antibiotics, vitamins and barbiturates.

Table 1.3: The functional group subjected to hydrolysis are given below

Drug type	Functional group	Examples
Esters	$RCOOR^1$ $ROPO_3Mx$	Aspirin, Aldehyde. Dexamethasone sodium phosphate
Amides	$RCONR^1_2$	Chloramphenicol
Imides		Glutethimide
Lactones		Pilocarpine
Oximes	$R_2C{=}NOR$	Steroids, Oximes
Lactams		Penicillin, Cephalosporins

1.4.2 Ester Hydrolysis

Drug that contains ester group, undergo hydrolysis to give acid and alcohols. This involves the rupture of a covalent linkage between a carbon atom and an oxygen atom. Catalyst is needed to promote the reaction, such as mineral acids, alkaloids, and some enzymes which are capable of supplying hydrogen or hydroxyl ions to the reaction mixture.

$$RCOO\text{-}R^1 + H_2O \longrightarrow \underset{\text{Acid}}{RCOOH} + \underset{\text{alcohol}}{R^1\text{-}OH}$$

Amide hydrolysis

Drugs containing an amide group undergo hydrolysis, hydrolytic cleavage of an amide resulting in the formation of an acid and an amine.

$$RCONH\text{-}R^1 + H_2O \longrightarrow \underset{\text{Acid}}{R\text{-}COOH} + \underset{\text{amine}}{R^1\text{-}NH_2}$$

1.4.3 Oxidation

Oxidation involves either the addition of oxygen or removal of electron. Auto-oxidation is the most common form of oxidative degradation that occurs in many of the pharmaceutical preparations, which involve a free radical chain process. Auto-oxidation may be defined as the reaction of any substance with molecular oxygen. The free radicals produced during the initial reaction are highly reactive and further catalyse the reaction to produce additional free radicals and causing a chain reaction.

Trace heavy metals such as copper, iron, cobalt and nickel catalyse the oxidative degradation. In the presence of catalyst like hydrogen peroxide and other oxides, the rate of reaction increases. Oxidation reactions are catalysed by H^+ & OH^- ions; hydroxyl ions catalyse oxidation faster than hydrogen ions. Steroids, vitamins, antibiotics and epinephrine undergo oxidative degradation.

Table 1.4: The functional group subjected to hydrolysis are given below

Drugs	Functional group	Example
Ethers	$R\text{-}O\text{-}R^1$	Diethyl ester
Aldehyde	RCHO	Paraldehyde
Thiols	RCH_2SH	Dimercaprol
Carboxylic acid	RCOOH	Fatty acid
Nitrites	RNO_2	Amylnitrite

Example 1:

Ascorbic acid ⟶ Dehydroascorbic acid.

- R-H ⟶ R-OH (hydroxylation): conversion of a hydrogen to a hydroxyl group.
- R-C-OH ⟶ R-C=O (dehydrogenation): conversion of hydroxyl groups to a carbonyl group.
- R-C=O ⟶ R-COOH (carboxylation): conversion of a carbonyl group to carboxyl group.
- R-C-NH_2 ⟶ R-C=O (deamination): conversion of an amino group to carbonyl group.

Example 2: Hydroxylation of amphetamine to 4-hydroxyamphetamine and norephedrine.

Reduction

It is the loss of oxygen atom from a molecule or the gaining of one or more electron/ addition of hydrogen.

- R-OH ⟶ R-H (dehydroxylation)
- R-C=O ⟶ R-C-OH (hydrogenation)
- R-NO_2 ⟶ R-NH_2 (amination)
- R-C-H ⟶ R-CH_3 (methylation)

Example: Inactivation of warfarin by the transformation of acetone group to a hydroxyl group (hydrogenation).

1.4.4 Racemisation Reaction or Optical Isomerisation

It is a reaction in which an optically active substance loses its optical activity without changing its chemical composition. The biological effect of the dextro form can be considerably less than that of the levo form, this reaction is important for the stability of drug.

Example: Levo-adrenaline is 15 to 20 times more active than dextro-adrenaline.

Since different isomers of a drug have different activities, such a conversion from one form to another may be regarded as a form of degradation resulting in serious loss of therapeutic activity. Most racemisation reactions are catalysed by an acid or a base. The racemisation reactions of drugs are those that involve epinephrine, pilocarpine, ergotamine and tetracycline.

Example: Epinephrine also shows acid-catalysed racemisation with loss of therapeutic activity.

1.4.5 Polymerisation

These types of reactions are not often the initial cause of drug decomposition. Primary decomposition product may react further and polymerise.

Adrenaline $\xrightarrow{\text{oxidation}}$ Adrenochrome polymerise $\xrightarrow{\text{polymerise}}$ Black brown pigment
(acid solution)

Dextrose $\xrightarrow{\text{auto cleaving}}$ 5-hydroxymethyl $\xrightarrow{\text{polymerise}}$ Straw coloured solution.
Injection

1.5 BIOPHARMACEUTICAL CLASSIFICATION SYSTEM (BCS)

BCS is a framework for classifying drug substances based on their aqueous solubility and permeability.

It is a drug classification scheme that provides a basis for establishing *in vitro-in vivo* correlation. It also takes into consideration gastric pH, gastric fluid volume and gastric emptying time, intestinal pH, intestinal fluid volume, intestinal transit time, and permeability.

Solubility and permeability are properties of a drug substance whereas dissolution is the property of a drug product. The drug absorption is primarily controlled by two factors, solubility in aqueous media coupled with permeability through the gastrointestinal membrane.

Biopharmaceutical classification system was introduced by Amidon, which classifies the drug into the following 4 groups based on solubility and permeability.

	High solubility	*Low solubility*
High Permeability	*Class 1* High solubility High permeability	*Class 2* Low solubility High permeability
Low Permeability	*Class 3* High solubility Low permeability	*Class 4* Low solubility Low permeability

Class I

- Drug dissolves rapidly.
- Rate limiting step is drug dissolution, if dissolution is very rapid then GI emptying rate becomes rate determining step.
- Drug is absorbed rapidly.
- Rapid therapeutic action.
- Rate of absorption is higher than rate of elimination.

Example: Metoprolol, Diltiazem, Propranolol

Class II

- Drug dissolves slowly.
- In vivo drug dissolution is the rate limiting step except at very high dose.
- Drug is absorbed rapidly.
- Bioavailability is controlled by dosage form and release rate of drug.
- Oral and IV routes for administration

Example: Mefenamic acid, Phenytoin, Ketoconazole

Class III

- Drug dissolves rapidly.
- Drug absorbance is limited.
- Permeability is the rate limiting step for drug absorption.
- Incomplete bioavailability.
- Oral or IV route for administration.

Example: Cimetidine, Acyclovir, Captopril.

Class IV

- Low dissolution rate.
- Low permeability property.
- Slow or low therapeutic action.
- Rarely developed and reach the market.

Example: Taxol, Griseofulvin.

1.5.1 Significance of BCS Classification

- Can be used as a basis for setting *in vitro* dissolution specifications.
- Provides a basis for predicting the probability of achieving a successful *in vivo-in vitro* correlation.

1.5.2 Application of Preformulation Considerations in the Development of Solid, Liquid Oral and Parenteral Dosage Form and Its Impact on Stability of Dosage Forms

- In any formulation design careful consideration of the preformulation data is the first step.
- The pharmaceutical research area is responsible for providing data on the drug substance.
- Experiments are designed to generate data characterizing specific, physico-chemical properties of the drug substance and its combination with selected solvents, excipients and packaging components.
- These studies are carried out under stressed conditions of temperature, light, humidity and oxygen in order to accelerate and detect potential reaction.
- To have an idea of what excipients to use and how best to put them together with the drug, it is necessary to know the inherent stability of the drug substance in designing a dosage form.

Stability studies are carried out under the following three categories.

1. Solid state stability of drug alone
   Stability under — Elevated temperature studies
   High humidity condition
   Photolytic stability
2. Stability in presence of excipients by — Differential thermal analysis
   Diffuse reflectance spectroscopy
3. Solution phase stability — Stability in gastrointestinal fluids
   Stability in solvents

- Before beginning a formulation development activity, the formulator should have a complete physicochemical profile of the active components.
- Preformulation data reduce the overall cost of product development by minimising problems in various phases of drug development and provide the foundation for successful formulation. It also provides key information necessary to guide the formulator towards the development of an elegant, stable dosage form with good bioavailability.

REVIEW QUESTIONS

Short Essays

1. Write the applications of preformulation consideration in the development of solid.
2. Write about BCS classification system with its significance.
3. Describe the importance of partition coefficient in the drug design with suitable example.

Short Answers

1. Application of partition coefficient.
2. BCS classification of drugs.
3. Write the importance of angle of repose in tableting.
4. What are hydrates and solvates. Give examples.

2

TABLETS

Learning Objectives

After going through this chapter, you would be able to:

1. Classify tablets and their ideal characteristics.
2. Understand the role of excipients in tablet formulation.
3. Learn the process and machines involved in tablet manufacturing.
4. Explain various types of tablet coating and their process.
5. Describe the quality control tests for tablets.

2.1 INTRODUCTION

The oral route is the most often used method of administering medicines for systemic effects. It is likely that at least 90% of all medications used to generate systemic effects are taken orally. When a new medicine is developed, one of the first things a pharmaceutical firm examines is whether the drug can be properly taken orally for the desired effect. If it cannot be, the medicine is generally administered in a hospital environment or in a physician's office. Solid oral dosage forms are the recommended class of product for medications that are taken orally.

Tablets are a unit solid dosage form of pharmaceuticals produced by compaction. The goal of the compressed tablet's design and production is to deliver the correct amount of medicine in the proper shape, at or over the suitable time, and in the intended area, while maintaining its chemical integrity until that point. Aside from the physical and chemical qualities of the medicinal agent(s) to be made into a tablet, the tablet's actual physical design, manufacturing method, and entire chemical makeup can all have a significant impact on the efficacy of the medication being delivered.

2.2 IDEAL CHARACTERISTICS OF TABLETS

- The tablet should include the correct dose of the drug.
- The appearance of the tablet should be elegant, and its weight, size and appearance should be consistent.
- The drug should be released from the tablet in a controlled and reproducible way.
- The tablet should be biocompatible, i.e., not include excipients, contaminants and microorganisms that could cause harm to patients.
- The tablet should be of sufficient mechanical strength to withstand fracture and erosion during handling.

- It must be able to release the medicinal agent(s) in the body in a predictable and reproducible manner.
- It must have a suitable chemical, physical, and microbiological stability over time so as not to allow alteration of the medicinal agent(s).

2.3 CLASSIFICATION OF TABLETS

Tablets can be classified as follows:

2.3.1 Tablets Ingested Orally

1. **Compressed tablet:** In addition to the medicinal agent or agents, compressed tablets usually contain several pharmaceutical adjuncts, including the following: diluents or fillers, binders or adhesives, disintegrants or disintegrating agents, anti-adherents, glidants, lubricants, or lubricating agents, colorants and flavouring agents.
2. **Multiple compressed tablet:** Multiple compressed tablets are prepared by subjecting the fill material to more than a single compression. The result may be a multiple-layer tablet or a tablet within a tablet, the inner tablet being the core and the outer portion being the shell. Layered tablets are prepared by initial compaction of a portion of fill material in a die followed by additional fill material and compression to form two-layered or three-layered tablets, depending on the number of separate fills. Each layer may contain a different medicinal agent, separated for reason of chemical or physical incompatibility and with different colour.
3. **Sugar coated tablet:** Compressed tablets may be coated with a coloured or an uncoloured sugar layer. The coating is water soluble and quickly dissolves after swallowing. The sugar coat protects the enclosed drug from the environment and provides a barrier to objectionable taste or odour. The sugar coat also enhances the appearance of the compressed tablet and permits imprinting of identifying manufacturer's information. Among the disadvantages to sugar coating tablets are size, weight, and shipping costs. Sugar coating may add 50% to the weight and bulk of the uncoated tablet.
4. **Film coated tablet:** Film coated tablets are compressed tablets coated with a thin layer of a polymer capable of forming a skin-like film. The film is usually coloured and has the advantage over sugar coatings in that it is more durable, less bulky, and less time consuming to apply. By its composition, the coating is designed to rupture and expose the core tablet at the desired location in the gastrointestinal tract.
5. **Chewable tablet:** Chewable tablets, which have a smooth, rapid disintegration when chewed or allowed to dissolve in the mouth, have a creamy base, usually of specially flavoured and coloured mannitol. Chewable tablets are especially useful for administration of large tablets to children and adults who have difficulty in swallowing solid dosage forms.

6. **Immediate release tablet:** Immediate-release tablets are designed to disintegrate and release their medication with no special rate-controlling features, such as special coatings and other techniques.

2.3.2 Tablets Used in Oral Cavity

1. **Buccal and sublingual tablets:** Buccal and sublingual tablets are flat, oval tablets intended to be dissolved in the buccal pouch (buccal tablets) or beneath the tongue (sublingual tablets) for absorption through the oral mucosa. They enable oral absorption of drugs that are destroyed by the gastric juice and/or are poorly absorbed from the gastrointestinal tract. Buccal tablets are designed to erode slowly, whereas those for sublingual use (such as nitroglycerin) dissolve promptly and provide rapid drug effects.
2. **Troches or Lozenges:** Lozenges or troches are disc-shaped solid dosage forms containing a medicinal agent and generally a flavouring substance in a hard candy or sugar base. They are intended to be slowly dissolved in the oral cavity, usually for local effects, although some are formulated for systemic absorption. An example would be Mycelex troches (Bayer).

2.3.3 Tablets Administered by Other Routes

1. **Vaginal tablets:** Vaginal tablets, also called vaginal inserts, are uncoated, bullet-shaped or ovoid tablets inserted into the vagina for local effects. They are prepared by compression and shaped to fit snugly on plastic inserter devices that accompany the product. They contain antibacterial elements for the treatment of nonspecific vaginitis caused by Haemophilus vaginalis or antifungals for the treatment of vulvovaginitis candidiasis caused by *Candida albicans* and related species.

2.3.4 Tablets Used to Prepare Solutions

1. **Effervescent tablets:** Effervescent tablets are prepared by compressing granular effervescent salts that release gas when in contact with water. These tablets generally contain medicinal substances that dissolve rapidly when added to water. The "bubble action" can assist in breaking up the tablets and enhancing the dissolution of the active drug.
2. **Dispensing tablets:** Dispensing tablets are no longer in use. They might better have been termed compounding tablets because the pharmacist used them to compound prescriptions. They were not dispensed as such to the patient. The tablets contained large amounts of highly potent drug substances, so the pharmacist could rapidly obtain premeasured amounts for compounding multiple dosage units. These tablets had the dangerous potential of being inadvertently dispensed as such to patients.
3. **Hypodermic tablets:** They were originally used by physicians in extemporaneous preparation of parenteral solutions. The required number of tablets was dissolved in a suitable vehicle, sterility attained, and the injection performed. The tablets were a convenience since they could be easily carried in the physician's medicine bag and injections prepared to meet the needs of the individual patients. However, the difficulty in achieving sterility and the availability of prefabricated injectable products, some in disposable syringes, have eliminated the need for hypodermic tablets.

4. **Tablet triturates:** Tablet triturates are small, usually cylindrical, moulded or compressed tablets containing small amounts of usually potent drugs. Today, only a few tablet triturate products are available commercially, with most of these produced by tablet compression. Since tablet triturates must be readily and completely soluble in water, only a minimal amount of pressure is applied during their manufacture. A combination of sucrose and lactose is usually the diluent. The few tablet triturates that remain are used sublingually, such as nitro-glycerine tablets.

2.4 TABLET EXCIPIENTS AND FORMULATION

Tablet formulation design starts with a predetermined value, which is the dose size. The amount of drug in a tablet can be a limiting step in formulation design.

All other tablet excipients must meet certain criteria in the formulation. These include the following:

1. They must be non-toxic and acceptable to the regulatory agencies in all countries where the product is to be marketed.
2. They must be commercially available in an acceptable grade in all countries where the product is to be manufactured.
3. Their cost must be acceptably low.
4. They must not be contraindicated by themselves (e.g., sucrose) or because of a component (e.g., sodium) in any segment of the population.
5. They must be physiologically inert.
6. They must be physically and chemically stable by themselves and in combination with the drug(s) and other tablet components.
7. They must be free of any unacceptable microbiologic "load".
8. They must be colour-compatible and do not produce any off-colour appearance.
9. If the drug product is also classified as a food, (certain vitamin products), the diluent and other excipients must be approved direct food additives.
10. They must have no deleterious effect on the bioavailability of the drug(s) in the product.

Tablet excipients can be classified on the basis of their functionality as listed below.

1. **Fillers/diluents:** Diluents are fillers designed to make up the required bulk of the tablet when the drug dosage itself is inadequate to produce this bulk. The dose of some drugs is sufficiently high that no filler is required (e.g., aspirin and certain antibiotics). Tablet formulations may contain a diluent for secondary reasons: to provide better tablet properties such as improved cohesion, to permit use of direct compression manufacturing, or to promote flow. Dibasic calcium phosphate and lactose are the commonly used diluents.
2. **Binders and adhesives:** These materials are added either dry or in liquid form during wet granulation to form granules or to promote cohesive compacts for directly compressed tablets. Acacia and tragacanth are natural gums and are employed in solutions ranging from 10 to 25% concentration, alone or in combination. These materials are much more effective when they are added as solutions in the preparation of granulations than when they are added dry to a direct compression formula.

Starch paste is one of the most common granulating agents. It is prepared by dispersing starch into water, which is then heated for some prescribed time. During the heating, the starch undergoes hydrolysis to dextrin and to glucose. Gelatin is a natural protein and is sometimes used in combination with acacia. It is a more consistent material than the two natural gums, is easier to prepare in solution form, and forms tablets equally as hard as acacia or tragacanth. Liquid glucose, which is a 50% solution in water, is a common wet granulating agent. These sugar solutions can produce wet granulations, which when tableted, produce hard but somewhat brittle compacts. These materials have the advantage of being low-cost adhesives. Unless the sugar solutions are highly concentrated, bacterial proliferation may be a problem.

Modified natural polymers, such as the alginates and cellulose derivatives (methylcellulose, hydroxypropyl methyl cellulose, and hydroxypropyl cellulose), are common binders and adhesives. Used dry for direct compression, they have some binder capabilities, while their aqueous solutions have adhesive properties. Hydroxypropyl cellulose may also be used as an alcohol solution to provide an anhydrous adhesive. Ethyl cellulose may be used only as an alcoholic solution, and it may bexpected to retard disintegration and dissolution time of drugs in the resulting tablets when wet granulation is employed. Polyvinylpyrrolidone is a synthetic polymer that may be used as an adhesive in either an aqueous solution or alcohol. It also has some capabilities as a dry binder.

3. **Disintegrants:** A disintegrant is added to most tablet formulations to facilitate a breakup or disintegration of the tablet when it contacts water in the gastrointestinal tract. Disintegrants may function by drawing water into the tablet, swelling, and causing the tablet to burst apart. Such tablet fragmentation may be critical to the subsequent dissolution of the drug and to the attainment of satisfactory drug bioavailability. Starch USP and various starch derivatives are the most common disintegrating agents. They also have the lowest cost. Starch is typically used in a concentration range of 5 to 20% of tablet weight. Various pregelatinized starches are also employed as disintegrants, usually in a 5% concentration.

   The cellulose class material, Ac-Di-Sol is effective in low concentration levels as a disintegrant. It is an internally crosslinked form of sodium carboxymethylcellulose. Another cross-linked polymer that is available as a disintegrant is cross-linked polyvinylpyrrolidone. Clays such as Vee gum HV and bentonite have been used as disintegrants at about a 10% level. Such use of these materials is limited unless the tablets are coloured since the clays produce an off-white appearance. The clays are typically less effective as disintegrants.

4. **Lubricants:** Lubricants are intended to reduce the friction during tablet ejection between the walls of the tablet and the walls of the die cavity in which the tablet was formed. Since lubrication is basically a coating process, the finer the particle size of the lubricant, the more effective the lubricant action is likely to be.

   Hydrocarbon oils such as mineral oil have been employed by application to granulation as a fine spray, either directly or in a solvent solution. The problem with using this type of lubricant is the production of oil spots. The most widely used lubricants have been stearic acid and various stearic acid salts and derivatives. Calcium and magnesium stearate are the most common salts employed. The higher-molecular-weight polyethylene glycols and certain polymeric surfactants have been used as water-soluble lubricants.

5. **Antiadherents:** Antiadherents have the purpose of reducing sticking or adhesion of any of the tablet granulation or powder to the faces of the punches or to the die wall. Talc, magnesium stearate, and starch as well as starch derivatives possess antiadherent properties. In addition, various colloidal silicas have been used as antiadherents.
6. **Glidants:** Glidants are intended to promote flow of the tablet granulation or powder materials by reducing faction between the particles. Materials used as glidants, or flow promoters, are typically talc at a 5% concentration, corn starch at a 5 to 10% concentration, or colloidal silicas such as Cab-O-Sil, Syloid, or Aerosil in 0.25 to 3% concentrations.
7. **Colours, Flavours and Sweeteners:** The use of colours and dyes in tablet making has served three purposes over the years: disguising of off-colour drugs, product identification, and production of a more elegant product. Two forms of colour have typically been used in tablet preparation. These are the FD&C and D&C dyes—which are applied as solutions, typically in the granulating agent—and the lake forms of these dyes. Lakes are dyes that have been absorbed on a hydrous oxide and usually are employed as dry powders for colouring. Flavours are usually limited to chewable tablets or other tablets intended to dissolve in the mouth. In general, flavours that are water-soluble have found little acceptance in tablet making because of their poor stability. Flavour soils are added to tablet granulations in solvents, are dispersed on clays and other absorbents, or are emulsified in aqueous granulating agents. Usually, the maximum amount of oil that can be added to a granulation without influencing its tabletting characteristics is 0.5 to 0.75%. The use of sweeteners is primarily limited to chewable tablets to exclude or limit the use of sugar in the tablets. Mannitol is reportedly about 72% as sweet as sucrose and is used commonly.

2.5 MANUFACTURING OF TABLETS

There are three methods used in the manufacture of tablets:

1. Direct compression
2. Compression granulation
3. Wet granulation

2.5.1 Direct Compression

In this method, the components of the tablet formula are directly compressed into tablets without a granulation stage. Crystalline materials such as sodium chloride, sodium bromide, and potassium chloride have the necessary flow properties and compressibility that make suitable for direct compression. However, such tablets may not disintegrate sufficiently. Most materials are not directly compressible since they may have weak intermolecular attraction or covered with films of adsorbed gases that interfere with compression. Thus, most large dose drugs with such properties cannot be made into tablets using this method. When a drug itself has poor compressible properties, it is possible to add a sufficient quantity of directly compressible (DC) diluents to make a formula suitable for tablet compression. With small dose drugs, however, a uniform blend of the drug and a coarser diluent is difficult to achieve and not practical. But with moderate dose drugs, it would be possible to prepare tablets by direct compression by using DC diluents such as spray-dried lactose and microcrystalline cellulose.

The steps involved in direct compression are weighing, dry blending with excipients (DC diluents, disintegrant, glidant and lubricants), compression to tablets. The scheme for this method is given in Fig. 2.1.

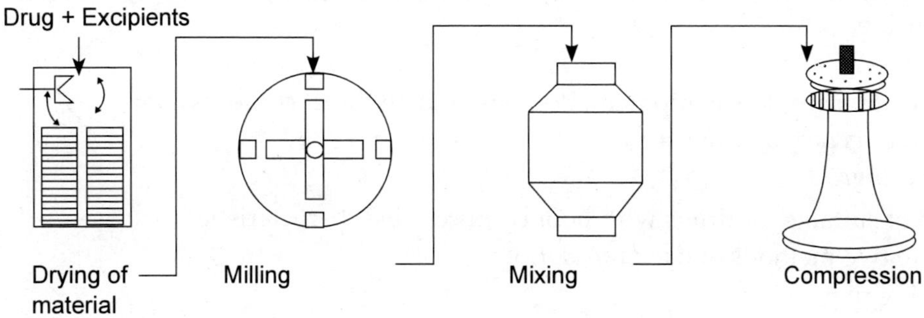

Fig. 2.1: Scheme for the manufacture of tablets by direct compression

Advantages

- Simple, economical.
- Fewer steps involved, less equipment, less floor space required, low labour input.
- Less risk of deterioration since it is a dry process.
- Faster drug release.
- E.g., vitamin B1 tablets, chlorpromazine tablets USP.

Disadvantages

- Stratification within granulation is possible.
- Large dose drugs if not directly compressible cannot be used (drug should not be more than 30% of formula).
- Not suitable for low dose drugs.
- Interaction between directly compressible diluent and drug possible. E.g., spray dried lactose.
- Dry nature of ingredients causes static charge buildup.

2.5.2 Compression Granulation

This method of tablet manufacture is also known as dry granulation, precompression or double compression. Compression granulation is used when (a) effective dose of the drug too high for direct compression, (b) when the drug is sensitive to heat/ moisture or both, e.g., aspirin, vitamins.

The components of the tablet formula are compacted by specially designed machines/modified tablet press, and the resulting compacts are milled, screened into a granulation that is finally compressed into tablets. E.g., aspirin tablets, effervescent aspirin tablets, vitamin C, B, magnesium hydroxide. By the dry granulation method, the powder mixture is compacted in large pieces and subsequently broken down or sized into granules. For this method, either the active ingredient or the diluent must have cohesive properties. Dry granulation is especially applicable to materials that cannot be prepared by wet granulation because they degrade in moisture, or the elevated temperatures are required for drying the granules.

The scheme for dry granulation methods is shown in Fig. 2.2. Steps involved are weighing, grinding/milling, blending, slugging, milling and screening, and mixing compression.

Advantages

- Fewer steps, less equipment, floor space than direct compression
- Avoids heat and moisture

Disadvantage

- Not suitable for drugs with poor compressible characteristics

There are two methods of dry granulation:

1. Slugging
2. Roller compactor or chilsonator

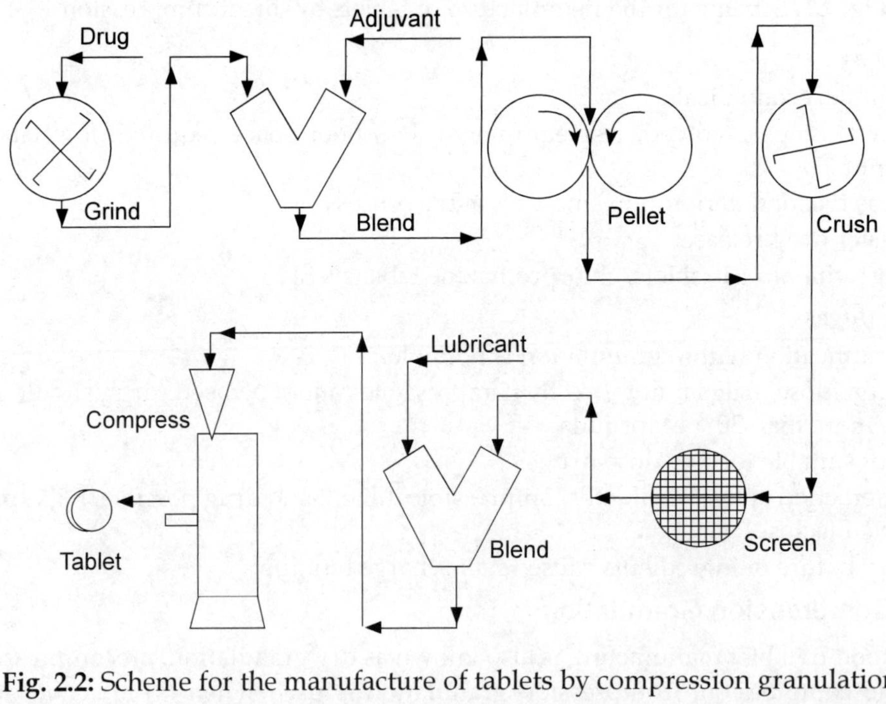

Fig. 2.2: Scheme for the manufacture of tablets by compression granulation

Slugging: After weighing and mixing the ingredients, the powder mixture is slugged, or compressed into large flat tablets or pellets about 1 inch in diameter. The slugs are broken up by hand or by a mill and passed through a screen of desired mesh for sizing. Lubricant is added in the usual manner, and tablets are prepared by compression. Aspirin, which is hydrolysed on exposure to moisture, may be prepared into tablets after slugging.

Roller Compaction: Instead of slugging, powder compactors may be used to increase the density of a powder by pressing it between rollers at 1 to 6 tonnes of pressure. The compacted material is broken up, sized, and lubricated, and tablets are prepared by compression in the usual manner. The roller compaction method is often preferred to slugging. Binding agents used in roller compaction formulations include methylcellulose or hydroxymethylcellulose (6% to 12%), which can produce good tablet hardness and friability. A schematic diagram of the Chilsonator roller Compactor is shown in Fig. 2.3.

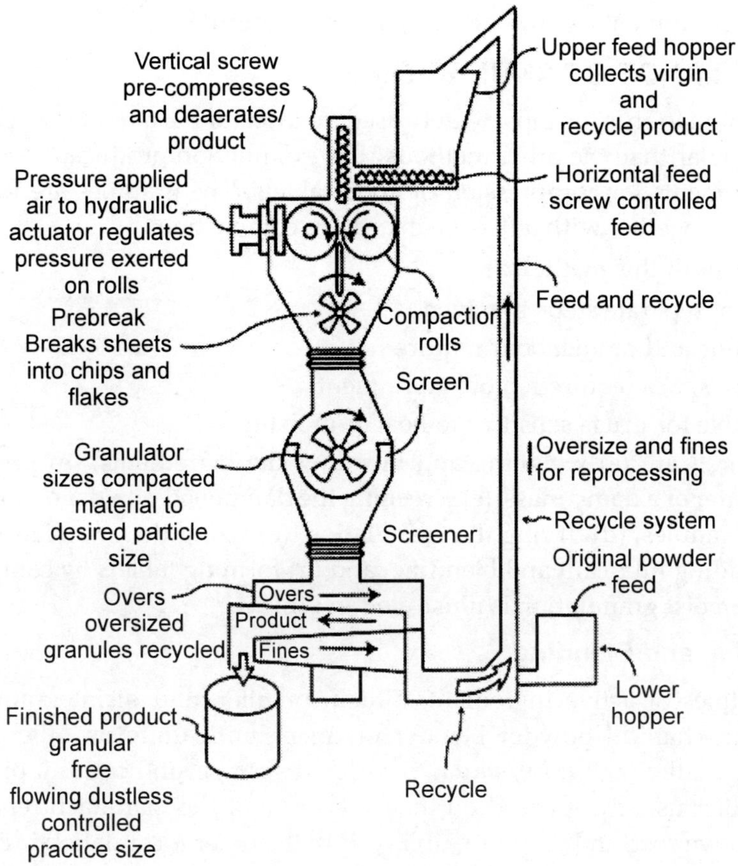

Fig. 2.3: Schematic diagram of a chilsonator roller compactor

Working of the Roller Compactor: The powder material (dry blend of drug, diluent, lubricant) from the hopper moves towards the screw conveyor and fed between the rollers by the screw conveyor. The horizontal screw picks up powder and conveys to the vertical screw, and the vertical screw delivers the powder mixture to the rollers.

Pressure is exerted by the rollers onto the powder material. The compacted mass resembling a wide ribbon break into large segments. The segments are milled and screened to produce granules.

The compaction force applied depends upon:

- Hydraulic pressure exerted on the rollers
- Rotational speed of the rollers
- Rotational speed of the feed screws

Advantages over the slugging process

- Increased production capacity
- Greater control over compaction pressure and dwell time
- No need of excessive lubrication
- Separate equipment for milling compacts not required

2.6 WET OR MOIST GRANULATION

Moist or wet granulation is the most widely used method for the manufacture of tablets and is more popular than the other methods. The granulation produced meets all the physical requirements for compression of good tablets. The granules are formed by binding powders together with adhesive instead of compaction.

The disadvantages of this method are:

- Number of separate steps involved
- Longer time and more labour required
- More floor space required, more equipment
- Not suitable for drugs sensitive to heat or moisture

The steps required are (a) weighing and blending the ingredients, (b) preparing a dampened powder or a damp mass, (c) screening the dampened powder or damp mass into pellets or granules, (d) drying the granulation, (e) sizing the granulation by dry screening, (f) adding lubricant and blending, and (g) forming tablets by compression. The scheme for moist granulation is illustrated in Fig. 2.4.

2.6.1 Weighing and Blending

Specified quantities of active ingredient, diluent or filler, and disintegrating agent are mixed by mechanical powder blender or mixer until uniform. Fillers include lactose, microcrystalline cellulose, starch, powdered sucrose, and calcium phosphate. The choice of filler usually is based on the experience of the manufacturer with the material, its relative cost, and its compatibility with the other formulation ingredients. For example, calcium salts must not be used as fillers with tetracycline antibiotics because of an interaction between the two agents that results in reduced tetracycline absorption from the gastrointestinal tract. Among the fillers most preferred are lactose, because of its solubility and compatibility, and microcrystalline cellulose, because of its easy compaction, compatibility, and consistent uniformity of supply.

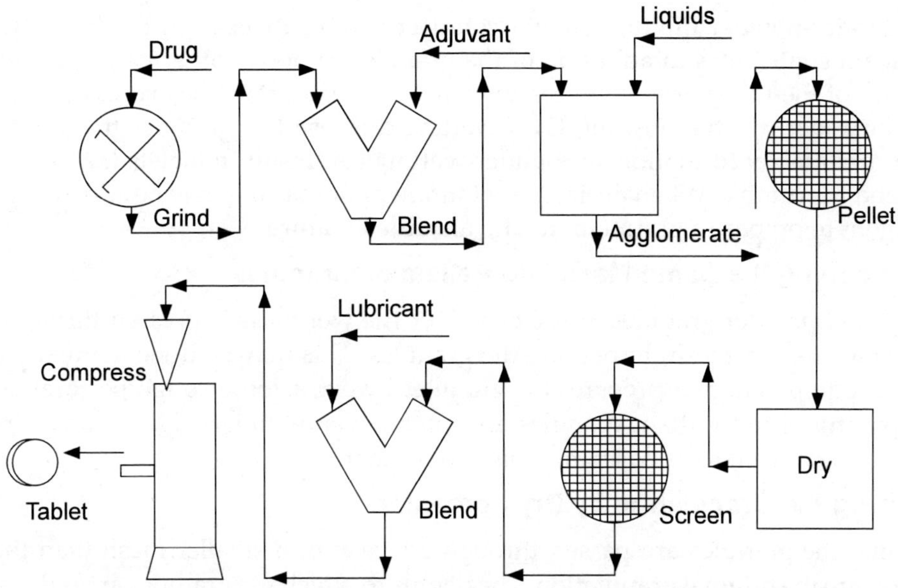

Fig. 2.4: Scheme for the manufacture of tablets by wet granulation

Disintegrating agents include croscarmellose, corn and potato starches, sodium starch glycolate, sodium carboxymethylcellulose, polyvinylpyrrolidone (PVP), crospovidone, cation exchange resins, alginic acid, and other materials that swell or expand on exposure to moisture and effect the rupture or breakup of the tablet in the gastrointestinal tract. Croscarmellose (2%) and sodium starch glycolate (5%) are often preferred because of their high-water uptake and rapid action. One commercial brand of sodium starch glycolate is reported to swell up to 300% of its volume in water. When starch is employed, 5% to 10% is usually suitable, but up to about 20% may be used to promote more rapid tablet disintegration. The total amount of disintegrant used is not always added in preparing the granulation. Often a portion (sometimes half) is reserved and added to the finished granulation prior to tablet formation. This results in double disintegration of the tablet. One portion assists in the breakup of the tablet into pieces and the other portion assists in the breakup of the pieces into fine particles.

2.6.2 Preparing the Damp Mass

A liquid binder is added to the powder mixture to facilitate adhesion of the powder particles. Either a dampened powder formed into granules or a damp mass resembling dough is formed and used to prepare the granulation. A good binder results in appropriate tablet hardness and does not hinder the release of the drug from the tablet.

Among binding agents are solutions of povidone, an aqueous preparation of corn starch (10% to 20%), glucose solution (25% to 50%), molasses, methylcellulose (3%), carboxymethyl cellulose, and microcrystalline cellulose. If the drug substance is adversely affected by an aqueous binder, a non-aqueous solution, or dry binder, may be used. The amount of binding agent used is part of the operator's art; however, the resulting binder-powder mixture should compact when squeezed in the hand. The binding agent contributes to adhesion of the granules to one another and maintains the integrity of the tablet after compression. However, care must be exercised not to over-wet or under-wet the powder. Over-wetting can result in granules that are too hard for proper tablet formation, and under-wetting can result in tablets that are too soft and tend to crumble. When desired, a colourant or flavouring may be added to the binding agent to prepare a granulation with an added feature.

2.6.3 Screening the Damp Mass into Pellets or Granules

The dampened powder granules are screened, or the wet mass is pressed through a screen (usually 6- or 8-mesh) to prepare the granules. This may be done manually or with special equipment that prepares the granules by extrusion through perforations in the apparatus. The resultant granules are spread evenly on large, lined trays and dried to consistent weight or constant moisture content.

2.6.4 Sizing the Granulation by Dry Screening

After drying, the granules are passed through a screen of a smaller mesh than that used to prepare the original granulation. The degree to which the granules are reduced depends on the size of the punches to be used. In general, the smaller the tablet to be produced, the smaller the granules. Screens of 12- to 20-mesh size are generally used for this purpose. Sizing of the granules is necessary so that the die cavities for tablet compression may be completely and rapidly filled by the free-flowing granulation. Voids or air spaces left by too large a granulation result in the production of uneven tablets.

2.6.5 Adding Lubrication and Blending

After dry screening, a dry lubricant is dusted over the spread-out granulation through a fine mesh screen. Lubricants contribute to the preparation of compressed tablets in several ways: They improve the flow of the granulation in the hopper to the die cavity. They prevent adhesion of the tablet formulation to the punches and dies during compression. They reduce friction between the tablet and the die wall during the ejection of the tablet from the machine. They give a sheen to the finished tablet. Among the more commonly used lubricants are magnesium stearate, calcium stearate, stearic acid, talc, and sodium stearyl fumarate. Magnesium stearate is mostly used. The quantity of lubricant used varies from one operation to another but usually ranges from about 0.1% to 5% of the weight of the granulation.

2.7 EQUIPMENT AND TABLET TOOLING

The size and shape of a tablet as well as certain identification markings are determined by the compression machine tooling. Each tooling set consists of a die and upper and lower punches. Since each tablet is formed by a tooling set, the tooling must meet many requirements to satisfy the needs of dosage uniformity, production efficiency, and aesthetic appearance. The terminology used with tooling is illustrated in Figs. 2.5 and 2.6.

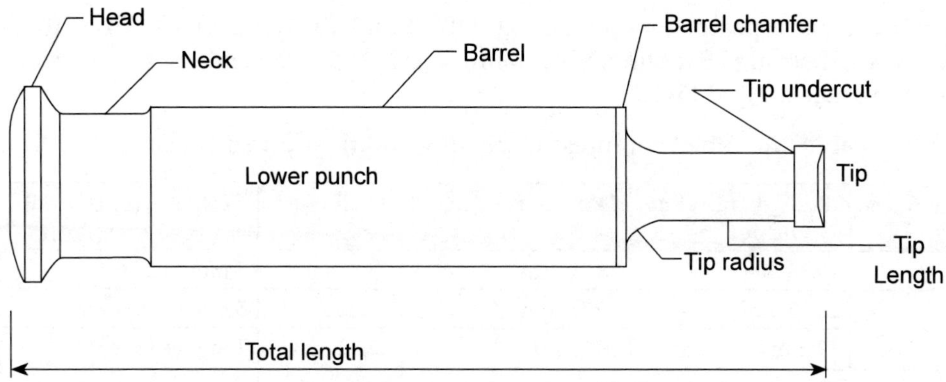

Fig. 2.5: Parts of a punch and its nomenclature

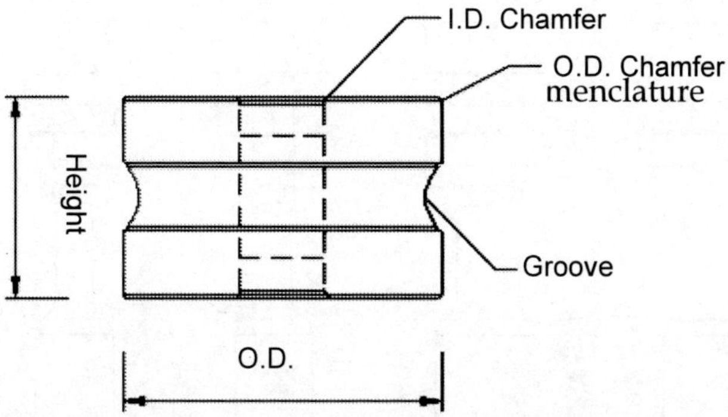

Fig. 2.6: Terminologies used to indicate the parts of a die

Upper punch: Upper punch is fitted in the turret bore and moves vertically in bores during compression. Upper punches make the upper cavity of the tablet. It is fitted with key for alignment with die bore in case of shape punches. For round punches, there is no need of key in upper punches. Upper punches travel 5-6 mm inside the die bore during compression and as per the penetration setting done in a compression machine. Tip length is shorter in the upper punch compared to the lower punch. Tip length of upper punch is generally 8-9 mm.

Lower punch: The lower punch is fitted in the turret bore and makes the lower cavity of the tablet during compression. Lower punch tip always stays inside the die bore hence there is no need of any key in case of lower punch. Tip length is relatively longer in the lower punch as it has to cover the entire height of the die and eject the tablet. The lower punch tip length is 25-28 mm.

Die: Die is fitted in the die plate. Die bore in the die is actually where the filling of powder is done. Upper punch tip and lower punch tip compress the powder in the die bore with the help of compression roller pressure applied on the head flat during compression to make the required shape of the tablet.

There are different types of tooling, i.e., D, DB, B and BB types. Apart from these standard types, there are FS tooling, BBS tooling. Various tooling and their dimensions are shown in Table 2.1 and Fig. 2.7.

Table 2.1: Tablet compression tooling and their dimensions

Tooling types	Body diameter of the punches	Die outer diameter	Die height	Tablet sizes (round)
D	25.35 mm	38.10 mm	23.81 mm	5 mm to 25 mm
DB	25.35 mm	30.16 mm	22.22 mm	5 mm to 19 mm
B	19 mm	30.16 mm	22.22 mm	4 mm to 16 mm
BB	19 mm	24 mm	22.22 mm	4 mm to 13 mm

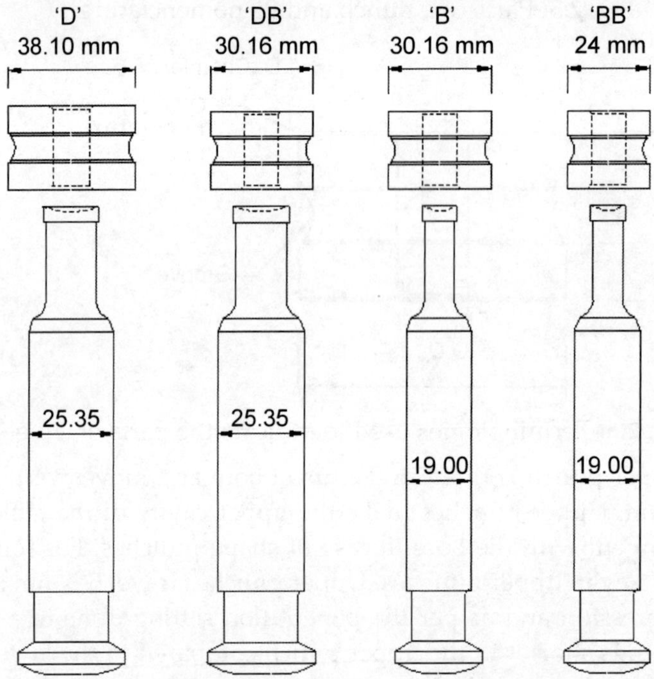

Fig. 2.7: Basic tooling types used in tablet compression machines

Several types of steel are normally used in the manufacture of compression tooling. These steels differ in toughness, to withstand the cyclic compacting forces, (ductility), and in wear resistance. Unfortunately, no single steel type has a high resistance to abrasive wear and high ductility.

2.8 TABLET COMPRESSION MACHINES

Tablets are made by compressing a formulation containing a drug or drugs with excipients by machines known as presses, whereby a tablet is formed by pressure exerted on granulation by punches within a die cavity.

The machines used for compression are of the following types:

1. Single punch/single station press
2. Multi-station rotary press
   (a) Single rotary tablet press
   (b) Double rotary tablet press

2.8.1 Single Punch Tablet Press

Single punch tablet press, also known as eccentric press or single station press, is the simplest machine for tablet manufacturing. This machine uses a single set of station tooling (a die and a pair of upper and lower punches).

The compaction force on the fill material is exerted by only the upper punch while the lower punch is static; such action is equivalent to hammering motion and as a result, the single punch press is referred to as stamping process. The single punch tablet press produces about 60-85 tablets/min.

2.8.2 Components/Functional Parts of a Single Punch Tablet Press

- Hopper - This is connected to the feed shoe, and it is where the granules/ powder mixtures are poured into prior to tabletting or compression. The hopper can be filled manually or by using mechanical equipment during subsequent tabletting.
- Die cavity is where the powder granules are compressed into tablets. The die determines.
  - ♦ The diameter of the tablet
  - ♦ The size of the tablet
  - ♦ To some extent the thickness of the tablet.
- Punches comprise upper and lower punches and they compress the powder into tablets of various shapes within the die.
- Tablet adjuster is used to adjust the volume of the powder to be compressed and so determines the weight of the tablet.
- Ejection adjuster facilitates the ejection of the tablet from the die cavity after compression.

The sequence of events involved in the formation of tablets.

1. Filling and metering

Position 1: The upper punch is raised, and lower punch drops to create a cavity in the die.

Position 2: The feed shoe moves over the die cavity and granules fall into the die cavity under the influence of gravity from the hopper.

Position 3: The feed shoe moves out of the way levelling the surface of the granules filled into the die.

2. Compression

Position 4: Punch descends to compress the granules/powder mixture into tablets by the progressive reduction of the porosity of the die content and forcing of the particles into close contact with one another.

3. Ejection

Position 5: The upper punch retracts, and the lower punch moves upwards to eject the compressed tablet. The whole events repeat until the feed material is exhausted.

Figure 2.8 shows the diagrammatic representation of the sequence of events.

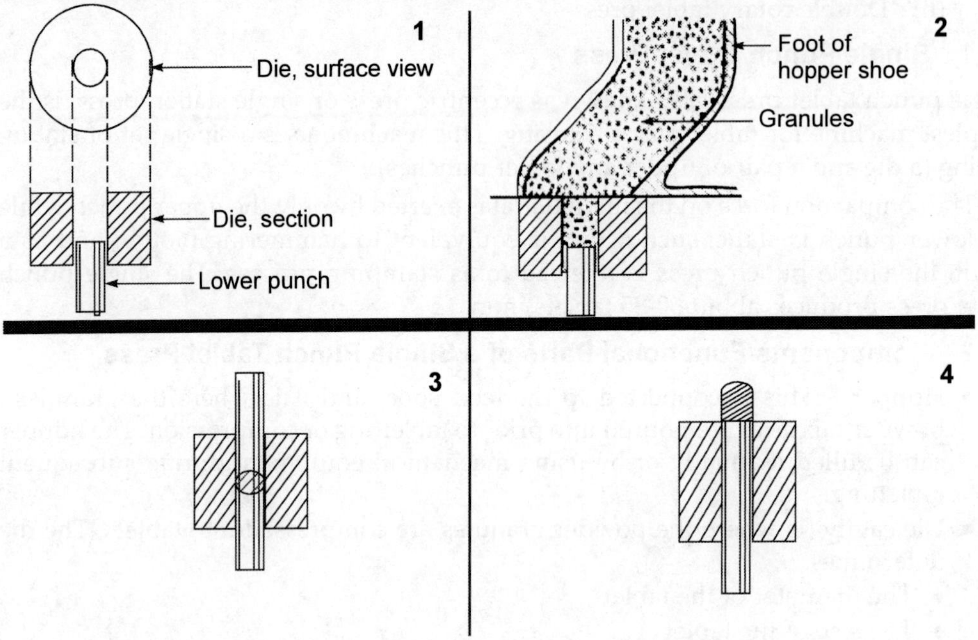

Fig. 2.8: The sequence of events involved in the formation of tablets

2.8.3 Advantages of the Single Punch Tablet Press

- The single punch structure is rational and small.
- Easy to operate and it operates at a high utilization ratio.
- It can manufacture odd-shaped products with a diameter of up to 20 mm.
- It is ideal for the development of tablets and small batch production.
- Single punch tablet press utilizes a high amount of pressure to reduce weight variations between tablets while maintaining a low noise level at the same time.

2.9 MULTI-STATION PRESS OR ROTARY TABLET MACHINE

Multi-station press is a mechanical device that unlike the single punch tablet press has several tooling stations which rotate to compress granules/powder mixture into tablets of uniform size, shape (depending on the punch design), and uniform weight. It was developed to increase the production of tablets.

2.9.1 Features of the Rotary Press

Components: Hopper, dies, punches, cam tracks, feed frame.

Upper turret: Portion of the head that holds upper punches.

Lower turret: Portion of the head that holds lower punches.

Die table: A large steel plate that holds the dies.

Fixed cam tracks: Guide the punches up and down which control sequence of filling, compression and ejection.

Feed frame: A feeding mechanism, has several interconnected compartments which help to spread the granulation over a wider area to provide time for the dies to fill.

In the rotary press, the compaction force on the fill material is exerted by both the upper and lower punches leaving the powder granules to be compressed in the middle. This is known as accordion type of compression.

The capacity of a rotary tablet press is determined by the rotation speed of the turret and the number of stations on the press. The tablet compression cycle in a multi-station machine is shown in Fig. 2.9.

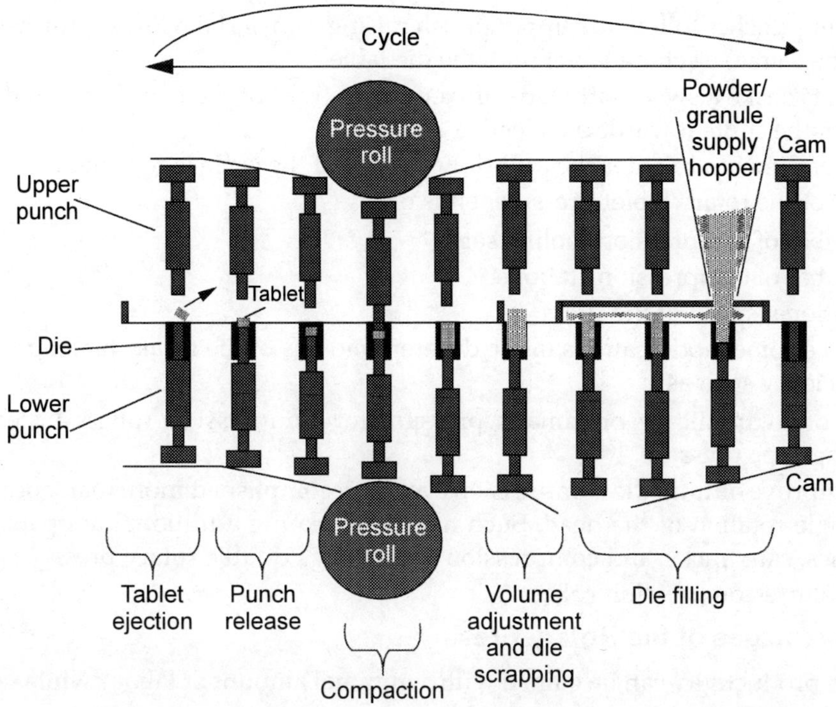

Fig. 2.9: Tablet compression cycle in a rotary tablet machine

2.10 WORKING OF THE ROTARY PRESS AND THE TABLET COMPRESSION CYCLE

1. Filling

- Granulation from the hopper moves into the feed frame.
- A pull-down cam guides the lower punches to the bottom allowing dies to overfill.

2. Weight adjustment

- Lower punches pass over the weight control cam which reduces the die fill to the desired amount.

- Wipe-off blades at the end of the feed frame to remove excess granules and move them back to the front of the feed frame.

3. Compression

- Lower punches travel over the lower compression roller and upper punches ride over the upper compression roller.
- Upper punches enter up to a fixed distance into the dies, the lower punches are raised to compact granulation within the dies (slow squeezing effect from top and bottom gives chance for the escape of entrapped air).

4. Ejection

- Upper punches follow the upper punch raising cam and the lower punches ride up the cam to eject the tablet onto the die table.
- Tablets strike a sweep-off blade affixed to the front of the feed frame and slide down the chute towards a collecting bin.
- Lower punches re-enter the pull-down cam and the cycle is repeated.

The output of the rotary tablet press depends on:

- Number of compression tooling sets
- Number of compression stations
- Rotational speed of the press

There may be some modifications in the different models of the rotary tablet press for greater efficiency such as:

- Use of hydraulic or pneumatic pressure for compression rollers instead of spring-type pressure.
- To improve output, the compression cycle is accomplished more than once with a single rotation of the head. Such machines require additional hoppers, feed frames, cam tracks, and compression rollers. E.g., double rotary press.
- Use of pre-compression rollers.

2.10.1 Advantages of the Rotary Press

- High productivity can be gained with a minimal amount of labour while saving money.
- The rotary press has an output of between 9000–234000 tablets/hour thus saving time and meeting up with the high demand of tablet dosage form.
- The powder-filled cavity can be automatically managed by a moving feeder.
- Rotary press decreases the waste of valuable formulation in non-specific tablets.
- The machine allows independent control of both weight and hardness.

2.11 COMPRESSION AND PROCESSING PROBLEMS IN TABLET MANUFACTURING (TABLET DEFECTS)

There are several types of tablet presses or tableting machines, each varying in productivity but similar in basic functions and operations. They all compress a tablet formulation within a steel die cavity by the pressure exerted by the movement of two steel punches: a lower punch, and an upper punch.

The operation of a single-punch tablet press describes the basic mechanical process. As the lower punch drops, the feed shoe filled with granulation from the hopper is positioned over and fills the die cavity. The feed shoe retracts, scrapes away the excessive granulation, and levels the fill in the die cavity. The upper punch lowers and compresses the fill, forming the tablet. The upper punch retracts as the lower punch rises with the formed tablet to the precise level of the stage. The feed shoe moves over the die cavity, shoves the tablet aside, and once again fills the cavity with granulation to repeat the process. The tablets fall into a collection container. Samples of tablets are assayed and tested for the various quality standards described earlier.

Rotary tablet machines equipped with multiple punches and dies operate via continuous rotating movement of the punches. A single rotary press with 16 stations (16 sets of punches and dies) may produce up to 1150 tablets per minute. Double rotary tablet presses with 27, 33, 37, 41, or 49 sets of punches and dies can produce two tablets for each die. Some of these machines can produce 10,000 or more tablets per minute of operation. For such high-speed production, induced die feeders are required to force the fill material into the dies to keep up with the rapidly moving punches. A consequence of high-speed production is the increased occurrence of lamination (horizontal striations) and tablet capping, in which the top of the tablet separates from the whole because the fill material does not have enough time to bond after compression. Reduced speed remedies the problem.

Multiple-layer tablets are produced by multiple feed and multiple compression of fill material within a single die. Tablets with an inner core are prepared by machines with a special feed apparatus that places the core tablet precisely within the die for compression with surrounding fill.

2.11.1 Processing Problems

In the normal process of developing formulations, and in the routine manufacture of tablets, various problems occur. Sometimes, the source of the problem is the formulation, the compression equipment, or a combination of the two.

Capping and Lamination: Capping is a term used to describe the partial or complete separation of the top or bottom crowns of a tablet from the main body of the tablet. Lamination is the separation of a tablet into two or more distinct layers. Figure 2.10 shows the capping and lamination of tablets.

Usually, these processing problems are readily apparent immediately after compression; however, capping and lamination may occur hours or even days later. Research has shown, however, that capping, and lamination are due to the deformational properties of the formulation during and immediately following compression.

Picking and sticking: "Picking" is a term used to describe the surface material from a tablet that is sticking to and being removed from the tablet's surface by a punch. Picking is of particular concern when punch tips have engraving or embossing. Small, enclosed areas such as those found in the letters "B," "A," and "O" are difficult to manufacture cleanly. Tablet materials that stick to the punches can accumulate to the point of obliterating the tip design.

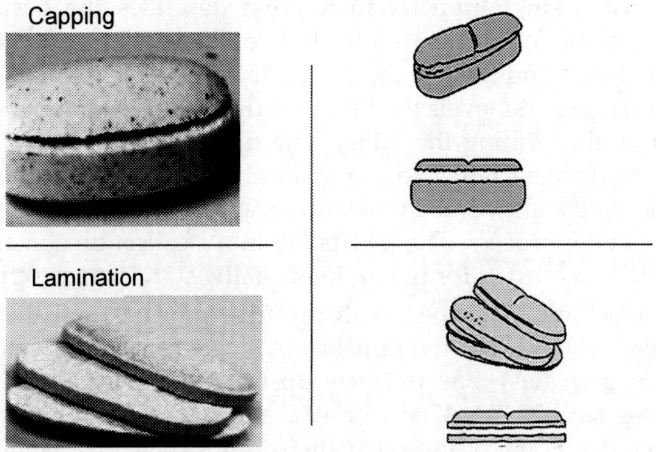

Fig. 2.10: Capping and lamination defects in tablet manufacturing

"Sticking" refers to tablet material adhering to the die wall. When sticking occurs, additional force is required to overcome the friction between the tablet and the die wall during ejection. Serious sticking at ejection can cause chipping of a tablet's edges and can produce a rough edge. The sticking and picking problems are represented in Fig. 2.11.

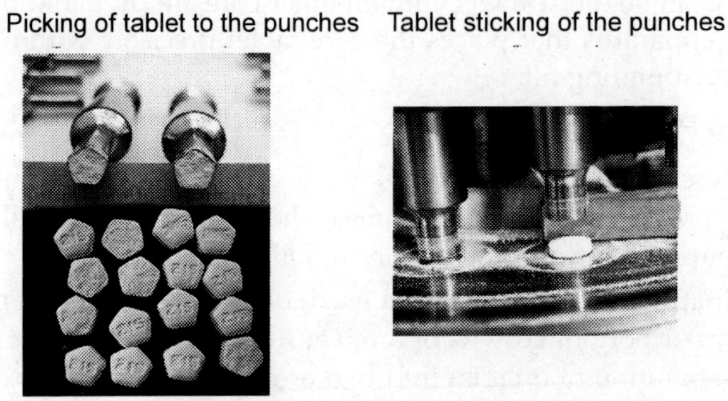

Fig. 2.11: Picking and sticking of tablets

In some cases, colloidal silica added to the formula acts as a polishing agent and makes the punch faces smooth so that material does not cling to them. On the other hand, the frictional nature of this material may require additional lubrication to facilitate release of the tablet from the die. Sometimes, additional binder or a change in binder may make the granules more cohesive, and therefore less adherent, than before.

Mottling: Mottling is an unequal distribution of colour on a tablet (as shown in Fig. 2.12), with light or dark areas standing out in an otherwise uniform surface. One cause of mottling is a drug whose colour differs from the tablet excipients or a drug whose degradation products are coloured. The use of colourants may solve the above problem.

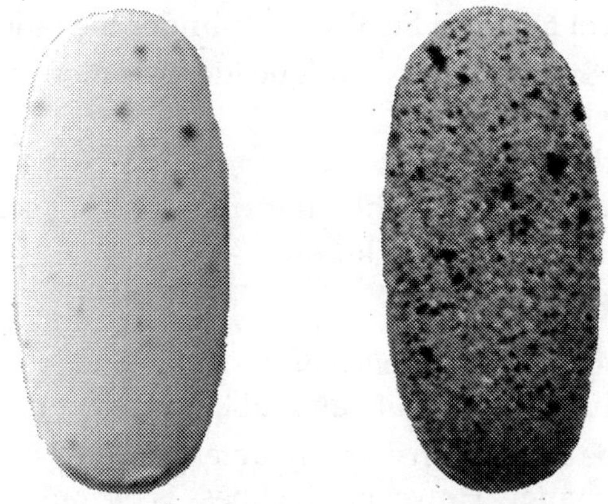

Fig. 2.12. Mottling in tablets

Weight Variation: Weight variation of tablets has been mentioned as an important in-process quality control measurement, and weight variation specifications have been given in pharmacopoeia. The weight of a tablet being compressed is determined by the amount of granulation in the die prior to compression. Therefore, anything that can alter the die-filling process can alter tablet's weight and weight variation.

Double Impression: The last problem for discussion is that of double impression. This involves only punches that have a monogram or other engraving on them. At the moment of compression, the tablet receives the imprint of the punch. On some machines, the lower punch is free to drop and then travel is uncontrolled for a short distance before it rides up the ejection cam to push the tablet out of the die. During its free travel, it rotates. At this point, the punch may make a new, although lighter, impression on the bottom of the tablet, resulting in a double imprint as shown in Fig. 2.13. Similar problems can be encountered with engraved upper punches and tablet machines that utilize two compression stages to compress a tablet.

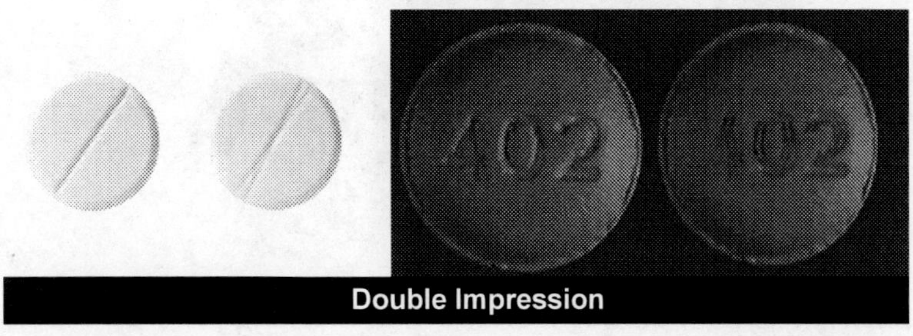

Fig. 2.13: Double impression problems occurring during tablet punching

2.12 QUALITY CONTROL TESTS FOR TABLETS: IN-PROCESS AND FINISHED PRODUCT TESTS

Evaluation of the quality of tablets takes place in three areas, i.e., raw material testing, e.g., identity tests for API, excipients; in-process testing, e.g., hardness, thickness, weight variation.

The various quality control tests can be discussed under the following headings:

1. *General appearance:* Size and shape, unique identification markings, organoleptic properties, physical defects
2. *Strength tests:* Hardness, friability
3. *Drug content:* Uniformity of weight, uniformity of drug content
4. *Drug release:* Disintegration, dissolution

2.12.1 General Appearance

General appearance is the overall elegance of the tablet and is essential for consumer acceptance, for batch-to-batch uniformity and tablet-to-tablet uniformity.

Size and shape: The shape and dimensions are determined by the tooling used during compression and do not change. However, thickness is the only variable and depends on (at constant compressive load) die fill, particle size distribution and packing and tablet weight. At constant die fill, thickness varies with compressive load (force). Thickness of individual tablets can be measured by a micrometer screw guage. A quicker method is to determine the total crown thickness of 5-10 tablets in a holding tray with a vernier calipers and determine the average. Tablet thickness should be controlled within a ± 5% of a standard value. Any variation in thickness should not be apparent to the unaided eye for consumer acceptance.

Unique identification markings: Unique markings are used by pharmaceutical manufacturers for rapid identification of their products. These markings may be embossed, engraved, or printed on the tablet surface. The type of marking used includes the company name/logo, product code, product name or product potency. Figure 2.14 illustrates tablets with such markings.

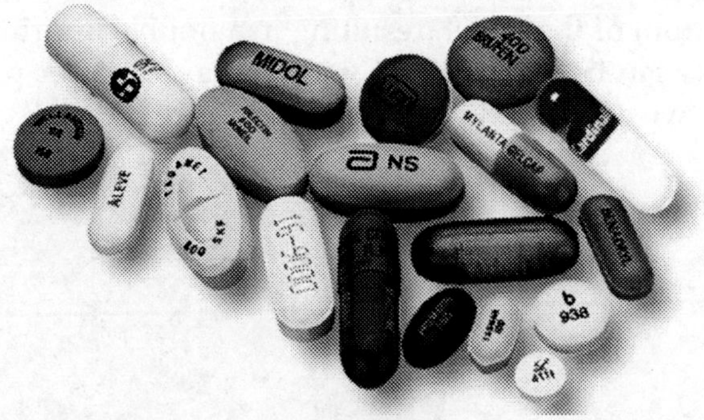

Fig. 2.14: Tablets with unique identification markings on their surfaces

2.12.2 Organoleptic Properties

Colour: Manufacturers use colour in their tablets for rapid identification and consumer acceptance. The colour of a tablet must be uniform within a tablet, from tablet to tablet, and from lot to lot. Colour evaluation may be visually done by comparing with colour standards; however, this may not be accurate. Instrumental methods such as reflectance spectrophotometry, tristimulus colorimetry, microreflectance photometry have been used to measure the colour uniformity and gloss on a tablet surface.

Odour: The presence of an odour in tablets maybe due to: a) stability problem, e.g., degrading aspirin tablets, (b) characteristic of drug, e.g., vitamin B, (c) added flavours, and (d) excipients, e.g., polymers for coating.

Taste: Taste is important for consumer acceptance of chewable and mouth dissolving tablets. Manufacturers may use taste panels to judge the preference of different flavours and flavour levels. The control of taste in such tablets is often the presence or absence of a specific taste.

Physical defects: Tablets in a batch are subjected to visual inspection for flaws such as chipping, cracks, contamination with foreign material, surface texture and appearance. Good tablets are collected and sent for packaging; the rejected tablets may be destroyed according to standard operating procedures.

2.12.3 Strength Tests

Hardness: Tablets require adequate hardness or strength to withstand mechanical shocks of handling in manufacture, packaging, shipping or in the hands of the consumer. In addition, tablet hardness affects tablet disintegration and drug dissolution and ultimately, drug bioavailability. Tablet hardness is defined as the force required to break a tablet in a diametric compression test and is also referred to as the crushing strength. Hardness can be measured using testers such as the Monsanto tester, Strong Cobb tester, Pfizer tester, Schleuniger tester, etc.

Principle of hardness testers: A tablet is placed between two anvils; force is applied to the anvils and the crushing strength or force required to break the tablet is recorded.

The Monsanto tester consists of a barrel containing a compressible spring between two plungers. The lower plunger is placed in contact with the tablet and a zero reading is taken. The upper plunger is forced against a spring by turning a threaded bolt until the tablet ruptures. As the spring is compressed, a pointer rides along a gauge to indicate the force.

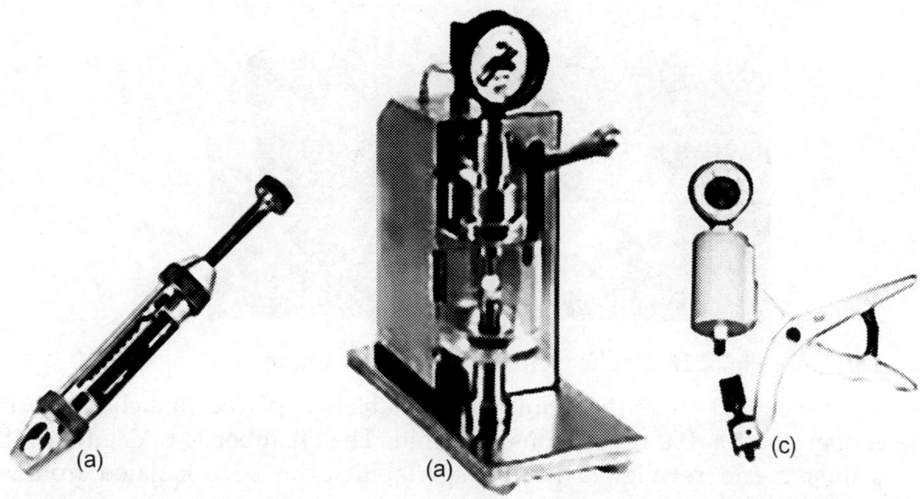

Fig. 2.15: (a) Monsanto tester (b) Strong Cobb tester (c) Pfizer tester

The Strong Cobb tester was developed to overcome the manual nature of the Monsanto tester. Air pressure is used to pump the lever arm, an anvil is forced against a stationary platform by hydraulic pressure. The force required to fracture the tablet is read from the hydraulic gauge.

Pfizer tester operates on the mechanical principle of a pair of pliers. As the handle is squeezed, the tablet is compressed between a holding anvil and a piston connected to a direct force reading gauge. These testers are shown in Fig. 2.15.

2.12.4 Friability

Tablet's hardness alone is not the only indicator of strength. Some hard tablets undergo chipping, capping, fragmentation on attrition. Such tablets lack elegance, affect consumer acceptance, create dirt due to powdering in coating or packaging which leads to significant weight variation, and content uniformity problems. Therefore, another measure of tablet strength that is considered, is its friability.

The objective of the friability test is to evaluate the ability of the tablet to withstand abrasion in packaging, handling, and shipping. Friability test is official in the USP but not the BP, and is now official in the IP (2014 edition).

The laboratory friability tester is known as the Roche friabilator (Fig. 2.16). This device subjects a number of tablets to the combined effects of abrasion and shock. It consists of a transparent, discoid plastic chamber with a curved partition and revolves at 25 rpm. The tablets are dropped from a distance of 6 inches at each turn of the chamber. There is also a timer to set the duration of the test.

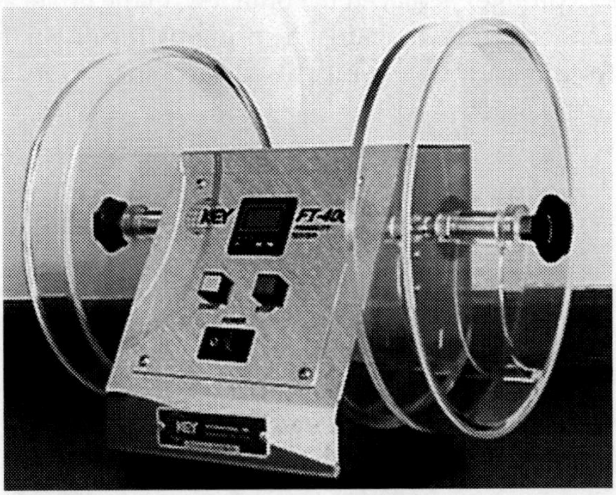

Fig. 2.16: Roche friabilator with two chambers

Method: A pre-weighed tablet (w_1) sample of 10 tablets is placed in a chamber. The machine is operated for 100 revolutions or 4 min. The chamber is opened, and the tablets are dusted and reweighed (w_2). The friability can be calculated from the formula:

$$F = 100 \times (w_1 - w_2/w_1)$$

To comply with the test, the calculated value should not exceed the limit of 1%. A particular sample of tablets is tested only once, if weight loss is greater than the targeted value, test is repeated twice and an average of 3 tests is taken.

Chewable and effervescent tablets tend to have greater friability. The friability can exceed limits due to 'whiskering', because of wear of concave faced punches and very dry granulations.

2.12.5 Drug Content Tests

Uniformity of weight: The weight of a tablet helps to ensure that it contains the specific amount or dose of the drug. The objective of this test is to determine whether the weight variation of tablets in a batch is within the prescribed limits.

Method: This test is run by weighing 10 or 20 tablets taken at random individually. The average weight of the tablets is determined. The percentage of deviation of its weight from the average weight was determined for each tablet. The deviation of the individual weight of each tablet from the average weight should not exceed the limits given in Table 2.2.

Table 2.2: Permissible limits for weight variation as per I.P.

Average wt. of tablets (mg)	Max. permissible limit for deviation (%)
80 or less	±10
More than 80 and less than 250	± 7.5
250 or more	± 5

The tablets comply with the test if no more than two tablets have a percentage deviation outside the permissible limit and if no tablet differs by more than twice this limit.

The weight variation test would be adequate for assessing the drug content uniformity, if the tablets contain 25 mg or more of the drug and comprises about 25% or more of the weight of one tablet. E.g., Paracetamol tablets usually contain more than 90% of the drug, hence the ± 5% weight variation will come close to its true potency or drug content.

2.12.6 Uniformity of Drug Content

The uniformity of weight test is not sufficient to assure uniformity of drug content or potency of tablets containing moderate or low dose drugs, in which excipients make up the bulk of the tablet weight. Such tablets require an additional test for evaluating the uniformity of drug content. The potency of a tablet is expressed in grams, milligrams, or micrograms of drug per tablet and is given as the label strength of the product.

Non-uniformity in drug content is due to:

- Non-uniform distribution of drug throughout powder/granulation
- Segregation of powder mixture/ granulation during manufacture
- Tablet weight variation

Method: About 30 tablets are taken at random from a batch. Out of these, 10 tablets are taken and the active content of each tablet is determined as per the assay given in the monograph or any other suitable method

Acceptance limits: The tablets comply with the test if the drug content in each tablet is 85 to 115 per cent of the labelled drug content.

The tablets fail if (a) more than one tablet test shows content outside above limits or (b) if one tablet shows content outside the limits of 75 to 125 per cent of the labelled content.

If one tablet is outside 85 -115% but within 75-125%, the test is repeated with the remaining 20 tablets. The tablets pass, if out of 30, not more than one shows drug content outside 85 -115% and none shows outside the limits of 75 to 125 % of the labelled strength.

2.12.7 Drug Release Tests

Disintegration: For a drug to dissolve adequately in the gastrointestinal fluids, from a tablet, the latter must disintegrate or break down into smaller particles or granules. Disintegration test determines whether tablets disintegrate within the prescribed time when placed in a liquid medium under the prescribed experimental conditions. The disintegration test can be used as an in-process control test to ensure lot-to-lot uniformity and as a guide to the formulator in the preparation of an optimum tablet formula. The apparatus used to evaluate disintegration of unit solid dosage forms is the USP disintegration test apparatus. A picture of the same is illustrated in Fig. 2.17.

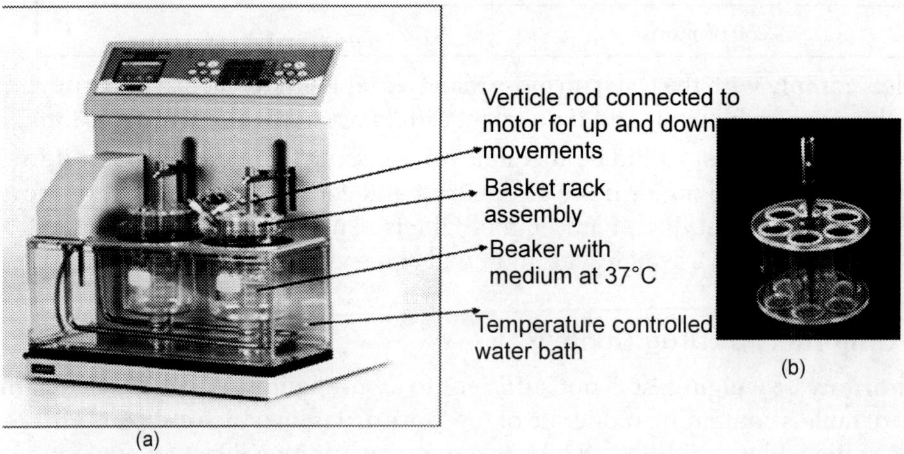

(a) (b)

Fig. 2.17: (a) USP disintegration apparatus (b) Basket rack assembly

Features of the USP disintegration test apparatus

- Consists of a basket rack assembly which has 6 glass tubes of3 inches length, held vertically between two transparent plastic plates.
- The plates have 6 holes to coincide with openings of the tubes (same diameter).
- Attached to the underside of the lower plate is a 10-mesh wire screen.

- There is a vertical metal rod fixed to the centre of the upper plate connected to a standard motor driven device for raising and lowering the assembly at a frequency of 28-32 cycles/min through a distance of 5-6 cm.
- The basket rack assembly is positioned in a 1 litre beaker containing distilled water/simulated gastric fluid/simulated intestinal fluid maintained at 37 ± 2°C by thermostatic arrangement (water bath).
- The volume of the medium should be such that the tablets remain 2.5 cm below the surface of the liquid on the upward movement and 2.5 cm from the bottom of the beaker on the downward movement.
- Perforated plastic discs are placed on top of the tablets to impart abrasive action and prevent tablets from floating.

Method as per the I.P. (2014)

Introduce one tablet into each tube of the basket rack assembly and add a disc to each tube. Suspend the assembly into a beaker containing the specified fluid. Operate the apparatus for the specified time. Remove the assembly from the liquid and observe for tablets that have completely disintegrated.

The pharmacopoeia gives procedures for running the disintegration test for uncoated tablets, film coated tablets, enteric coated tablets, buccal, sublingual tablets, and fast mouth disintegrating tablets. The time limits for some of these are given in Table 2.3.

Table 2.3: Disintegration time limits

Type of tablet		**Disintegration time**
Uncoated Tablets		15 minutes
Coated Tablets	Film-coated	30 minutes
	Other coated tablets	60 minutes
Enteric coated Tablets	0.1 M hydrochloric acid	Should not disintegrate in 120 minutes
	Mixed phosphate buffer pH 6.8,	60 minutes.
Dispersible and soluble tablets		within 3 minutes
Effervescent tablets		5 minutes

Acceptance criteria: To comply with the test (pharmacopoeial standards), all tablets must disintegrate, and all particles must pass through the screen within the time specified. If any residue remains, it must have a soft mass with no palpably firm core.

If 1 or 2 tablets fail to disintegrate, repeat the test with an additional 12 tablets. Not less than 16 of a total of 18 tablets should disintegrate within the prescribed time to comply with the test.

Dissolution: The disintegration test does not give assurance that the tablet particles after disintegration will dissolve at the appropriate rate. Drug absorption and bioavailability depend on the rate and extent of drug dissolution at the site of absorption. Therefore, suitable dissolution characteristics are important properties of a satisfactory tablet, and the dissolution test can be considered an indirect method for the measurement of bioavailability of the drug, provided there is good in vitro-in vivo correlation.

Objectives

- To show that the release of the drug from the tablet is as close to 100% as possible.
- Rate of drug release is uniform from batch to batch and same as the release rate from proven bioavailable and clinically effective batches.

The apparatus used is the USP dissolution test apparatus 1 and 2. The USP specifies that either of the two apparatuses be used for determining dissolution rates.

2.13 FEATURES OF THE USP DISSOLUTION TEST APPARATUS

Apparatus 1 as per the I.P.

- It consists of a transparent cylindrical vessel with hemispherical bottom, made of borosilicate glass or plastic of 1000 mL capacity (Fig. 2.18).
- The stirring element is a paddle formed from a blade and shaft connected to the motor with a speed regulator.
- Flask or vessel containing the dissolution medium is maintained at 37°C ± 0.5°C by a constant temperature bath.
- The lower edge of the paddle blade is 2.5 cm from the inside bottom of the vessel.

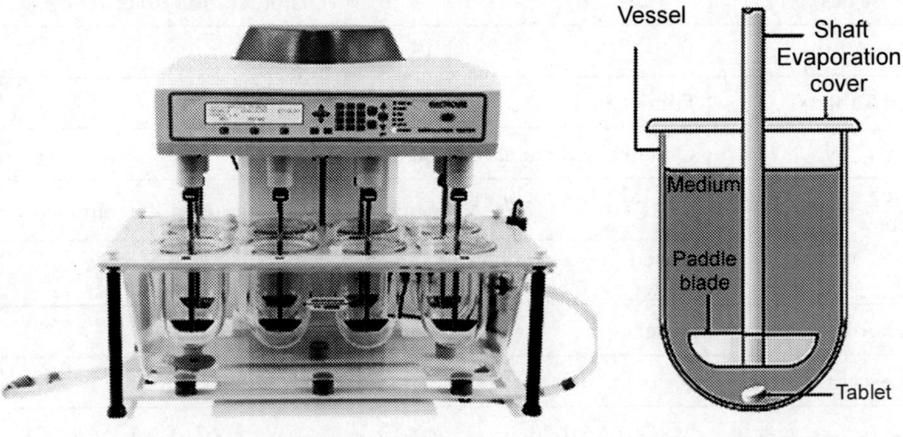

(a) (b)

Fig. 2.18: USP Dissolution Test Apparatus 1 (a) Schematic representation of dissolution vessel with paddle (b)

Apparatus 2 as per the I.P.

- Features are the same as Apparatus 1, but the stirring element consists of a stainlesssteel wire mesh basket (Fig. 2.19).

- The basket consists of a top part with a vent attached to the shaft and has 3 spring clips, the lower detachable part made of wire mesh cloth and cylindrical in shape into which the dosage form to be tested is placed. Alternatively, instead of the spring clips, some models use baskets with screw threads that can be used to fix them onto the shaft.
- The tablet is placed in the basket before immersion in the medium.

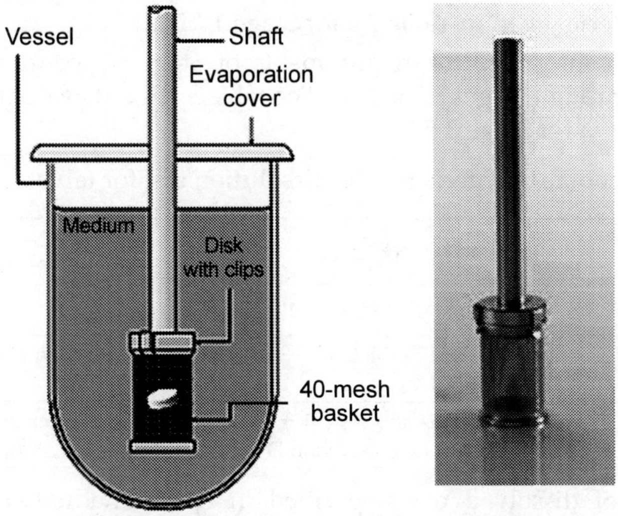

Fig. 2.19: Schematic representation of dissolution vessel with basket in the USP dissolution test apparatus 2 (a) wire mesh basket with shaft (b)

2.14 DISSOLUTION PARAMETERS

The individual monograph for the dissolution study of tablets specifies:

- Type of apparatus to be used
- Type of dissolution medium, e.g., simulated gastric or intestinal fluid
- Volume of dissolution medium
- Speed of paddle or basket in rpm, e.g., 50 or 100 rpm
- Time limit of test, e.g., 30 min
- Assay procedure, e.g., HPLC
- Test tolerance expressed as percentage of labelled amount of drug dissolved (D value)

Method: The stated volume of the dissolution medium is placed into the vessel. The apparatus is assembled, and the medium is warmed to 37.5°C. The tablet is placed in the medium and allowed to sink to the bottom (for Apparatus 1) or placed in the basket prior to immersion in the medium (for Apparatus 2). The apparatus is operated immediately at the speed of rotation specified. At time/time intervals specified, a sample of the medium is removed midway between the surface of the dissolution medium and the top of the rotating blade but not less than 10 mm from the wall of the vessel. In case of multiple-point analysis, the sample taken can be replaced with equal volume of fresh dissolution medium to keep the volume of the latter constant. Analysis for the drug is performed as per the assay specified. The entire operation is repeated 5 more times. For each tablet tested, the amount of dissolved drug is calculated as a percentage of the stated amount.

Acceptance criteria: Tablets comply with the test if the quantity of the drug dissolved conforms to the criteria given in Table 2.4 for Stage 1 (S1).

If they do not conform to the requirements of Stage S1, continue testing with additional tablets through stages S2 and S3. The tablets fail if they do not comply with the acceptance criteria for Stage 3 (S3).

Table 2.4: Acceptance criteria for the dissolution test for tablets in 3 stages

Level	Number tested	Acceptance criteria
S1	6	Each tablet is not less than D + 5%
S2	6	Average of 12 tablets (S1 + S2) is = or greater than D and no tablet is less than D - 15%
S3	12	Average of 24 tablets (S1 + S2 + S3) is = or greater than D, not more than 2 tablets are less than D - 15% and none is less than D - 25%

D is the amount of dissolved drug specified in the individual monograph and expressed as percentage of the labelled content.

REVIEW QUESTIONS

Short Answers

1. What are the types of tablets?
2. Discuss the advantages of tablets over other dosage forms.
3. Write a note on binders used in tablets.
4. Discuss the dissolution testing of tablets.
5. Write a note on granulation techniques.
6. Discuss the tooling of tablet compression equipment.
7. What are the defects of tablets?

Short Essays

1. Explain the formulation of tablets.
2. What is the quality control tests for tablets? Explain.
3. Describe the tablet compression cycle.

3

TABLET COATING

Learning Objectives

After going through this chapter, you would be able to:

1. Discuss the different types of coating.
2. Describe different steps in each coating process.
3. Explain the general formulation of the coating solution.
4. Give examples of polymers used in coating solutions.
5. Understand the working process of a coting pan.
6. Discuss the coated film defects.

3.1 INTRODUCTION

Tablet coating is the process of applying a coating solution to a moving bed of tablets with the use of hot air to facilitate evaporation of the solvent. Covering the tablet surface by a suitable material and methods and equipment. The coating of the tablet is an additional process that also raises the cost of the tablet.

Objectives of tablet coating are:

1. To mask the unpleasant taste, odour and colour of the drug.
2. To provide physical and chemical protection for the drug.
3. To control the drug release.
4. Protecting drug from gastric environment by applying enteric coating (acid resistance)
5. To incorporate another drug in the form of coating or any adjuvant to avoid chemical incompatibility.
6. To improve aesthetic qualities of the product.

There are three different types of coating:

(a) Sugar coating
(b) Film coating
(c) Enteric coating

3.2 SUGAR COATING

It has multiple steps and takes anywhere from a few hours to a few days to complete. The good quality coating depends on the skill of the coating operator. The coating operator decides on the amount of solution to apply, method and rate of solution pouring, the time of dry air application, and how long or how fast the tablets must tumble in the pan.

Sugar coating process involves the following steps:

(a) Sealing
(b) Subcoating
(c) Syruping (smoothing)
(d) Finishing
(e) Polishing

(a) ***Sealing (seal coating):*** To prevent moisture from penetrating the tablet core, a seal coat is applied. During the pan ladling procedure tablets are over-wetted, without seal coat tablet absorbs excess moisture, becomes soft, even disintegrates, even affects the physical and chemical properties of the product. Seal coat prevents the above problem. Sealing coats usually consist of alcoholic solutions of resins such as shellac, zein, hydroxyl propyl methyl cellulose (HPMC), polyvinyl acetate phthalate (PVAP), cellulose acetate phthalate (CAP).

Shellac is a good sealer; however, the polymerization of shellac may cause it to take longer to disintegrate and dissolve with age. By introducing PVP into the shellac composition, this problem can be reduced.

Zein is also a sealant, alcohol soluble protein derivative obtained from corn. As shellac, Zein does not lengthen dissolution rate. When water insoluble polymer is used as a seal coat formulation, it is applied in minimum quantity to give the appropriate protection.

(b) ***Subcoating:*** It is the most important step in the sugar coating process. Subcoating is applied to cover and round the edges of the tablet, resulting in a 50-100 per cent increase in tablet weight. Subcoating involves applying sticky binder solution and then applying dusting subcoating powder and then drying. This process is repeated until the tablet's edges are covered and the appropriate tablet thickness is reached. The spray process is used for this step consist subcoating suspension containing both binder solution and insoluble powder. The critical step is controlling drying rate. Fillers like talc, calcium sulphate, calcium carbonate, kaolin, and titanium dioxide are commonly used in subcoating compositions. Auxiliary film formers, such as acacia, gelatin, and cellulose derivatives, may also be used to improve the coating's structural integrity.

(c) ***Syruping/Syrup coating, smoothing and colouring:*** Syruping is applied to cover imperfect surface of the tablet caused during subcoating, as well as at this stage colour is applied on the tablet surface.

First syrup containing suspended powder such as talc, calcium carbonate, starch is called as "grossing syrups"(bulky).To achieve a smooth surface, the final few applications might be applied with a syrup free of suspended powder. If the tablets are to be coloured, the colourants are usually put in these clear syrup layers, which helps to ensure that the colour on the tablet surface is uniform. Colour is not applied till tablet surface is not sufficiently smooth otherwise may lead to mottling effect at final stage. In this stage coloured syrup solution is used until final size and colour is not achieved. In the final finishing step, one or two layers of clear syrup may be applied. Coloured syrup solution is utilized at this stage until the ultimate size and colour are not reached. One or two layers of clear syrup may be added at the final stage.

(d) ***Polishing and Finishing:*** Since freshly colour coated tablets are typically dull, it is necessary to polish them. It is the final step where tablets are polished to give gloss (shine) on the tablet surface. To polish the tablet coating pan or canvas lined polishing pan, powdered wax (bees wax/carnauba wax) or warm solution of these waxes in naphtha or another suitable solvent (volatile) is applied on the surface of the pan or canvas on which the tablets are tumbled.

3.2.1 Sugar Coating Process

1. Materials and equipment

- ***Stainless steel coating pan:*** 40-inch diameter with variable speed control.
- ***Accela-Cota pan system:*** 48-inch diameter with 2-3 air atomizing nozzles having 0.40 to 0.30-inch diameter nozzle. The air is set at 30 to 40 psig, capacity 55 to 70 kg of tablet load having 3/8-inch standard convex tablet. Solution for coating can be poured on the tablet bed or ladled onto the tablets (with spoon with long handle) for even distributing of coating solution the steady state solution is applied.

2. Process

- ***Seal coat:*** Spray system provides even distribution and process is faster. Place tablet load in rotating pan at 10 rpm. set air to 30°C. Apply 800 mL of zein solution in 3 applications (3 times) and at each application allow tablet to dry for 15-20 minutes. If the tablets are sticky, use enough talc to keep them from sticking together.
- ***Subcoat:*** Use gelatin or acacia solution. Turn on the heat, turn off the inlet air, and maintain pan speed at 10 rpm. Apply 3-9 coats of warm solution of gelatin or acacia solution and ensure edges are covered and tablet gets desired thickness checked volumetrically. Allow 20 minutes for drying, ensure uniform distribution of coating, dust with subcoating powder if tackiness develops till tablets rolls freely. After last coat, run or shake the pan periodically for 2-4 hours for uniform and complete drying.
- ***Syruping- Smoothing and Colour Coat:*** It involves 3 types of syrup coating

  (a) Grossing syrup to attain gross weight of tablet

  (b) Heavy syrup

  (c) Regular syrup

1. Remove any excess dust, turn on the exhaust outlet air, set the temperature inlet air to 45-480°C, and set the pan speed to 12 rpm.
2. Apply 5-15 coats of grossing syrup to wet entire tablet bed and ensure uniform and rapid distribution. Apply grossing syrup immediately, after each application drying.

3. Apply coloured heavy syrup with several coats till tablet gets desirable volume.
4. Turn off the heat and reduce the amount of inlet and exhaust air.
5. Apply several coats of coloured syrup to the tablet to achieve the desired smoothness, size, and colour.
6. Apply coloured syrup coat (regular syrup coat) when tablet exhibits frosty appearance and does not allow tablet to become dusty.

- ***Finishing:*** Make sure of clean pan.

1. Set pan speed at 12 rpm, turn off heat, reduce exhaust air.
2. Apply 3-4 coats of coloured regular syrup quickly, then inspect the tablet for frostiness or dustiness.
3. Apply final coat of regular syrup without colour, tablet attains depth of colour and increases elegance of coat.
4. Shut off exhaust before application of last coat, tablet remains damp, shake at every 15-30 minutes to prevent sticking of tablets. Leave the tablet to dry slowly overnight.

- ***Polishing:*** Although polishing can be done in the same coating pan, but the good results are obtained by canvas lined pans. Supply air and exhaust air but heat must be turned off, and the pan speed must be set at 12 rpm. Apply 3-4 coats of warm polishing solution, 300 mL/application. Allow the solvent to completely evaporate between coats.

3.3 FILM COATING

The technique of film coating includes depositing a thin, uniform film on the surface of tablets, granules, and capsules.

Film coating offers many advantages:

- Minimal weight increase - compared to sugar coating, film coating causes only a minimal weight increase in the product usually about 2 to 4%.
- Reduced processing time and process efficiency is increased.
- Facilitates product identification.
- Formulation flexibility is improved.
- The coating's resistance to chipping has been increased.

3.3.1 Types of Film Coating Methods

1. **Pan pour method / ladle application:** It is an old method used for film coating. This old technique is now displaced by new techniques, which are faster and more reproducible. Usually carried out in conventional pans equipped with baffles. Film coating solution is too viscous, necessary to spray effectively, which involves application of solution, mixing, drying. It is a slow method and the operator must be skilled to produce good and acceptable product. Additional drying is required to eliminate the latent solvent. Aqueous based film coating solutions are not suited for the pan pour method as it shows inherent localized over wetting of tablets causes tablet surface erosion, product instability and unacceptable high moisture content in the tablet core.

2. **Pan spray method:** Newly developed method for application of coating solution by spraying, to improve efficiency of film coating process. Spraying allows for automated control of liquid application. Flat spray patterns with appropriate nozzle systems are chosen to cover the entire tablet bed; typically, 1-5 nozzles cover the full tablet bed.

   Process variables: Some of the factors to be controlled and monitored to produce good quality product. The following are a few of the spray pan film coating parameters that can be modified.

   Pan variables: Pan shape, baffling, rotational speed, pan load affects the mixing and coating of the tablet. Tablet uniform mixing enhances deposition of good film. Tablet coating adds 2-5% of weight gain by film coating. Poor tablet movement in coating pan may lead non-uniformity of film coating over tablet.

   Tablet shape affects the coating, particular shaped tablet mixes freely and helps in uniform coating. The other tablet shape resist to mix, then baffles arrangement is provided, even baffles must be such that it must not cause chipping and breaking of tablets.

   Not only pan speed affects mixing even tablet passing under the spray at particular velocity affect mixing. Slow speed may result in over-wetting, while rapid speed may not provide enough time for tablets to dry before being reintroduced to the spray, resulting in a rough appearance. For non-aqueous coating solutions, a big coating pan with a speed of 10 to 15 rpm is frequently used, while for aqueous film coating solutions, a small coating pan with a speed of 3 to 10 rpm is commonly employed.

   Spray variables: Variation in spray is controlled by controlling rate of coating liquid application, spray pattern and degree of atomization. Fluid pressure and nozzle design influence all three variables, which are interconnected. Atomizing air pressure, air volume, and the form and design of the air jets' relationship to the fluid stream all affect the spray pattern and degree of atomization. The rate at which the coating solution is applied is determined by the mixing of the tablets, the drying efficiency of the coating, as well as the coating formula and tablet features.

   To spray coating solution evenly on tablet, more number of nozzles is used in larger pans. Coating solution should be applied only on tablet bed and not on pan surface which may waste solution. Moving the nozzles closer or further away from the tablet bed can change the spray width. The distance between the nozzles and the tablet bed influences not only the spray width but also the amount of coating liquid applied to individual tablets. Each coating solution requires a different orifice size, nozzle design, fluid pressure, atomizing, air pressure, air volume, and fluid viscosity.

   Process air variables: To obtain the optimum drying of tablet, air temperature, air volume, and air quality should be controlled. Higher temperatures in the tablet bed and coating chamber are more important for solvent evaporation and subsequent faster coating rate. Balance between inlet air and exhaust air must be maintained.

Fluidized bed process: Used for rapid tablet coating, granules and capsules are coated. Same as pan process, use of particular chamber design mainly depends on process air; fluidization pattern control. Tablet mass to be fluidized is affected by tablet shape, size, density, and load quantity. The pace of the process air is regulated by a variable speed blower or dampers to keep the tablet mass in continual fluid motion, which ensures adequate fluidization and drying.

3.4 COATING EQUIPMENT

Three types of coating pans are used.

- Standard coating pan
- Perforated coating pan
- Fluidized bed coater or air suspension coater

1. **Standard coating pan or conventional coating pan:** It consist a circular metal pan mounted angularly on a stand. The pan has a diameter of 8 to 60 inches and revolves on a horizontal axis. The tablet bed's pan is filled with heated air, which is then exhausted through ducts in the front of the pan.

   The coating solution is applied to the tablet bed using a pan ladling method or a spray system. The use of an atomizing device to spray the coating solution on to the tablet bed results in a faster process, even distribution of coating solution and reduce the drying time.

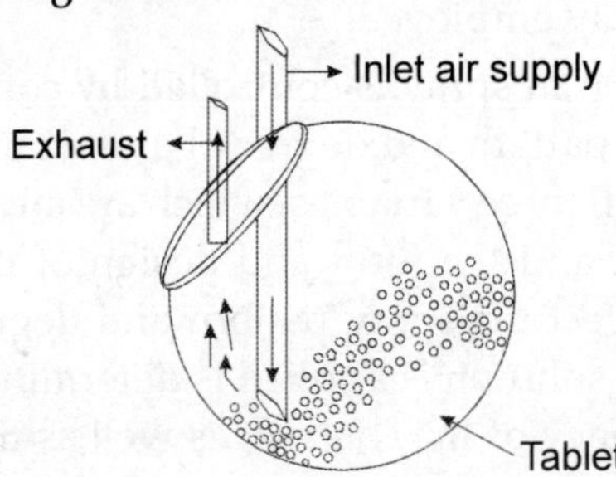

Fig. 3.1: Standard coating pan or conventional coating pan

Examples of standard coating pan

- Pellegrini coating pan
- Immersion sword coating pan
- Immersion tube system
- ***Pellegrini system***: It has an inbuilt baffle system that ensures consistent mixing and a diffuser that evenly distributes drying air over the tablet bed surface. Newer versions in the Pellegrini system are closed, which boosts drying efficiency and influences automated controls. Pellegrini pans are available with capacities ranging from 10 kg to 1000 kg.

- ***Immersion sword system*: Glatt immersion sword coater**
- The drying air is introduced via a perforated metal sword that is submerged in the tablet bed. Dry air rushes upwards from the sword through the tablet bed, making intimate contact with the wet tablets and therefore improving drying efficiency. The coating solution is applied by atomized spray system directly on tablet surface which are rotated.

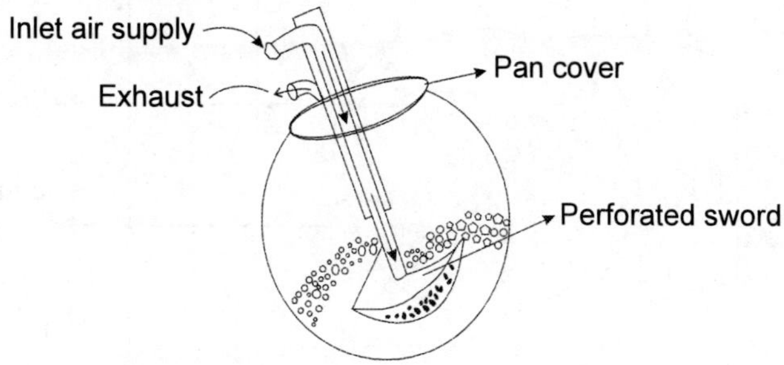

Fig. 3.2: Glatt immersion sword coater

- ***Immersion tube system*:** The immersed tube consists of hot air inlet and a spray nozzle delivers coating solution built at the tip of the tube. When the coating solution is applied, hot air is blown via a tube to dry the tablet bed. The exhaust drying air flows upwards and is evacuated through the output duct (conventional duct). It is a rapid process, takes less time for sugar and film coating processes.

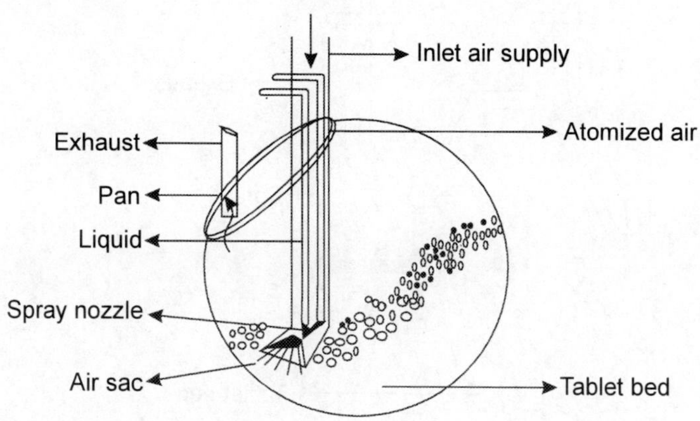

Fig. 3.3: Immersion tube coater

2. **Perforated coating pan:** It consists perforated or partially perforated pan, pan rotates in an enclosed housing on its horizontal axis.

- ***Accela-cota and Hi-coater system*:** Drying air is introduced into the tablet bed and exhausted air is taken out from perforated bottom of pan.

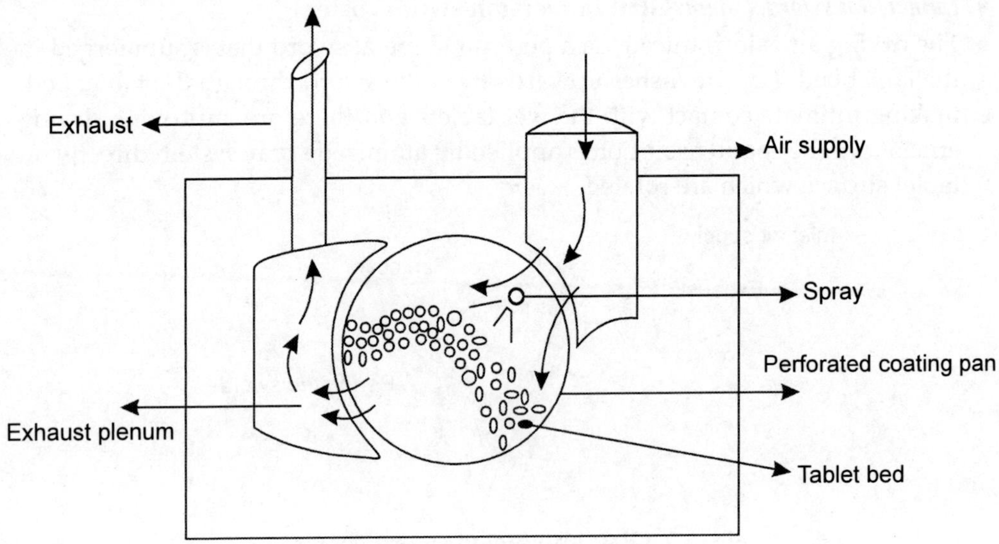

Fig. 3.4: Accela-cota system

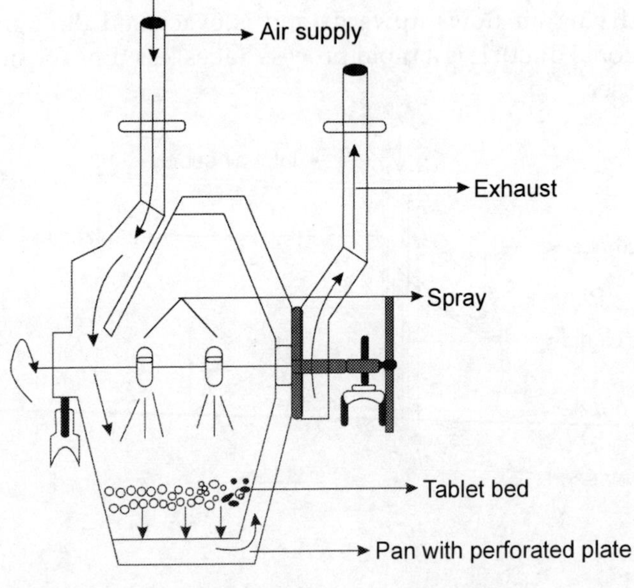

Fig. 3.5: Hi-coater system

- ***Driacoater system***: Hot air is introduced into the drum through hollow perforated ribs on the inside periphery. The coating pan rotates the ribs into the tablet bed, drying air travels up through and fluidizes the tablet, and the exhaust air is drawn out of the back of the pan when the tablet has dried.

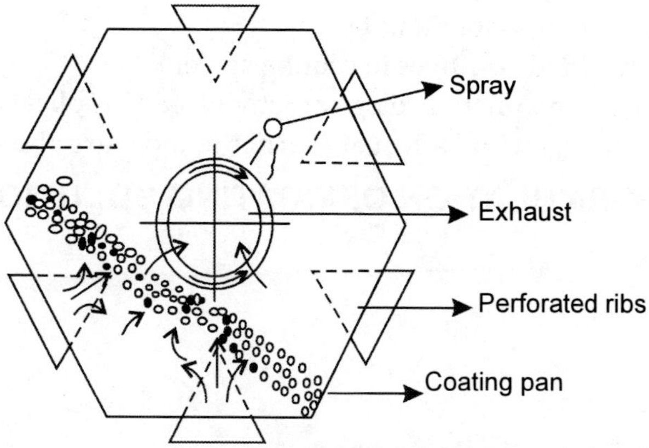

Fig. 3.6: Driacoater system

- *Glatt coater:* Inside the drum, drying air is introduced through the tablet bed, and exhaust air is taken out through the exhaust duct. Spraying nozzles positioned inside the drum apply the coating solution to the tablet bed. It is an efficient drying system with high coating capacity, useful in film and sugar coating.

3. **Fluidized bed system/air suspension coater** is a highly efficient drying system. The upward movement of drying air is used to fluidize the tablet mass in a columnar chamber. As more air enters the column's centre, the tablet rises in the centre. The tablets ascend through the chamber's centre. They then fall towards the chamber wall and descend to re-enter the air stream at the chamber's bottom. Coating solutions are continually applied through a spray nozzle at the chamber's bottom or top region.

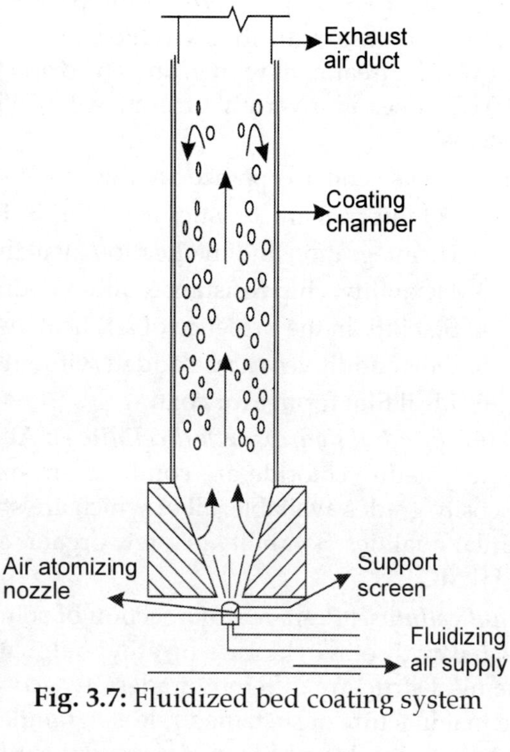

Fig. 3.7: Fluidized bed coating system

3.4.1 Materials Used for Film Coating

The coating materials must have following properties.

- Ingredients must have solubility in selected solvent.
- Should produce elegant looking product.
- Heat, light, moisture, air, and the substrate being coated do not affect the stability of the coating. The qualities of the film must not alter as it ages.

- Should not have colour, odour and taste.
- Compatible with added additives in coating solvent.
- Should be non-toxic, no pharmacological activity, easy application to the tablet.
- Should be crack resistant and adequate barrier to moisture absorption, light.

3.5 GENERAL FORMULATION OF COATING SOLUTION

- Film formers
- Solvents
- Platicizers
- Colourants
- Opaquant

3.5.1 Film Formers: Synthetic Polymers

(a) Non-enteric materials: Following are the commonly used film formers.

***HPMC (hydroxy propyl methyl cellulose)*:** HPMC polymer is made by treating alkali-treated cellulose with methyl chloride to form the methoxy group, which is then followed by treatment with propylene oxide to form the propylene glycol ether group. HPMC comes in a variety of grades, but it's best for air suspension and pan spray systems.

The wide use and acceptance are due to:

1. Solubility characteristics in GI fluids, in organic solvents and aqueous solvents.
2. Disintegration and medication availability are unaffected.
3. Flexibility, chip resistance, and no odour or taste.
4. Stability in the presence of air, heat, light, and a sufficient amount of moisture.
5. Other additives can be added without any difficulties.
6. Ideal film former for coating.

***MHEC (Methyl hydroxy ethyl cellulose)*:** Alkali-treated cellulose and ethylene oxide-treated methyl chloride are combined to make this product. There are a variety of viscosity grades available, all of which are structural similarity with HPMC and have similar qualities. Solubility in a few organic solvents, MHEC is not used as frequently as HPMC.

***Ethyl cellulose*:** Prepared by reaction of solution of cellulose with sodium hydroxide treated with ethyl chloride or ethyl sulphate. As a number of ethoxy group in the chemical structure different grades of viscosity available and used commercially. For the manufacture of sustained release granules and tablets, a mixture of ethyl cellulose and water-soluble additives is commonly utilised. Colourless, odourless, and tasteless, soluble in a wide range of organic solvents, stable under physical conditions, and are non-toxic.

***Hydroxypropyl cellulose* (HPC):** The HPC is prepared by treating cellulose first with sodium hydroxide then reaction with propylene glycol at an elevated temperature and pressure. Soluble in water below 40°C temperature (and insoluble above 45°C), GIT fluids and many polar organic solvents. Once it dries form a tacky film and useful for subcoat but not suitable for colour or gloss (shine) coat. Produce flexible film, to improve film property used in combination with other polymers.

***Povidone*:** It is a synthetic polymer consisting 1-vinyl -2- pyrrolidon groups. Povidone polymerization depends on various molecular weights range. Povidone is available in four different viscosity grades. K-15, K-30, K-60, and K-90 have molecular weights of 10,000, 40,000, 160,000, and 360,000, respectively. In pharmaceutical industry povidone K-30 is used as binder and tablet coating. Povidone is soluble in water, as well as a variety of organic solvents, gastric and intestinal fluid, produce clear, glossy and hard film. Material is tacky, it is modified by using plasticizers or polymers, as it is soluble in acidic and basic fluids can be cross-linked with other materials to produce enteric properties. To produce uniform coloured film povidone with colourant dispersion used.

***Sodium carboxymethyl cellulose*:** It is a sodium salt of carboxymethyl cellulose. It is prepared by the reaction of cellulose with sodium salt of monochloroacetic acid. Low, medium, high, and very high viscosity grades are available. Insoluble in most organic solvents yet easily dispersed in water to produce colloidal solution. Films formed are brittle but adhere well on tablet surface, after drying film becomes tacky but modified by use of additives.

***Polyethylene glycols*:** It is prepared by ethylene glycol reacting with ethylene oxide in the presence of sodium hydroxide at elevated temperature and pressure. In the tablet coating, different molecular weight PEGs are utilized. PEGs are white solids at room temperature, 200-600 molecular weight PEGs are liquid at room temperature, 900-8000 molecular weight are higher molecular weights PEGs are waxy. To modify film properties used in combination with other polymers. PEGs and cellulose acetate phthalate film dissolves in gastric fluid. PEG coats produced hard, smooth, tasteless and non-toxic film but sensitive to elevated temperature.

***Acrylate polymers*:** These polymers are marketed under trademark "Eudragit". Eudragit-E is a cationic copolymer based on dimethyl aminoethyl methylacrylate and other neutral methacrylic acid esters freely soluble in gastric fluid up to pH 5. Available in:

1. Organic solution 12.5% in isopropanol/acetone
2. Solid materials
3. 30% aqueous dispersion

Eudragit RL and RS synthetic copolymer from acrylic and methacrylic acid esters with low content of quaternary ammonium groups. These polymers film produce delayed release actions (pH independent).

(b) Enteric materials: Enteric coated pills and compressed tablets are in existence for more than a century, important reasons for entry coating.

1. Protect acid labile drugs, certain antibiotics.
2. Prevent nausea, gastric distress, vomiting due to irritation.
3. Intended for local action in intestine.

4. Optimum absorption in the small intestine at high concentration.
5. Provide delayed release.

Ideal enteric coating properties:

- Resistance to dissolve in gastric fluid.
- Readily available in intestinal fluid.
- Compatible with most of the coating solvent components and drug.
- Stable and properties should not change of aging.
- Should form continuous film.
- Nontoxic and low cost.
- Easy application without specialized equipment.
- Allow coating to form uniform film on debossed tablets.

Polymers

1. Cellulose acetate phthalate (CAP)
2. Acrylate polymer
3. Hydroxypropyl methyl cellulose phthalate
4. Polyvinyl acetate phthalate (PVAP)

***Cellulose acetate phthalate* (CAP):** Is widely used, the only disadvantage it dissolves above pH 6 and delays absorption, as compared to other enteric polymers it is hygroscopic. Change in film properties due to hydrolytic removal of phthalic and acetic acid. It is combined with other enteric polymers because it forms a brittle film.

Acrylate polymers: There are 2 acrylic resins having enteric property. Eudragit-L & Eudragit-S are available, produce gastric fluid resistance film, soluble in intestinal fluid, Eudragit -L at pH 6 & Eudragit-S at pH7.

Hydroxypropyl methyl cellulose phthalate: Three enteric polymers available are derived from HPMC by esterification with phthalic anhydride and marketed as HPMC-50, 55 and 55s also known as HP-50, HP-55 & HP-55s. HPMC is its trade name of HPMC phthalate, dissolves at lower pH 5 to 5.5 as compared to previous two polymers.

***Polyvinyl acetate phthalate* (PVAP):** Manufactured by esterification of partially hydrolyzed polyvinyl acetate with phthalic anhydride, it is stable and has pH dependent solubility.

3.5.2 Solvents

Is a medium for dissolving or dispersing the polymer and other additives so that a film can be formed over the substrate (tablet surface).

Ideal properties of solvents:

1. It should either allow to dissolve or disperse polymer system.
2. It should easily disperse other coating solution.
3. 2-10% of polymers concentration should not result viscous solution.
4. It should be colourless, odourless, tasteless, and odourless, as well as inexpensive, non-toxic, inert, and nonflammable.
5. Rapid drying rate for 300 kg load should dry in 3 to 5 hours.

Commonly used solvents are ethanol, methanol alone or in combination with water, isopropanol, chloroform, acetone, methylethyl ketone and methylene chloride. As environmental and economic considerations water is the choice of coating solvent. But drug may hydrolyze in presence of water thus first non-aqueous based solvents seal coat is applied to prevent hydrolyzation of the drug.

3.5.3 Plasticizers

Plasticizers are film forming agents added to the polymers in order to make the polymer flexible and soft, enhancing the flexibility and plasticity of the films.

- The quality of the film is modified by the use of internal and external plasticizers technique that changes physical properties of the polymers.
- More often external plasticizers are used as additives to the coating solution for desired enteric effect, which when incorporated with primary polymeric film former changes flexibility, tensile strength or adhesion property of the film.
- The type of plasticizer and its ratio to the polymer can be optimized to achieve the desired film properties.
- The viscosity of plasticizers can affect film permeability, tackiness, flexibility, solubility, and taste, as well as its toxicity, compatibility with other coating solution components, and the film's and final coated product's stability.
- Combination of plasticizers may be needed to achieve the desired effect.
- Castor oil, propylene glycol, and glycerin are commonly used plasticizers. PEG -200 and 400 series are low molecular weight PEGs. Polysorbate (tweens), sorbitan esters (spans), and organic acid esters are examples of surfactants.

3.5.4 Colourants

Colourant may be soluble or dispersed as insoluble powders in a coating solution, provide distinct colour, elegancy to dosage forms.

- To provide uniform distribution of colour it must be a fine powder of less than 10 micro-particle size.
- To get uniform dispersion colourants must be milled in coating solvent or solution to avoid colour variation.
- Certified FD&C or D&C colourants are used commonly. These are synthetic dyes or lakes of dyes.
- Lakes are derived from dyes by precipitating with carrier's example talc or alumina.
- Colourants are commonly used for sugar/film coating systems.
- Concentration of colour depends on the type of shade required.
- Inorganic materials: Iron oxide.

Natural colours: Caramel, carotenoids, chlorophyll, indigo, flavones, turmeric and carminic acids.

Commercially available colours:

Opalux: Opaquant colour for sugar coating.

Opaspray: Opaquant colour for film coating.
Opadry: Film coating.

3.5.5 Opaquant Extenders

To provide more pastel colours and increase film coverage, fine powders of inorganic substances used in the coating solution formulation, provide white coating on the surface of tablet or mask the odd colours of the tablet core. Colourants are more expensive, when opaquants are used less colourant are required.

Examples:
Titanium dioxide,
Silicates: talc, aluminium silicates
Carbonates: magnesium carbonates,
Sulphate: calcium sulphate

3.6 QUALITY CONTROL TEST FOR COATED TABLET

1. General appearance: Size, colour, defects in coating.
2. *In vitro* tests: Dissolution, disintegration, mechanical strength, chipping and cracking.
3. Stability testing: Physical and chemical stability.

3.6.1 Film Defects

1. ***Sticking and picking:*** Over-wetting or film tackiness may cause tablet to stick to another tablet or tablet stick to coating pan.
   On drying at the point of contact a piece of film may remain adhered to another tablet or pan surface, resulting in a small exposed area of the tablet surface.
   - Reduce application rate of coating solution and increase drying air temperature and air volume solve this problem.
2. ***Roughness:*** Gritty or rough surface of a tablet is due to early drying of a coating solution droplet before reaching to tablet bed during spraying. The spray dried particles deposit on a tablet surface instead of finely divided coating solution droplets. Roughness may occur due to the pigment concentration and polymer concentration in coating solution.
   - Move the nozzle closer to the tablet bed, reduced degree of atomization can decrease the roughness.
3. ***Orange peel effects:*** Inadequate spreading of coating solution before drying causes bumpy or orange peel effect. It occurs due to rapid drying or too viscous coating solution.
   - By decreasing the viscosity of coating solution and decreasing the rate of drying temperature may solve this problem.
4. ***Bridging and filling:*** During drying film may shrink and pull away from the corners of a tablet surface or it may bisect resulting in bridging. It occurs in tablets consisting of monogram or bisection.
   Bridging can be decreased by increasing the plasticizer content or changing the plasticizer.

Filling is caused by applying too much of solution and if the solution applied too fast resulting in a thick film that fills and retained in the monogram narrows the monogram or bisect. Filling is prevented by monitoring the mixing of the tablets in the pan and the fluid application.

5. ***Blistering***: It is a unsmooth film surface shows a number of uneven spots. When coated tablets require further drying, too rapid evaporation of the solvent from the coated tablets and the effect of high temperature on the strength, elasticity and adhesion of the film may result in blistering.
6. ***Hazing/dull film (blooming)***: It occurs when too high temperature is used for a particular formulation, if the coated tablet is exposed to high humidity conditions and partial solvation of film.
7. ***Colour variation***: Migration of soluble dyer, plasticizers and other additives during drying may give the coating a mottled or spotted appearance. Improper mixing, uneven spray pattern and insufficient coating may result in colour variation.
    - Proper mixing of coating solution, uniform spray of coating solution, use of lake dye eliminate dye migration. A reformulation with different plasticizers and additives is the best way to solve film instability caused by the ingredients.
8. ***Cracking***: If the internal stress in the film exceeds the tensile strength of the film cracking occurs.
    - By using higher molecular weight polymers or polymers blends, tensile strength of the film can be increased.
    - By adjusting the plasticizer type and concentration, and the pigment type and concentration, internal stresses in the film can be minimized.
9. ***Twinning***: Twinning is a two or more tablets' cores are stuck together. Higher rate of application of coating solution, insufficient drying causes twinning.
    - Controlling the drying rate and rate of movement of pan. Adjusting the coating solution concentration can prevent twinning.

3.7 SPECIALIZED COATING

1. **Compression coating:** The finished product is a tablet within a tablet. Compression coating requires specialized tablet machine and is not widely used but it has advantages.
    - Compression coating is done to a tablet core that cannot tolerate organic solvents or water and to mask the taste.
    - Provide delayed or enteric properties.
    - Incompatible ingredients can be separated by this process.
2. **Electrostatic coating:** Electrostatic coating is a method of applying coating to conductive substrates. A strong electrostatic charge is applied to the substrate. The coating material containing conductive ionic species of opposite charge is sprayed onto the charged substrate. Complete and uniform coating of corners is achieved.
3. **Dip coating:** Coating is applied to the tablet cores by dipping them into the coating liquid. The wet tablets are dried in a coating pan, dipping and drying

steps may be repeated several times to obtain the desired coating. This dip coating process lacks speed, versatility and reliability of the spray coating techniques.

4. **Vacuum film coating:** Coating is carried out in a specially designed baffled pan. The pan consists of hot water jacketed and vacuum system is achieved by sealing the pan. In the sealed baffled pan, the tablets are placed and the nitrogen is used to displace the air in the pan before the desired vacuum level is obtained. The airless spray system is used to apply coating solution. The evaporation is caused by the heated pan and the vapours are removed by the vacuum system.

REVIEW QUESTIONS

Long Essays

1. Define tablet coating. Enlist tablet coating equipment. Explain the different steps involved in the sugar coating of tablets. Write the advantages and disadvantages.
2. Mention the desired features for a core tablet to undergo coating process. Discuss in detail about the formulation and coating process for film coated tablets with its merits and demerits.
3. Explain in detail film coating of tablets giving details of the equipment used.
4. Compare and contrast sugar coating and film coating of tablets.
5. Describe perforated coating pans. Explain steps in sugar coating process of tablets.

Short Essays

1. Explain different steps involved in sugar coating of tablets.
2. Describe the ingredients required for film coating process.
3. Write a note on sugar coating of tablets and its advantages.
4. Explain compression coating technique.
5. Explain the formulation and manufacturing technique for film coating process.
6. Film defects of coated tablets.
7. Discuss the steps involved in sugar coating with suitable examples of ingredients uses in each step.

Short Answers

1. Advantages of film coating of tablets.
2. Differentiate between enteric and film coating.
3. Enumerate the defects in tablet coating.
4. Write the ingredients used for sugar coating of tablets.
5. Objectives of tablet coating.

4

LIQUID ORALS

Learning Objectives

After going through this chapter, you would be able to:

1. Make a list of different types of liquid orals.
2. Discuss general formulation of liquid orals.
3. List out the excipients used in liquid orals.
4. Explain manufacturing requirements.
5. Describe the filling process for liquid orals.

4.1. INTRODUCTION

Liquid orals are homogeneous liquid solutions containing one or more active ingredients that have been dissolved in a suitable solvent or a mixture of solvents that are mutually miscible. They are prepared for oral administration either undiluted or after dilution. They may contain other substances such as dispersing, emulsifying, suspending, wetting, solubilizing, thickening, and stabilizing agents and anti-microbial preservatives. They also contain suitable sweetening agents, flavouring agents and permitted colouring agents.

Advantages

- Ease of use for those who have difficulty in swallowing solid dose forms.
- A drug given as a solution is instantly available for absorption, and it is absorbed more quickly and efficiently than the same amount of drug given as a tablet or capsule.
- Use of flavours and sweeteners make them palatable, especially for children.
- Because a solution is a homogeneous system, the drug gets dispersed evenly throughout the preparation.

CLASSIFICATION OF LIQUID ORALS

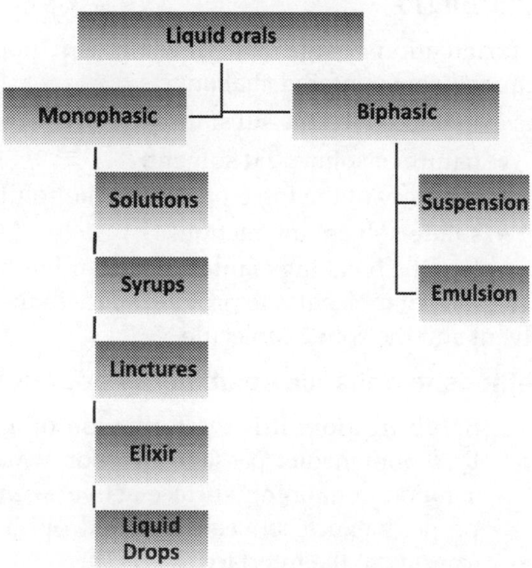

Solubility

1. Solubilisation
2. pH
3. Dielectric constant
4. Co-solvency
5. Hydrotrophy
6. Chemical modification of the drug
7. Salt form

Stability

1. Chemical stability
2. Physical stability

Formulation components

Monophasic

1. Sweetening agents
2. Viscosity controlling agents
3. Buffers
4. Antioxidants
5. Flavours
6. Preservatives

Biphasic

Flocculating agents
Wetting agents
Deflocculants
Dispersing agents
Protective colloids
Formulation adjuvents
1. Preservatives
2. Colour
3. Perfume
4. Flavour

Emulsifying agents
Surface active agents
Viscosity modifiers
Anti-oxidants

SOLUBILITY

In formulation design and development poorly soluble drugs solubilization is a frequently encountered challenge.

The extent to which the substance dissolves depends largely on the:

- nature of solute and solvent;
- intensity of the force present in the solute and solvent; and
- solute-solvent interaction.

It involves the breaking of intermolecular bonds in the solute, as well as the separation of the solvent molecules to provide space in the solvent for the interaction between the solvent and the solute molecule.

Methods to enhance solubility of poor soluble compounds

1. **Solubilization:** It is the formation of a thermodynamically stable solution by the spontaneous passage of poor water-soluble molecules into an aqueous solution containing surface-active agents. Most surface-active agents have a proper balance between their hydrophilic and lipophilic properties so that they can stay at the interface.

When a surface-active agent is added to water, it gets adsorbed at airawater interface. In water at low concentration, surface-active agents exist individually as monomers. As the concentration of surfactant increases, molecules get accumulated progressively at the interface, some of them go into solution. As the concentration increases the monomers aggregate themselves, these aggregates are called micelles. Each micelle may contain around 50 or more than 50 monomers and size may be around 50A°. Critical micelle concentration (CMC) is defined as the concentration range of surfactants at which micelles start forming.

Micellar solubilization: Above the CMC, i.e., when micelles are formed poor water-soluble drugs can be solubilised, this phenomenon is called micellar solubilisation.

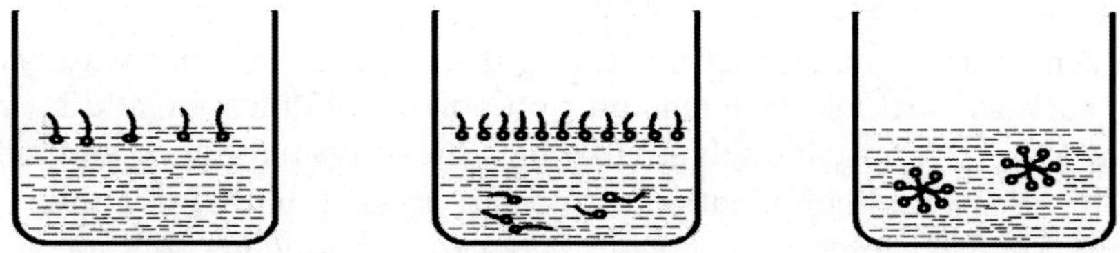

Fig. 4.1: Micellar solubilization of drugs

Surfactant solution's ability to solubilize water-insoluble compounds starts at critical micelle concentration and increases with the concentration of the micelles.

Generally, lypophilic surface active agents with higher HLB values are the best solubilizing agents but selection is done based on phase solubility studies.

Classification of surfactants

(i) Ionic surfactant
  - Anionic surfactant: Sodium lauryl sulphate, potassium stearates
  - Cationic surfactant: Cetrimide
  - Ampholytic surfactant: polypeptides, lecithin

(ii) Nonionic surfactants: Tweens and spans

2. **pH modification**: Since most drugs are weak acids or weak base, pH is helpful in enhancing solubility, their degree of ionisation depends on the pH of the biological fluid.

   Depending on the pH, the drug undergoes dissociation at dissociation equilibrium. The drug is present in unionised as well as ionised forms in the solution. If pH of the medium favours the formation of unionised species, the drug can be rapidly diffused across the lipoidal bio-membrane.

The drugs are either weak acid or weak base and are poorly soluble in water. The solubility of such drug is markedly affected by change in pH. If the pH of a solution is reduced, the solubility of weak acidic drug or its salts decreases with a decrease in pH.

Solubility of weak basic drug or their salts increases with a decrease in the pH. The relationship between the pH, solubility and pk_a value of an acidic drug is given by

$$pH_p = pK_a + \log S\text{–}S_0 / S_0$$

$$pH_p = pK_a + \log S_0 / S\text{–}S_0$$

where,

pH_p = pH below which the drug precipitates from solution.

S = overall solubility of the drug.

S_0 = solubility of its unionized form.

3. **Co-solvency**: It is a method of increasing the solubility of poor water-soluble drugs, such as weak electrolytes and non-polar molecules, by adding a little amount of a water miscible solvent to which the drugs have good solubility.

   The solvents used in combination to increase the solubility are known as co-solvents. Reduced interfacial tension between the aqueous solution and the hydrophobic solute is the mechanism for solubility enhancement through co-solvency.

   The most commonly used co-solvents are glycerin, ethanol, propylene glycol, sorbitol, polyethylene glycol. Co-solvents are used to
   - enhance the solubility of the drug, and
   - improve the solubility of volatile constituents used to impart a desirable flavour and odour to the product.
4. **Hydrotropy:** It is defined as the increase in solubility of poor water-soluble drugs in water due to the addition of large amount of additives. The agents which are responsible for hydrotropy are called hydrotropes. Hydrotropes are amphiphilic substances composed mainly of hydrophilic functional groups. Hydrotropes are organic salts and can enhance the solubility of a variety of hydrophobic organic substance when present in aqueous solution. These substances include aryl sulfonic acid their potassium, sodium, calcium and ammonium salts, some typical hydrotropes are hydroxyl benzenes, hydroxybenzoates and benzene sulfonates which can enhance the solubility of hydrophobic drugs when present in significant concentration in water.

Table 4.1: Various agents used for hydrotropic solubilization of drugs

Drugs	Additives used to exhibit hydrotropism
Paracetamol, diclofenac sodium	Sodium acetate, urea
Cefadroxil	Potassium acetate, potassium citrate, sodium acetate, urea
Theophylline	Sodium salicylate
Nifedipine	Sodium salicylate

5. **Complexation:** The use of complexing agents is one of the several methods for improving the water solubility of poorly soluble drugs.

Complexation is the process of making a compound form a complex with another (complexing agents). Complexation is the association between two or more molecule to form a non-bonded entity with a well defined stiochiometry. Complexing agents are the substances capable of forming a complex with another compound in solution. Formulation of water-soluble complexes improve drug dissolution. A common example of a complexing agents is EDTA, cyclodextrine. Complex formation techniques have been used to improve the aqueous solubility, dissolution rate, and bioavailability of weak water-soluble medicines among all the solubility improvement techniques.

Every substance has a specific equilibrium solubility in a given solvent at a given temperature. Deviation from this inherent solubility must be due to the formation of a new species in solution. When complex formation occurs, the inherent solubility of the uncomplexed medication plus the concentration of drugs complex in solution equals total solubility.

The interaction between a drug D and a complexing agent C.

$$xD + yC \rightleftharpoons DxCy$$

x & y are stoichiometry of the interaction

The total solubility of drugs is

$$ST = [D] + X\,[DxCy]$$

D is the solubility of uncomplexed = ks

X [DxCy] is the concentration of drugs in complexed form.

By use of the solubility analysis technique the stiochiometry of this interaction and its equilibrium constant can be determined. An excess quantity of drugs is placed together with solution containing various concentration of complexing agents, in closed containers. The containers are agitated at a constant temperature until equilibrium is achieved. Then remove the aliquot samples of the suspernatant liquid and assayed for total concentration of drug.

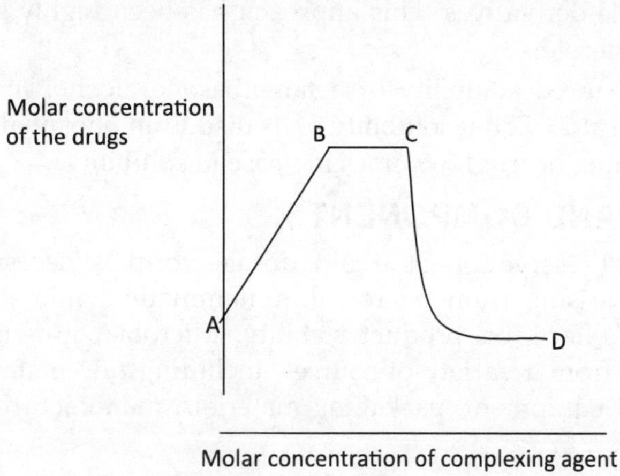

1. Initially, solubility of drug increases due to complex formation from point A to B.
2. The solution is saturated with both the drug and complex at point B.
3. At point C, the drug remaining in the system is entirely converted to complex.

Further, there is no increase in solubility with increase in concentration of complexing agent after point 'c' due to unavailability of drug.

6. **Dielectric constant:** The dielectric constant is a feature of a solvent that describes how much energy it takes to separate two oppositely charged molecules in the solvent.
   The dielectric constant (κ) of a solvent is a measure of its polarity. The higher the dielectric constant of solvents, the more polar it is. At specific dielectric constant, every solute shows a maximum solubility in any given solvent system, the dielectric constants tell us how well the solvent is able to separate ions. Molecules dissolve in the liquid when the solute-solute interaction forces are greater than the force holding the material in its original stalk.
   Water has a very high dielectric constant and this allows salts to dissolve in water with dissociation. The dielectric constant of water at 25°C is 78.5 co-ordination of water molecules around the anion and the cation greatly reduces the ion-ion contraction in the salt. In polar solvents, polar molecules dissolve best. Molecules that are non-polar dissolve well in non-polar solvents.
7. **Salt formation:** It is the most popular and successful way to boost the solubility and dissolution rates of acidic and basic drugs, which are converted into salt forms. Generally, with weak acidic drugs, a strong base salt is prepared such as the sodium and potassium salts of barbiturates and sulphonamides. For weak basic drugs a strong acid salt is prepared like the hydrochloride or sulphate salts of several alkaloid drugs.
   Example: The sodium salt of a non-steroidal anti-inflammatory drugs naproxen has a better solubility profile if compared with the free acid form.
8. **Chemical modification of the drugs:** Poor soluble drugs can chemically modify to water-soluble derivatives. This approach has been highly successful in the case of corticosteroids.
   Examples: Enhanced solubility of betamethasone alcohol in water which is 5.8 mg/100 mL at 25°C, but solubility of its disodium phosphate ester is greater than 10 g/100 mL, nearly 1500 times increase in solubility.

4.2 ADDITIVES AND COMPONENTS

1. **Preservatives:** Preservation of liquid dosage form is necessary because of complications arising from microbial contamination; microbial growth can cause marked effects on product stability. Microbial growth is a result of contamination from a variety of sources, including raw materials, processing containers and equipment, packaging materials, manufacturing environment and the operator.

An ideal preservative must be:

- Physically, chemically and microbiologically stable for the life time of the product.
- Effective against a broad spectrum of microorganisms.
- Non-toxic, non-sensitizing, adequately soluble, compatible with other components of formulation.
- Taste and odour are acceptable at the concentration used.

No single preservative exists that satisfies all of these requirements for all formulations. A combination of two or more preservatives is needed to achieve the desired antimicrobial effect.

Preservatives are classified into four major groups:

1. Acidic
2. Neutral
3. Mercurial
4. Quaternary ammonium compounds

Acidic:

For oral preparation concentrations

Phenol	:	0.2-0.5
P-hydroxybenzoic acid	:	0.001-0.2
Salts of benzoic acid	:	0.5-1.0
Salts of sorbic acid	:	0.05-0.2

Phenols are the oldest and best known pharmaceutical preservatives, but are less used in oral pharmaceuticals owning to their characteristic odour and instability when exposed to oxygen.

A combination of two or more esters of parahydroxy benzoic acid are used to achieve the desired antimicrobial effect.

Example: Methyl and propyl parahydroxy benzoic acid are often used together in a ratio of 10:1.

Neutral:

- Used in ophthalmic, nasal, parental products.
- Less used in oral pharmaceuticals.
- The neutral preservatives are volatile alcohols, and their volatility introduces odour problem and preservatives less on aging.

Benzyl alcohol	: 1.0%
Chlorbutanol	: 0.5%

Mercurials

- Used in ophthalmic, nasal, parenteral products.
- Excellent preservatives.

- Incompatibility problem arises as they are readily reduced to free mercury.

Phenyl mercuric acetate & nitrate	:	0.002-0.005%
Nitromersol	:	0.001-0.1%
Thimersol	:	0.001-0.1%

Quaternary ammonium compounds:

- Used in ophthalmic, nasal and parenteral products.
- Excellent preservatives.
- Incompatibilities arises as they get inactivated by a variety of anionic substances.

Cetylpyridinium chloride	:	0.01–0.02%
Benzalkonium chloride	:	0.004–0.02%

Syrups containing 85% sugar resist bacterial growth by their exosmotic effects on microorganisms. Syrups containing less than 85% sucrose must contain sufficient concentration of polyol, such as sorbitol, glycerine, propylene glycol, or polyethylene glycol, to have an exosmotic impact on microbes and resist bacterial growth.

2. **Viscosity controlling agents/viscosity inducing agents:** Viscosity controlling agents increase the viscosity of the liquid, and improve palatability. Viscosity controlling agents are polyvinylpyrrolidone and various cellulosic derivatives like methylcellulose, sodium carboxymethyl cellulose, available in different viscosity grades.

   Viscosity inducing agents should be used with caution, since they form molecular complexes with a variety of organic and inorganic compounds which may influence the activity of these compounds.

3. **Sweetening agents:** Agents which impart sweetness to the formulation.
   - Sucrose is the most widely used sweetening agent. It is available in highly purified form, it is soluble in aqueous media, in pH range of 4-8 it is chemically and physically stable.
   - 80% w/v sucrose solution acts as self-preservatives.
   - One of the main disadvantages of sucrose is crystallization which leads to cap locking, that occurs when the product crystallizes on the threads of the bottle cap and interferes with cap removal.
   - Sucrose is combined with glycerin, sorbitol and other polyols to minimize the tendency of sucrose to crystallize.
   - Liquid glucose is an extremely viscous substance that imparts sweetness and consistency to liquid formulations. It is prepared by the partial hydrolysis of starch with strong acid and contains dextrose as main component and small amount of dextrin.
   - Saccharin is used to supplement polyols and sugar as sweeteners. It is 250 to 500 times as sweet as sugar, if it is not used properly in the formulation, it can have a bitter after taste.
   - Aspartame is a synthetic sweetener. It is 200 times sweeter than sucrose. Aspartame is the methyl ester of aspartic acid and phenylalanine. Sweetness is enhanced when aspartame is added with saccharin, sucrose, and glucose.

4. **Flavouring agents:** These are the substances added to the formulation to improve the taste and improve patient compliance.
   Four basic taste sensations are sweet, salty, bitter, and sour.
   Selection of flavour

Table 4.2: Taste sensation and recommended flavour

Sweet	vanilla, berry
Salt	vanilla, peach
Bitter	chocolate, mint
Sour	raspberry, citrus flavour

A combination of flavouring agents is required to mask these taste sensations effectively. Evaluation of flavours has progressed to a greater extent than selection of flavour. Evaluation is done by preparing flavoured vehicles and incorporating the medicament or components of formulation responsible for the unpleasant taste. The concentration at which the taste of the medicament is noticeable is referred to as the minimum threshold level.

Appearance: The appearance of liquid dosage forms depends on their colour and clarity.

- Colour selection is based on the flavour. Example: blue or green for mint, red for berry.
- Maximum clarity may be achieved through purification that involves removal of all particulate matter that may come from formulation components. Removal of particulate matter is called 'polishing' and is achieved by **filtration, settling and subsequent decantation**, and **centrifugation**. Filtration is the only pratical method when large volume of liquids is involved.
- Studies should be carried out before and after filtration to ensure any preservative, flavour, colourants other components of product are adsorbed. If there is any adsorption from filter pads, it may affect the physical and chemical stability of the product.

Stability: Is the quality of being stable, it includes physical and chemical stability throughout its shelf life.

Chemical stability: It is accomplished by the use of chemical kinetics to the study of the degradation of an active drug in solution, as well as the determination of the mechanism that causes the degradation.

Drug undergoes chemical reactions like degradation, hydrolysis, oxidation, reduction, photolysis, and racemization. Therefore, drug content will get diminished or there may be formation of toxic compounds.

Since the liquid formulation consists of several active ingredients, it is difficult to check the degradative characteristics of each ingredient. It is possible to evaluate the stability by determining some property of degradation as a function of time. Stability of package in which the liquid is filled is very important. Both, effect of package on drug content and effect of system on the package have been studied.

Physical stability: A physically stable oral liquid should retain its colour, viscosity, taste, clarity and odour throughout its shelf life. All these characteristics are evaluated during the course of stability assessment. A freshly made sample should serve as a reference standard for evaluation.

Colour: It is measured by spectrophotometric method. The absorbance of aged samples is compared with the initial value to determine the extent of colour change.

Clarity: Determined by passing a beam of light through the solution. Undissolved particles scatter the light if present, the solution appears cloudy.

Taste and odour: Evaluated by a panel of unbiased, taste-sensitive individuals.

Viscosity: Determined by viscometer.

Colouring agents: These are added to liquid preparation to improve their oraganoleptic properties.

Colouring is required for the following reasons:

1. For identification and to improve acceptability to patients. Example: cherry red cough mixtures for paediatric use.
2. To produce standard preparation. Example: natural calamine does not have constant colour and has been replaced with artificially prepared material tinted with ferric oxide.
3. To maintain uniformity.

Classification of colouring agents is based on their source.

(a) Mineral colour: Rarely used, replaced by synthetic colours. Example: ferric oxide.

(b) Plant and animal colour:
- Plants. Examples: indigo, chlorophyll, carotenoid.
- Animals. Example: cochineal

(c) Synthetic colours
- Toxic, therefore not used in pharmaceutical products. Example:
  (i) Coal tar colours: napthol blue, brilliant blue, fast green, fast red, amaranth, sunset yellow.

4.3 FORMULATION COMPONENTS OF SUSPENSION

1. **Wetting agents:** These are used for modifying the wetting characteristics of hydrophobic drugs.

   The degree to which water wets the materials is determined by their hydrophilicity. Less difficulty in wetting by water if the substance is more hydrophilic. Wetting difficulty is due to a higher interfacial tension between the drug and the liquid. Wetting agents decrease the solid-liquid interfacial tension and contact angle between solid particle and liquid vehicle. Commonly used wetting agents are surfactants. Surfactants with HLB values higher than 10 are often used.

(a) Non-ionic type: Polyoxyalkyl ethers, polyoxyalkyl phenyl ethers, polyoxy hydrogenated castor oil, sorbitan esters and polyoxysorbitan esters.

(b) Anion type: Docusate sodium, sodium lauryl sulphate.

2. **Suspending agents:** Suspending agents are substances that are used to prevent finely divided insoluble materials from settling and to keep them suspended in a liquid media by imparting viscosity to the dispersion media and prevent agglomeration by reducing interparticle attraction.

   Suspending agents include:

   1. *Viscosity enhancers* are used to make the dispersion medium more viscous.
   2. *Surfactants* reduce the surface tension between the liquid medium and solid particles by getting adsorbed strongly at the interface by bringing down the surface-free energy.
   3. *Protective colloids* decrease interparticle attraction by forming film around particles.

   Suspending agents:

   (a) Natural suspending agents:

   Animal source: gelatin

   Plant source: acacia, tragacanth, starch

   Mineral source: bentonite, kaoline

   (b) Semisynthetic agents:

   Modified cellulose polymers: sodium carboxy methyl cellulose (CMC), methyl cellulose (MC), hydroxy propyl methyl cellulose (HPMC) is widely used in oral, topical and parentral dosage form.

   (c) Synthetic agents: carbopol

3. **Emulsifying agents** prevent the coalescence of the globules of the dispersed phase. They act by reducing the interfacial tension between the two phases and form a stable interfacial film.

   Emulsifying agents:

   Carbohydrates: acacia, tragacanth, agar

   Protein: gelatin, eggyolk

   High mol.wt alcohols: stearyl alcohol, cetyl alcohol

   Surfactants: span, tween

4.4 MANUFACTURING CONSIDERATIONS

1. Raw material
2. Equipment
3. Manufacturing procedures

4.4.1 Raw Materials

The raw material used in formulation should conform to standard specification. Identity, purity, uniformity, and freedom from microbial contamination should be assured by these specifications.

- Before being released for manufacture, incoming raw materials should be thoroughly tested.
- Water is the most important constituent in liquid products obtained by distillation or ion exchange treatment. Techniques employed to make water free from microbial contamination are reverse osmosis purification, membrane filtration, ultraviolet sterilization.
  Factors should be emphasized for ultraviolet sterilization.
- The flow rate of the water should not exceed the capability of the sterilizing unit.
- A filter should be used downstream to remove the dead microorganisms and particulate matter.
- The use of ion-exchange resins in the water system is important to maintaining low bacterial counts.
  Ambergard X^E – 352: Large pore, macro reticular, Type 1 quaternary ammonium anion exchange resin.
  Amberlite IR-120: Strongly acidic, cation exchange resin that balances the chemical equilibrium of the water.

4.4.2 Equipment

Equipment used in the manufacture of liquid orals:

- Measuring devices for large and small amounts of solids.
- Mixing tanks equipped with agitator.
- Filtration system for the final polishing and sterilization of the solution.
- For emulsion, homogenizer, ultrasonifiers, colloid mills are used to reduce particle size.

4.4.3 Manufacturing Procedure

Simple liquids

Solutions are prepared by adding solute to the solvent and agitated until the solution is homogeneous. It may be helpful to use heat when the solute is less soluble.

- All equipment must be thoroughly cleaned and sanitized before use by using disinfectants like dilute solution of hydrogen peroxide, phenol derivatives.
- All equipment and lines can be sterilized by using alcohol, boiling water, autoclaving, steam or dry heat.
- Tanks are usually constructed of polished stainless steel and for heating and cooling of the contents, tanks are usually jacketed.
- Until released by the QC department, the prepared liquid is stored in an adjacent tank.
- The liquid may then be transported to the filling line, the distance the product travels between the holding tank and the filling line should be minimum to reduce the chance of microbial contamination and should be easy to disassemble, clean and sanitize.

4.5 FILLING AND PACKING OF LIQUID ORALS

Filling a pharmaceutical liquid varies depending on the characteristics of the liquid such as viscosity, surface tension, foam producing qualities, compatibility with the construction material of the filling machine, type of package into which liquid is placed.

Three basic filling methods

1. Gravimetric filling
2. Volumetric filling
3. Constant level filling

1. **Gravimetric filling:** Containers are filled with liquid to a given weight.
    - Limited to large container or highly viscous products.
    - Higher cost.
    - This process does not have high speed and automatic equipment.
2. **Volumetric filling:** Containers are filled with liquid to a given volume.
    - Volumetric filling is achieved by positive displacement piston action. Each filling station consists of a measuring piston and a cylinder.
    - The fill amount is measured by the stroke of the piston.
    - This device is capable of accuracy to within fractions of millilitres.

Problems of volumetric filling

- Highly viscous liquid may cause the pistons to seize leads to loss of fill accuracy.
- Thin liquids may flow past the piston, causing uncontrollable dripping from the filling spout and associated fill inaccuracies.
- When containers are used that are not dimensionally uniform. Even though the fill amount is accurate, fill height varies, i.e., an oversized package appearance to have a slack fill, whereas an undersized package appears to have an excessive fill. Problems may be prevented by proper engineering of filling machine.

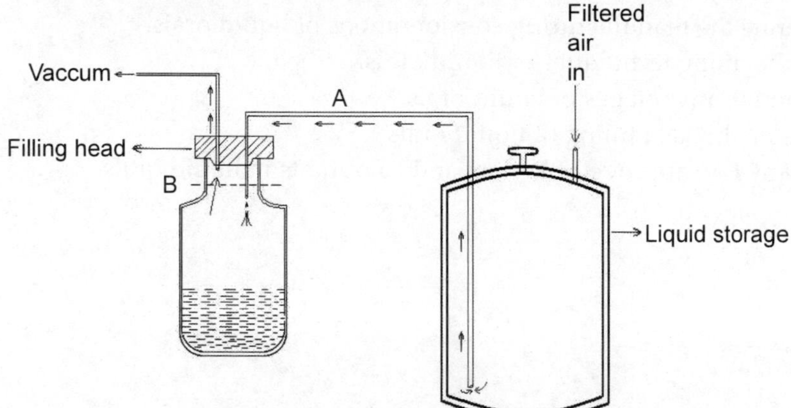

Fig. 4.2: Vacuum filling process

3. Constant level filling: Containers are used to control fill of each unit.

- Fill amount is varied by adjusting the height to which container is filled.
- Dimensional variations in containers result in variation in net fill per unit.
- Constant level filling machines in use today are high speed, and automated.

Widely used methods of constant level filling are given below.

(*a*) *Vacuum filling:* The vacuum reduces pressure in the container. Pressure differential causes liquid in the storage tank to flow through tube A into the container. When the liquid level reaches point B, excess is carried out through tube C and recycled to liquid storage tank.

(*b*) *Gravity vacuum filling:* The bottom of the liquid storage tank is at a level above the filling head. Force of gravity can be used to move the product into the container.

(*c*) *Pressure vacuum filling:* A positive pressure is applied to the liquid in storage tank to fill the container.

REVIEW QUESTIONS

Long Essays

1. Define and classify oral liquid dosage forms. Discuss the general formulation and evaluation of suspension.
2. Explain in detail about manufacture of liquid orals.
3. Define and classify oral liquid dosage forms. Discuss the general formulation and filling of monophasic liquid orals.

Short Essays

1. Explain significance of solubility in formulating liquid orals.
2. List out approved colourants and flavourants in liquid orals.
3. Explain formulation of liquid orals.
4. Discuss in detail about various factors affecting formulation of liquid orals.
5. Explain in brief the general formulation and filling of monophasic liquid orals.
6. Explain filling and packing of liquid orals.
7. Enumerate the manufacturing considerations of liquid orals.
8. Name the filling techniques of liquid orals.
9. Mention the advantages of liquid orals.
10. List the methods of filling of liquid orals.
11. Name any two approved flavours and colourants in liquid orals.

5

HARD GELATIN CAPSULES

Learning Objectives

After going through this chapter, you would be able to:

1. List out the types of capsules and their applications.
2. Describe the formulation of capsules and the challenges.
3. Explain the manufacturing techniques of hard and soft gelatin capsules.
4. Compare the capsules with other dosage forms.
5. Quality requirements of capsules.

5.1. INTRODUCTION

Capsules are unit solid dosage forms in which the drug substance and excipients are enclosed in either a hard or soft soluble shell of a suitable form of gelatin. Most filled capsules are intended to be swallowed whole.

Although gelatin is the most popular capsule shell material; capsules can be made using methylcellulose, calcium alginate, and polyvinyl alcohol.

Advantages of capsules

- Capsules are a popular dosage form due to their smooth, slippery, and easily swallowable shell.
- Capsules can mask the taste, colour, and odour of drug substances filled inside.
- They are elegant in appearance.
- They can be economically produced in large quantities in a wide range of colours.
- The capsules make the drug readily available as it uses the minimum amount of excipients and little pressure used for compaction.
- Capsules allow modification of drug release by coating them with suitable polymers.

Disadvantages of capsules

- Capsules cannot be used for the administration of highly soluble materials such as potassium chloride, potassium bromide or ammonium chloride.
- Capsules are not suitable for highly efflorescent or deliquescent material.

5.2 HARD GELATIN CAPSULES

Hard gelatin capsule shells are used in most commercial medicated capsules in the industry. These capsules may consist of two sections, one slipping over the other and the surrounding the drug formulation. The capsule is filled by introducing the powdered drug along with excipients in the longer end of the body of capsule and then slipping on the cap. Hard gelatin capsule shells are made mainly from gelatin, colours and opacifying agents.

5.2.1 Production of Hard Gelatin Capsule Shells

Preparation of gelatin

Gelatin is a heterogeneous substance of animal collagen hydrolytic extraction. Its physicochemical properties are mainly decided by the parent collagen, method of extraction, pH value, thermal degradation and electrolyte content. Familiar sources of collagen are animal bones, head portions, and frozen pork skin.

Gelatin is a long polypeptide obtained by the hydrolysis of 18 amino acids in which glycine and alanine are prominent. The process involves acidic or alkaline hydrolysis of collagen that is obtained from connective tissues such as bone and skin of animals. Depending on the sources and the method of extraction, the physical and chemical properties of gelatin may vary.

There are two types of gelatin prepared based on the method of extraction.

Type A gelatin is produced by acid treatment of pork skin majorly. This type exhibits an isoelectric point of pH 9. The acid extraction process takes lesser time in comparison with alkaline treatment.

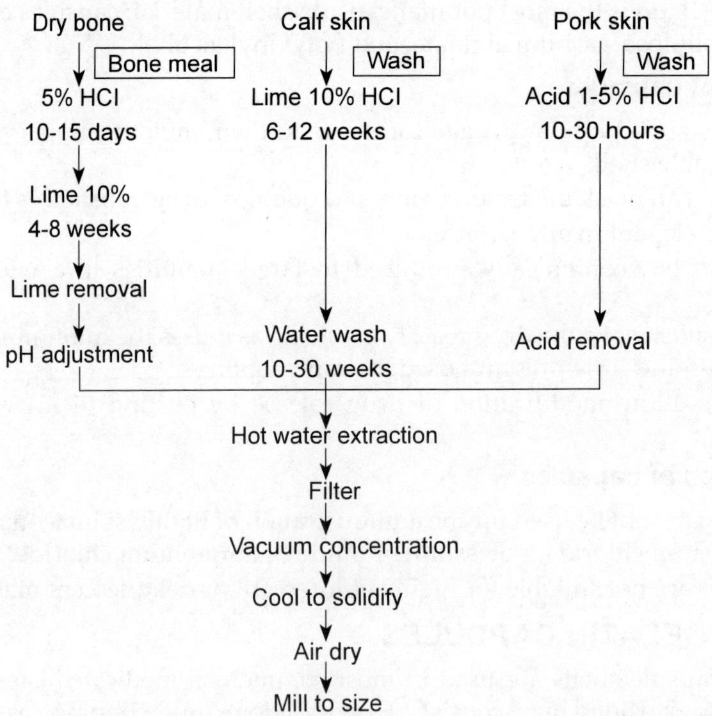

Fig. 5.1: Steps involved in the production of gelatin

Type B gelatin is prepared by alkaline treatment of animal skin and bones and has an isoelectric region of pH 4.7.

Because of their difference in viscosity and film-forming characters, a mixture of type A and B gelatin is usually used to manufacture capsule shells. The steps involved in the production of gelatin is shown in Figure 5.1.

5.2.2 Other Capsule Shell Components

Other than the suitable mixture gelatin grade, the capsule shells will contain colourants, either soluble coal tar dyes or insoluble pigments like iron oxides.

Opaquing agents like titanium dioxide are included to conceal the content and for elegancy.

Antimicrobial preservatives such as methyl and propyl parabens are employed to prevent gelatin degradation by microbial attack. Plasticizers such as glycerine and polyethylene glycol are added to gelatin to make them flexible.

5.2.3 Production of Capsule Shells

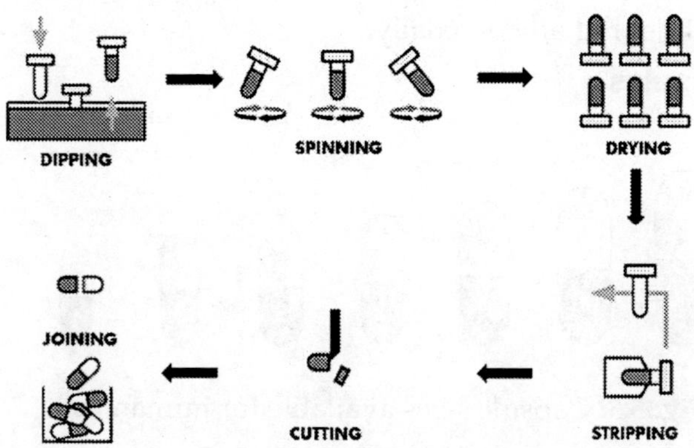

Fig. 5.2: Steps in the production of hard gelatin capsule shells

Caps and bodies of capsules are formed simultaneously on fully automatic machines. It involves the following stages:

1. **Dipping:** Pairs of 150 stainless steel pins for the cap and the body are dipped simultaneously into gelatin sol of a controlled viscosity. The gelatin sol is prepared in demineralized water at a concentration of 30-40% gelatin. The pins are lubricated prior with a mould release agent before dipping. The pins will be maintained at an ambient temperature of 22°C, whereas the dipping solution will be at a temperature of 50°C in a heated jacketed dipping pan. The dipping time for the casting of the film is approximately 12 seconds.
2. **Rotation or spinning:** After spinning, the pins are elevated and rotated 2½ times. The gelatin gets distributed uniformly on the pins, avoiding forming a bead at the tip of the capsule. The pins are inverted and exposed to a blast of cool air for setting the gelatin film.
3. **Drying:** The racks of pins coated with gelatin are passed through a series of drying chambers where dry air is blown for dehumidification. Only warm air

will be used to prevent the melting of gelatin, and a gradual drying will be executed to prevent 'case hardening' and over-drying. Over-dying may result in brittle gelatin shells, whereas under-drying will leave them sticky and soft.

4. **Stripping:** Using a series of bronze jaws that are softer than stainless steel, the formed capsule shells are gently stripped from the pins.
5. **Trimming:** The stripped caps and body are trimmed to the proper length by holding them firmly and rotating against knives in the machine.
6. **Joining:** The caps and the body of capsules are arranged concentrically and pushed to each other gently to join them.
7. **Sorting:** The capsules produced in the above steps will be having a moisture content varying from 15-18% w/w. Additional adjustments in moisture content are made during sorting. Moisture content below 12% will make the capsule shell too brittle, and above 18%, the shell becomes softer. Additionally, the capsule shells are visually examined on a moving conveyor for any defects or imperfections.
8. **Printing:** Any printing of brand name or required information should be carried out before filling. Automatic offset rotary presses are used to print on the capsules either radially or axially.

5.2.4 Sizes of Capsules

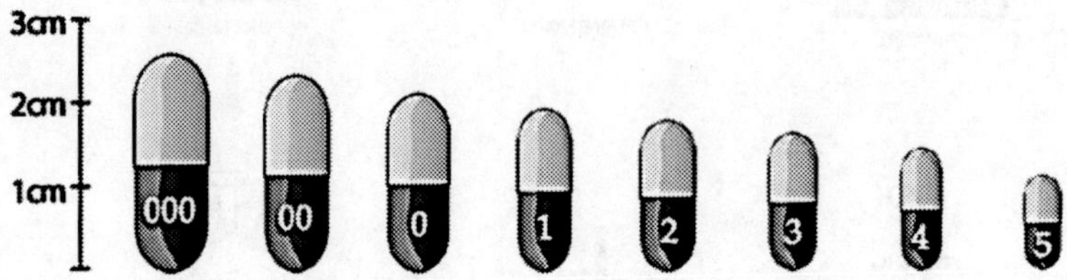

Fig. 5.3: Capsule sizes available for human use

Capsules of human use vary from sizes 000, 00, 0, 1, 2, 3, 4 and 5, where 000 is the largest and 5 is the smallest. The capacities of these capsules are shown in the Table 5.1.

Table 5.1: Capsule sizes available for human use and their fill volume and capacity

Size	Volume (mL)	Approx. fill weight (mg) of a powder with a density of 0.8 g/cc
000	1.37	1096
00	0.95	760
0	0.68	544
1	0.50	400
2	0.37	296
3	0.30	240
4	0.21	168
5	0.13	104

5.2.5 Formulation of Hard Gelatin Capsules

The hard gelatin capsule contains not only the active ingredient but necessary excipients will also be added. The general composition of a hard gelatin capsule will be as follows:

1. **The active ingredients:** A capsule formulation is developed to deliver a drug with an accurate dose with good bioavailability, ease of manufacture, better stability, and elegant appearance. While mixing the powdered drugs with excipients, a thorough blending must be ensured to uniform powder mixing for the capsule filling. Mixing is critical in low dose drugs, where a lack of homogeneity will result in significant dose variations. Preformulation studies help to determine the bulk powder properties and help in assessing the effectiveness of blending and particle size requirements.
2. **Diluents/fillers:** Suitable diluent or filler is added to the powder mix so as to produce sufficient volume to fill the body of the capsule. Partial filling of capsule shells can result in dose variations and weight variations which are critical quality considerations. Microcrystalline cellulose, starch and lactose are popular fillers employed in capsules. In addition to providing the volume, they are beneficial in transferring powder blend to capsule shells in the machine filling.
3. **Lubricants/glidants:** Glidants are finely divided dry powders added to the formulations in small quantities to improve their flow properties. When capsules are filled in high-speed automated machines, the powder mix or granules must be free-flowing to allow steady passage from the hopper to fill plates and then into the capsule shell. In order to enhance the flow properties, lubricants and glidants such as silicon dioxide, magnesium stearate, calcium stearate, stearic acid or talc are used at 0.25 to 1 % w/w.
4. **Surfactants:** When inorganic materials like magnesium stearate are used as a lubricant, and its waterproofing behaviour can retard the penetration of gastrointestinal fluids and reduce the powder wetting. Poorly water-soluble drugs may suffer bioavailability problems due to low absorption. In order to improve wetting of the drug material and the solubility, a surfactant such as sodium lauryl sulphate is added to the powder mix.
5. **Disintegrants:** Disintegrants are often added in capsules for easy breakup and distribution of the contents in GI fluid. Croscarmellose sodium, pregelatinizes starch and sodium starch glycolate are popular choices.

5.2.6 Filling of Hard Gelatin Capsules

Several types of filling machines are used in the industry for capsule filling. The machines vary from manual, semi-automatic or fully automatic. Examples of capsule filling machines are Lilly capsule filling machine, Rotofil from Eli Lilly, Farmatic, and Osaka.

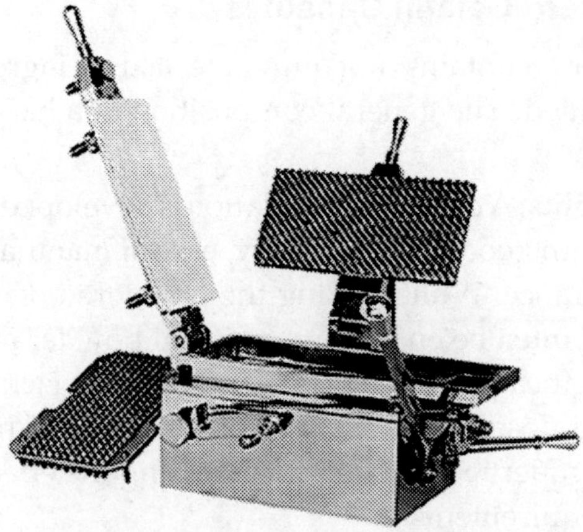

Fig. 5.4: Manual capsule filling machine

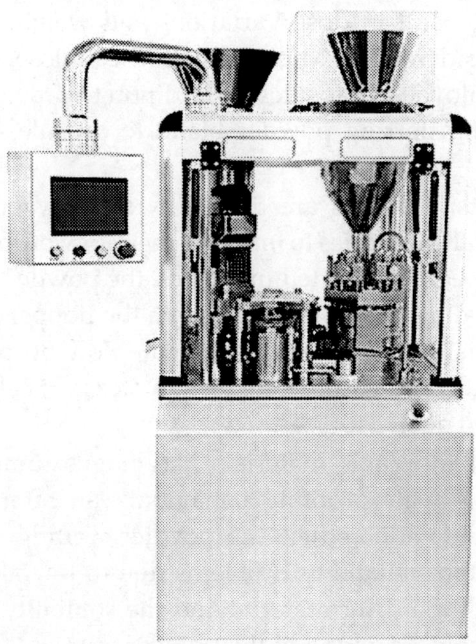

Fig. 5.5: Automatic capsule-filling machine

The general steps involved in filling in any of these machines are as follows.

1. **Rectification:** Rectification involves the orientation of empty capsules in the same direction so that body is oriented down and the cap upwards. For this, the capsules pass one at a time through a channel and are pushed to align vertically.
2. **Separation of caps from body:** The separation of caps depends upon the diameter difference between that of the cap and the body. The body end of the rectified capsules is pushed into the upper portion of the split filling rings. A vacuum applied from the bottom holds the body firmly thereby pulling it

downward. As the vacuum pulls the body of the capsule towards the lower portion of the split filling rings, the cap fails to follow the body due to its higher diameter. Then the upper and lower split rings are separated to open up the capsules exposing the body for filling.

3. **Dosing of the fill material:** Various mechanisms are used to fill the material into the capsule body. Some primary techniques are Augur fill principle, vibratory filling, piston-tamp filling and non-powder filling.
   Using suitable mechanisms, the fill material is added and levelled on the filling ring so that the body is completely filled with the material. Excess materials are removed by suitable blades automatically.
4. **Replacement of caps:** The caps and body portions are joined by bringing the upper filling ring on the top of the lower ring and pushing the filled body into the caps using suitable pins.
5. **Ejection of capsules:** Closed capsules are ejected by compressed air or pushing gently with pins at the bottom. Ejected capsules are collected and taken for dusting and polishing.
6. **Finishing:** Filled capsules are taken for dusting and polishing face in order to remove any adhering materials. Pan polishing, brushing, or cloth dusting methods are used to polish the capsules.

Pan polishing: Accela Cota tablet coating pan may be used to dust and polish capsules. Polyurethane or cheesecloth liner in the pan helps to trap dust imparting gloss to the capsules.

Cloth dusting: Here, the bulk of filled capsules is rubbed with a cloth that may or may not be impregnated with an inert oil. This procedure is manual, and it imparts a somewhat improved gloss to the capsules.

Brushing: In this procedure, capsules are fed under rotating soft brushes, which serve to remove the dust from the capsule shell. Vacuuming for dust removal must accompany this operation. Some materials are tough to remove by brushing, even to the point of impregnating the brushes and causing scratches or deformation of the capsules.

5.2.7 Special Techniques in Capsules

Some special techniques that may be applied to the capsules as a dosage form include the following.

1. Imprinting is a convenient method of placing the company or product identification information upon each capsule. The imprinting operation is best performed on the empty capsules, although filled capsules can be printed. The preference for imprinting empty capsules arises because the imprinting operation may occasionally damage some capsules. When filled capsules are imprinted, contamination, poor print quality, and actual damage to the imprinting equipment result. All imprinting machines operate on a rotogravure process, and a wide variety of colours of edible inks, both water- and solvent-based, are commercially available.

2. Special purpose capsules are capsules to which a particular treatment has been given to retard the solubility in some manner. This may be done in an attempt to delay the absorption of the active ingredient or to provide enteric properties. Various coatings have been used to provide similarly modified solubility characteristics. These coatings include salol, shellac, cellulose acetate phthalate, and particular resins that usual pan coating techniques have usually applied. Gelatin capsules are a convenient way to deliver pellets or granular material when delayed or prolonged release properties have been incorporated in all or portions of the material to be filled.
3. Separation of incompatible materials is carried out by the use of a two-phase fill in the capsule. One phase consists of either a soft capsule, a smaller hard capsule, a pill, or a suitably coated tablet that is filled into each capsule shell. Following this, a powder fill is added in the usual manner as a second phase. If this technique is used on commercial filling equipment, modifications must be made to the filling cycle of the machine.

5.2.8 Quality Control Tests for Capsules

Major quality control tests for capsules include the weight variation test, content uniformity test, dissolution testing. The procedure is similar to tablets which can be referred to in the section of quality control tests for tablets. A disintegration test may not be necessary as the capsules are not compressed by force.

REVIEW QUESTIONS

Short Answers

1. Explain the composition of hard gelating capsule shells.
2. Discuss the process of capsule filling.
3. Explain the quality control tests for capusles.

Short Essays

1. Eplain the process of production of capsule shells.
2. Explain the formulation of hard gelatin capsules.

6

Soft Gelatin Capsules

Learning Objectives

After going through this chapter, you would be able to:

1. Learn the differences in formulation of soft and hard gelatin capsules.
2. Explain the technology behind the production of softgels.
3. List of the properties of materials to be filled in soft gelatin capsules.
4. Understand the quality requirements for soft gelatin capsules.

6.1. INTRODUCTION

Soft gelatin capsules are composed of gelatin with the addition of water, plasticizer and some other excipients. Soft gelatin capsules, which contain more moisture than hard capsules, may include a preservative, such as methylparaben and/or propylparaben, to retard microbial growth. Soft gelatin capsules are widely used in pharmaceutical industries, and millions of capsules are marketed in various sizes and shapes. Shape of the soft gelatin capsules may be oblong, oval, or round in shape. Soft gelatin capsules can be easily swallowed. They can also be used in cosmetic industries for the package of breadth inhalers, perfumes, bath oils and various skin creams.

6.1.1 Advantages

1. Soft gelatin capsules can be used as an oral dosage form for human or veterinary use.
2. They can be used as a suppository dosage form for rectal use, or for vaginal use.
3. As a speciality package in tube form, for human and veterinary single dose application of topical, ophthalmic preparations, and rectal ointments.
4. Higher degree of reproducibility is possible since soft gelatin capsules are derived via encapsulation process.
5. Rapid release of content from liquid fill capsules ensures greater bioavailability.
6. Many of the drugs that are subjected to oxidative degradation can be successfully formulated in this dosage form by lipid vehicles and soft gel capsule shells.
7. Easy to swallow. Convenient administration of a liquid-drug dosage form.

6.1.2 Disadvantages

1. When compared to dry filled hard gelatin capsules, there is much chemical interaction between the capsule shell and the liquid content.
2. Solutes can migrate into outer shells, and hence can be easily washed off or get eroded.

6.1.3 Composition of Soft Gelatin Capsules

Nature of the capsule shell

The basic components of soft gelatin shells are gelatin, plasticizer and water. Other ingredients include preservatives, colouring agents, opacifying agents, flavouring, sugars, acids, and medicaments to achieve desired effects. Molecular weight or the cohesive strength determines the gelatin strength or bloom of the capsule shell. And it is proportional to the molecular weight of the gelatin. Bloom is determined by measuring the weight in grammes required to move a plastic plunger that is 0.5 inches in diameter 4 mm into a 6%% gelatin gel that has been held at 10°C for 17 hours. Cost of the capsule depends on the bloom of the product.

Viscosity of gelatin, is determined on a 6% concentration of gelatin in water at 60°C. It helps to determine the molecular characteristic of the gelatin thin film. Usually, low viscosity, i.e., 25-32 millipoise, and height bloom of 180 to 250 gm gelatins are used with the capsulation of vehicles and solids.

Iron is usually present in raw gelatin. Gelatins used in the manufacture of soft gelatin capsules should not contain more than 15 ppm of this element, because it may cause colour reaction of the oraganic compound.

Nature of capsule content

Soft gelatin capsules are prepared to contain a variety of liquid, paste, and dry fills. Water-immiscible volatile and nonvolatile liquids such as vegetable and aromatic oils, aromatic and aliphatic hydrocarbons, chlorinated hydrocarbons, ethers, esters, alcohols, and organic acids can be filled in soft gelatin capsules. Water-miscible nonvolatile liquids, such as polyethylene glycols, and nonionic surface active agents, such as polysorbate 80 are also filled in soft gelatin capsules.

Liquids that can easily migrate through the capsule shell are not suitable for soft gelatin capsules. These materials include water above 5% and low molecular-weight water-soluble and volatile organic compounds such as alcohols, ketones, acids, amines, and esters.

Solids may be encapsulated into soft gelatin capsules as solutions in a suitable liquid solvent, suspensions, dry powders, granules, pellets, or small tablets.

6.1.4 Formulation of Soft Gelatin Capsules

Gelatin

Gelatin is the basic core material for the preparation of soft gelatin capsules. Various gelatin shell formulations are available, depending on the nature of liquid fill matrix. Most commonly the gelatin is alkali processed (type B) and it normally constitutes 40% of the wet molten gel mass. Type A acid-processed gelatin can also be used.

Plasticizers

Plasticizers are used to make the soft gel shell elastic and pliable. They account for 20-30% of the wet gel formulation. Frequently used plasticizers are glycerol. Sorbitol and propylene glycol can also be used in fusion with glycerol. Choice of plasticizer accounts for the hardness of the final capsule and thus may affect its dissolution and disintegration properties. However, plasticizers should not alter the physiochemical characteristics of the shells, and it should achieve minimum interaction between the capsule shell and liquid fill matrix. The choice of plasticizer type and concentration is important in ensuring optimum compatibility of the shell with the liquid fill matrix.

Water

Water usually accounts for 30-40% of the wet gel formulation and it is necessary during gel preparation and soft gel encapsulation. Following encapsulation, excess water is removed from the soft gels through controlled drying. In dry soft gels the equilibrium water content is typically in the range 5-8% w/w, which represents the proportion of water that is bound to the gelatin in the soft gel shell. Level of water should be in this range for better physical stability.

Colourants/opacifiers

Colourants (soluble dyes, or insoluble pigments or lakes) and opacifiers are typically used at low concentrations in the wet gel formulation. Usually, synthetic or natural colourants are used to provide necessary colour for the capsule shell. Colourants can be either synthetic or natural, and are used to impart the desired shell colour for product identification. An opacifier, usually titanium dioxide, may be added to produce an opaque shell when the fill formulation is a suspension, or to prevent photo degradation of light-sensitive fill ingredients. Titanium dioxide can either be used alone to produce a white opaque shell or in combination with pigments to produce a coloured opaque shell.

6.1.5 Manufacturing of Soft Gelatin Capsule

1. **Plate process:** By the plate process, a warm sheet of plain or coloured gelatin is placed on the bottom plate of the mould and the medication-containing liquid is evenly poured on it. Then a second sheet of gelatin is carefully placed on top of the medication and the top plate of the mould is put into place. Pressure is then applied to the mould to form, fill, and seal the capsules simultaneously. The capsules are removed and washed with a solvent harmless to the capsules.
2. **Rotary die process:** Most soft gelatin capsules are manufactured by the rotary die process, a method developed in 1933 by Robert P. Scherer. Rotary die process involves the rapid formation of a heat seal among two ribbons of gelatin, simultaneous with dosing of the fill liquid into each capsule. By this method, liquid gelatin flowing from an overhead tank is formed into two continuous ribbons by the rotary die machine and brought together between twin rotating dies. At the same time, metered fill material is injected between the ribbons precisely at the moment that the dies form pockets of the gelatin ribbons. These pockets of fill-containing gelatin are sealed by pressure and heat and then severed from the ribbon. Use of ribbons of two different colours results in bi-coloured capsules. A schematic representation of this process is shown in Fig. 6.1.

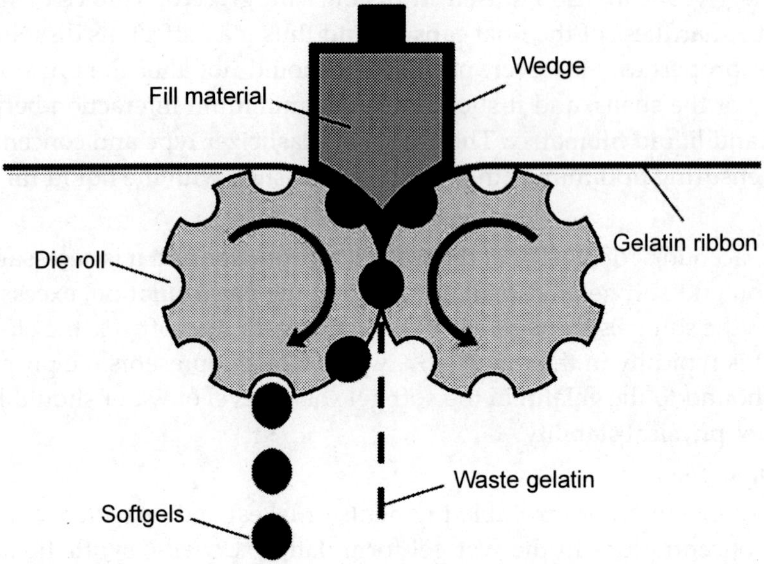

Figure 6.1: Rotary die process in the manufacture of soft gelatin capsules

3. **Accogel process:** Beneficial method for those capsules filled with powders or granules. Main parts include a measuring roll, a die roll and a sealing roll. Measuring roll rotates directly over the die roll and the pockets in the two rolls are aligned with each other. The powder is held in the pockets of measuring roll under the vacuum. A plasticized sheet is drawn into the die pockets of the die roll under vacuum. As the measuring roll and die rolls rotate, the measured doses are transferred to the gelatin lined pockets of the die roll. The continued rotation of the filled die converges with the rotating sealing roll where a second gelatin sheet is applied to form the other half of the capsule. Pressure developed between the die roll and sealing roll seals and cuts out the capsules.
4. **Bubble method:** Truly seamless, one piece of soft gelatin capsules can be made by a "bubble method". A concentric tube dispenser simultaneously discharges the molten gelatin from the outer annulus and the liquid content from the inner tube. The liquids are discharged into chilled oil as droplets, which consist of liquid medicament core within a molten gelatin envelop. The droplets assume a spherical shape under surface tension forces, and the gelatin congeals on cooling. The finished capsules then must be degreased and dried.

6.1.6 Quality Control Test for Capsules

Dissolution test for soft gelatin capsules

The apparatus used, dissolution medium and the procedure is similar to the procedure used for the dissolution test of uncoated and plain-coated tablets. If the capsule shells react during the chemical analysis, then empty capsules are dissolved in the dissolution medium by removing the contents within the capsules before the chemical analysis.

Weight variation

Weight variation mainly determines the uniformity of the dosage unit. Approximately 10 intact capsules are measured individually. Contents from the capsules are removed by washing with the solvent. The solvent is allowed to evaporate at room temperature over about 30 minutes, with precautions to avoid uptake or loss of moisture. The individual shells are weighed and the net contents calculated. From the results of the assay directed in the individual monograph, the content of the active ingredient in each capsule is determined.

Content uniformity

Unless otherwise stated in the USP monograph for an individual capsule, the amount of active ingredient, determined by assay, is within the range of 85% to 115% of the label claim for 9 of 10 dosage units assayed, with no unit outside the range of 70% to 125% of the label claim.

6.1.7 Packaging and Storage Stability for Capsules

Liquid filled soft gels are more susceptible to oxidative degradation rather than dry form. The liquid is prepared and encapsulated under a protective nitrogen atmosphere and the subsequently dried shell has very low oxygen permeability. To protect the drugs from moisture, they are packed in blister packs using materials of low moisture transmission. In harsh storage conditions soft gels will become either too soft and fuse together, or too hard and embrittled.

REVIEW QUESTIONS

Short Answers

1. What are the components of capsules.
2. Explain the rotary die process in the manufacture of soft gelatin capsules.

Short Essay

1. What are the advantages of soft gelatin capsules? Explain the methods of manufacture of soft gelatin capsules.

7

Pellets

Learning Objectives

After going through this chapter, you would be able to:

1. Define pellets as a pharmaceutical dosage form.
2. Understand the various types of pellets.
3. Describe the various pelletization processes.
4. Explain various applications of pellets in drug delivery.
5. Explain different equipment used in manufacturing of pellets.

7.1. INTRODUCTION

Pellets are small, free-flowing, spherical-shaped units made using a group of fine powders or granules of drugs through pelletization. Over the years, pelletization has gained popularity across the pharmaceutical industry owing to its various advantages over other oral medicines.

Pellets are small, free flowing, systematically produced, spherical or semi-spherical solid units, geometrically defined agglomerates of about size ranging from 0.2 mm to 2.0 mm, obtained from diverse starting materials of fine powders or granules of bulk drugs and excipients utilizing different pelletization techniques. Pellets offer various types of drug releases such as controlled release, immediate release, and sustained release. They also offer site-specific drug delivery that is necessary, in certain cases. Pellets intended for oral use are administered in the form of hard gelatin capsules or disintegrating tablets which quickly liberate their contents in the stomach and gets distributed throughout the gastrointestinal tract without loss of the depot effect, as the subunit acts as self-contained depots.

7.1.1 Advantages of Pellets

Pellets offer a significant number of advantages over conventional unit dosage forms.

7.1.2 Technological Advantages

1. Uniformity of dose layering techniques and extrusion spheronization technique offers great accuracy with uniform drug delivery to the pellets.
2. Spheres have excellent flow properties, which is very useful in automated processes or in process where exact dosing is required such as tableting, moulding operations, capsule filling, and packing.
3. Prevention of dust formation resulting in an improvement of the process safety as fine powders can cause dust explosions and the respiration of fines can cause health problems.

4. Controlled release application of pellets due to the ideal low surface area to volume ratio that provides an ideal shape for the application of film coatings.
5. They can be blended to deliver incompatible drugs simultaneously in a single dosage form, each providing same or different release profile at same of different sites in the GI tract.

7.1.3 Therapeutic Advantages

1. Pellets can disperse freely throughout the GIT after administration and consequently the drug absorption is maximized.
2. The wide distribution of spherical particles in the GI tract limits the localized build-up of the drug avoiding the irritant effect of some drugs on the gastric mucosa.
3. Reduce inter- and intra-patient variability.
4. Modified release multi-particulate delivery systems are less susceptible to dose dumping than single unit dosage forms.

7.1.4 Limitations of Pellets

1. It is difficult to compress pellets into tablets as they are too rigid. Therefore, they are often delivered encapsulated in hard gelatin capsule shells.
2. Pelletization demands highly sophisticated and specialized equipment, thereby increasing the cost of manufacturing.
3. The control of manufacturing process is complicated with too many process variables as well as formulation variables.

7.2 PELLETIZATION TECHNIQUES

The most commonly used and intensively investigated pelletization techniques include extrusion/spheronization, powder layering and solution or suspension layering. There are other methods available which can be used for preparing pellets. However, practical applicability of this method is often very limited.

7.2.1 Extrusion/Spheronization

Extrusion/spheronization is a multistage process for obtaining pellets with uniform size from those granules called extrudates. The method involves the following main steps.

- Dry mixing of ingredients, to achieve homogeneous powder dispersions.
- Wet massing, in which the powders are wet mixed to form a successfully plastic mass.
- An extrusion stage, in which the wet mass is shaped into cylindrical segments with uniform diameter.
- The spheronization stage, in which the small cylinders are rolled into solid spheres, called spheroids.
- The drying of spheroids, to achieve the desired final moisture content.
- Screening, to achieve the desired narrow size distribution.

Extrusion consists of applying pressure to Everett Mars until it passes through the calibrated openings of a screen or die played of the extruder and further shaped into small extrudate segments. The extrudates must have enough plasticity to deform, but an excessive plasticity may lead to sticking each other. The diameter of the segments and the final size of spheroids depend on the diameter of the openings in the extruder screen.

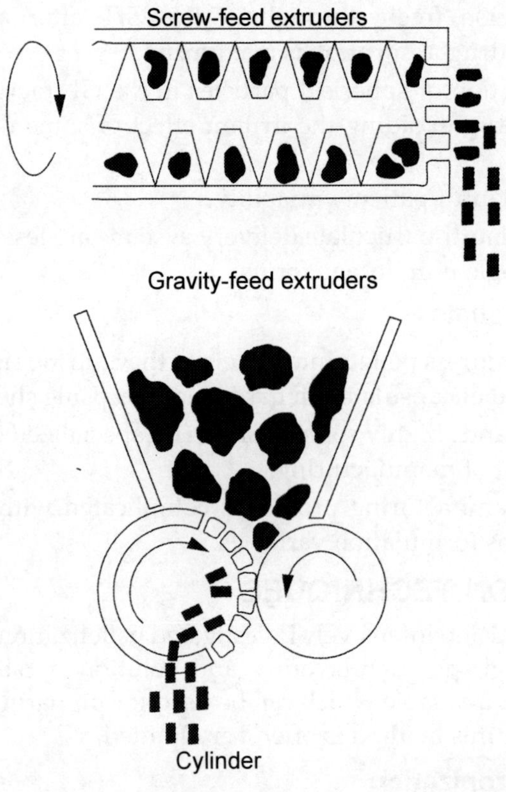

Figure 7.1: Representation of various extruders used in the manufacturing of pellets

Spheronization refers to the formation of spherical particles from the small roads produced by extrusion. The essential part of the spheronizer is the friction played. The indentation pattern on the plate can have various designs, which correspond to specific purposes. The most common design is crosshatch pattern with grooves intersecting each other at 90-degree angles.

To form spheroids, the extrudates are brought on to the rotating friction plate of the spheronizer, which imparts rolling motion to the material. Following the collisions between the extrudates with each other and with friction plate and stationary valves of spheronization chamber the cylindrical segments change their shape and size. The movement of the product along the chamber and transition from almost cylindrical segments to spheres during the spheronization process occurs in several stages as shown in Fig. 7.3.

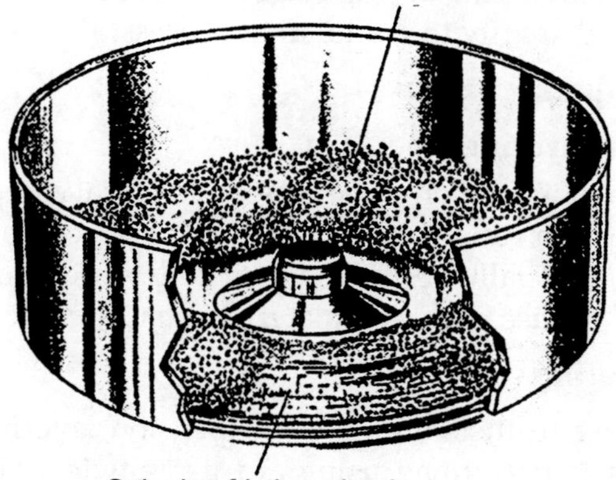

Figure 7.2: Spheronizer showing toroidal (rope-like) motion of pellet forming material during operation

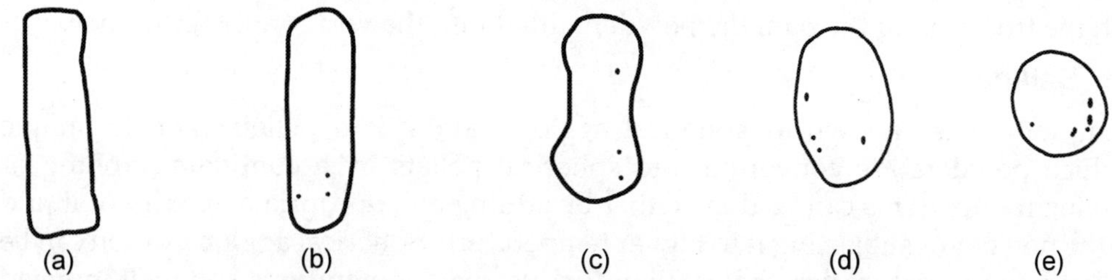

Figure 7.3: Mechanism of spheronization showing the transition of cylindrical particles to spheres

Extrusion spheronization is a versatile process for producing pellets with useful properties. Microcrystalline cellulose is extensively used for preparing the above-mentioned wet mass from which the pellets are to be prepared. microcrystalline cellulose is considered a golden standard for extrusion spheronization. Based on its good binding properties, it is able to provide the appropriate rheological conditions the process needs. Moreover, by controlling the movement of water through the plastic mass, it prevents phase separation during extrusion or spheronization.

7.2.2 Hot Melt Extrusion

This is a newly modified variation of extrusion spheronization method. Here a drug substance and excipients are converted into a molten or semi-molten state and subsequently shaped using appropriate equipment to provide solid spheres or pellets.

This is a simple, efficient and continuous process which requires fewer processing stages. It does not require along the drying stage since it does not involve addition of water or other solvent, in disparity to granulation process.

7.2.3 Layering Techniques

Solution and suspension layering

A solution or suspension of a drug on a starter seed material can produce pellets that are uniform in size distribution and generally possess very good surface morphology. These characteristics are especially desirable when pellets are quoted for the purpose of achieving a controlled release. The seed material usually is a coarse crystal.

7.2.4 Dry Powder Layering

Powder layering is similar to the solution or suspension layering. Instead of these dispersions, the layering is performed using a drug powder. The process involves the deposition of successive layers of dry powder of drug or experience or both on preformed nuclei or cores with the help of a binding liquid. Usually, the process is carried out in conventional coating pans. Initially, the start are seeds are charged into a rotating pan, and then wetted by spraying an adhesive solution. As the wet seeds reach the front end of the pan, the powder added into the vortex adheres to them.

7.2.5 Balling

Balling, otherwise known as spherical agglomeration, is a pelletization technique in which powders are converted into spherical pellets by a continuous rolling or tumbling motion. This can be done either by adding an appropriate amount of liquid into the powder or subjecting it to higher temperature. Spherical agglomeration can be divided into two categories, that is, liquid induced agglomerations and melt induced agglomerations. Various instruments are used ranging from conventional horizontal drum palletizers, inclined dish palletisers or tumbling blenders to more advanced rotary fluid bed granulators and high shear mixers. This technique is popularly used in iron ore fertiliser industries and its pharmaceutical applications are very limited.

7.2.6 Compression

Compression is one type of compaction technique for preparing pellets. Pellets of definite size and shape are prepared by compacting mixtures or blends of active ingredients and excipients under pressure. The formulation and process variables controlling the quality of pellets prepared are similar to those used in tablet manufacturing.

7.2.7 Globulation

Globulation or droplet formation consists of two related processes, spray drying and spray congealing. Nation of hot melt, solutions, or suspensions to generate spherical particles or pellets.

7.2.8 Spray Drying

During spray drying the entities in solution or suspension are spread with or without exceptions into a hot stream of air to generate dry, highly spherical particles. As the atomised droplets come into contact with hot air evaporation. Of the application medium occurs. This drying process continues through a series of stages whereby the viscosity of the droplets constantly increases until finally almost the entire application medium is evaporated, and solid particles are obtained.

Of controlled release pellets, it is generally employed to improve the dissolution rates and the bioavailability of poorly soluble drugs. Also, for processing, heat-sensitive pharmaceuticals such as amino-acids, antibiotics, ascorbic acid, liver extracts, pepsin and similar enzymes.

The spray dried particles are homogeneous with approximately spherical shape and uniform in size. The design and operation of spray dryer can influence a great number of characteristics of the final product such as particle size, size distribution, bulk density, porosity, moisture content, flour ability and friability.

7.3 DESIRABLE PROPERTIES OF PELLETS

Uncoated pellets

- Uniform spherical shape
- Uniform size
- Good flow properties
- Reproducible packing (into hard gelatin capsules)
- High strength
- Low friability
- Low dust
- Smooth surface
- Ease of coating

Coated pellets

- Maintain all the above properties
- Have desired drug release characteristics

REVIEW QUESTIONS

Short Answers

1. Define pellets and explain their advantages.
2. Explain the extrusion/spheronization method in the manufacture of pellets.
3. Discuss the desirable properties of pellets.

Short Essay

1. Explain the pelletization process and various techniques used in manufacture of pellets.

8

PARENTERAL DOSAGE FORMS

Learning Objectives

After going through this chapter, you would be able to:

1. List out the advantages and disadvantages of parenteral dosage forms.
2. Explain the various routes of injection.
3. Classify parenteral dosage forms.
4. Describe the characteristics of parenteral solutions, suspensions, emulsions, sterile solids and subdermal implants.
5. Elaborate on the types of vehicles and added solutes used in the formulation of parenteral preparations.
6. Describe the infrastructure of the functional areas and the facilities required for parenteral manufacture.
7. Explain the steps involved in the manufacture of sterile dosage forms.
8. Describe the quality control tests for parenteral dosage forms.

8.1 INTRODUCTION

Parenteral dosage forms can be defined as sterile pyrogen-free solutions, suspensions, or emulsions of one or more drugs in an aqueous or oily vehicle meant to be administered by injection (using syringe and needle) through one or more layers of skin or mucous membrane into internal body compartments.

The administration of such medications will therefore require to circumvent the body's highly efficient first line of defence, i.e., skin or mucous membrane and so these dosage forms must be free from microbial contamination, toxic components, and must have exceptionally high level of purity in terms of chemical or microbial contaminants

All components and processes involved as well as the environment in which these products are prepared must be selected and designed to eliminate all types of physical, chemical or microbiological contaminants.

Advantages

1. Useful when quick onset of action is required (in emergency situations, IV injection can be given).
2. Accurate dose of the drug can be administered.
3. The parenteral route avoids problems related with oral administration such as gastric irritation, degradation of drug by GI fluids or enzymes, etc.
4. Avoids first pass metabolism and enhances the bioavailability of the administered drug.

5. Convenient for administration to unconscious, uncooperative patients, nausea and vomiting.
6. Modification of drug release (prolonged action) is possible by formulation as suspensions, emulsions, microspheres and such preparations are known as repository or depot injections.

Disadvantages

1. There is a requirement of asepsis at the site of administration.
2. Possible risk of tissue toxicity from local irritation.
3. Administration by injection will be associated by the pain factor (real or psychological).
4. There is a difficulty in correcting any errors such as by overdose unless a direct pharmacological antagonist is available.
5. Poor patient compliance if frequent administration is required.
6. Administration through the wrong route may be fatal, e.g., administration of suspensions by the intravenous route.
7. Administration of the medication requires skilled or professionally trained persons.

8.2 ROUTES OF INJECTION

The most common routes of injection are:

1. Subcutaneous (SC) or hypodermic
2. Intramuscular (IM)
3. Intravenous (IV)

The less commonly used routes of injection are:

Intradermal (ID), intra-arterial, intrathecal, intracardiac, intracisternal, intraperitoneal and intra-articular

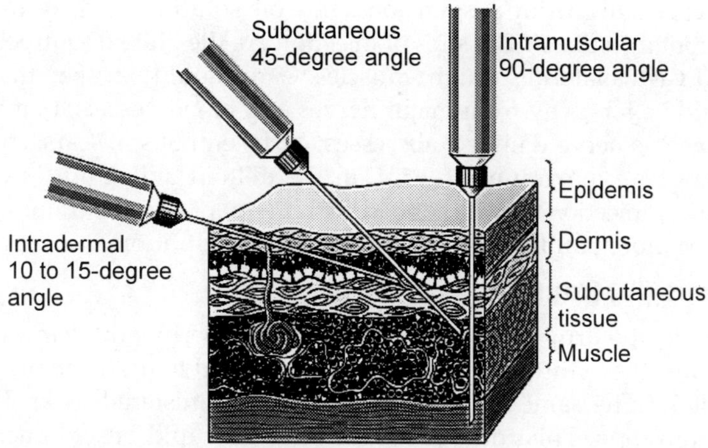

Fig. 8.1. Common routes of injection

8.2.1 Intradermal Route

The injection is made into the vascular layer of skin beneath the epidermis. This route is mainly used for diagnostic, desensitization or immunization purposes, e.g., allergen testing, mantoux test for tuberculosis, vaccines, etc. The site of injection is the anterior surface of forearm and the volume administered does not exceed 0.1 mL.

8.2.2 Subcutaneous (SC) or Hypodermic Route

Formulations administered by the subcutaneous or hypodermic route are usually injected into the subcutaneous tissue. This route can be used for both short-term and long-term therapies. The common site is the skin of the outer upper arm, front of the thigh or of the abdominal area. Volumes of not greater than 2 mL are usually administered and the site of injection is usually rotated when frequent administration is required. This route requires absorption via simple diffusion and is somewhat slower than the IV route. Vascularity in the SC tissue is less than that of muscle tissue, and therefore absorption may be slower than IM but faster than by the oral route.

SC injection minimizes the risks of haemolysis or thrombosis associated with IV injection and may provide constant, slow, and sustained effects. This route should not be used with drugs that cause tissue irritation, or thick suspensions because severe pain and necrosis may occur, however, it is suitable for administration of depot injections.

8.2.3 Intramuscular Injection (IM)

The intramuscular route is used to refer to the injection of sterile formulations deep into the skeletal muscle. It is considered to be less hazardous and easier to use than the intravenous route. The onset of action is typically longer than with IV administration, but shorter with SC. Aqueous or oleaginous solutions or suspensions of drug substances may be administered intramuscularly. However, the absorption rates vary with the type of preparation. As a result of slow absorption of the drug from the site of injection, more sustained blood concentrations are produced than after intravenous administration, especially from suspensions and oil solutions which are therefore referred to as 'depot injections'. The sites of injection are the gluteal (buttocks), deltoid (upper arm), and vastus lateralis (thigh) muscles. Care should be taken that the point of injection should be far away from major nerves and blood vessels, to minimise the risk of injuries such as nerve damage, abscesses, cysts, embolism, scars, etc. Volumes administered may be a maximum of 2 mL in the deltoid and 4 mL in the gluteus maximus. The site of injection may be rotated with frequent administration. This route is considered to be more painful than intravenous administration.

8.2.4 Intravenous (IV) Route

IV injection requires the drug to be administered into a peripheral vein as a bolus or infusion. As a bolus, the 'entire dose' of a drug is delivered to the systemic circulation almost immediately. The same dose could also be administered as an IV infusion but for a longer duration. This route provides the most rapid onset of action of any parenteral route since absorption is not a factor. Optimum blood levels may be achieved with accuracy and immediacy not possible by other routes because the drug is completely available to the body. Therefore, the IV injection of drugs can be a life-saving procedure in emergency situations.

Drugs that are too irritating for IM or SC (e.g., chemotherapy agents) can be given by this route. As with all parenteral routes, once administered the drug cannot be retrieved in case of overdose or the wrong drug being administered. The site of injection is actually any superficial vein, e.g., veins of antecubital area, the back of the hand (basilic), and some of the larger veins in the foot. The basilic and cephalic veins (dorsal forearm) are the best peripheral veins. The volumes administered may be both small and large (of 100 mL or more as in IV infusions). The formulations must be aqueous solutions and miscible with blood. Suspensions, oily preparations and emulsions cannot be administered except INTRALIPID

8.3 PREFORMULATION

Preformulation studies are critical for the injectable solution development, which covers the measurement of solubility/stability as a function of pH, pKa, partition, moisture sorption/desorption, polymorphism and crystallinity by differential scanning calorimetry (DSC), thermogravimetric analysis (TGA) and powder X-ray diffraction, salt form screening, stability of drug substance, assessing the compatibility of API and excipients using stress testing, and forced degradation to evaluate the effect of pH, temperature, humidity, light, and oxidizing agents. In addition, compound solubility in commonly used solvent, cosolvent, surfactant, solubilizer, and complex agents will be useful in setting the direction of formulation development.

The aqueous solubility of a compound depends on its state of ionization, including the ratio of ionized to unionized fraction. The degree of ionization can be estimated using the Henderson-Hasselbach equation. For weak acidic compounds, (HA) is:

$$pH = pKa + \log[A-]/[HA];$$

for weak basic compounds, (BH) is:

$$pH = pKa + \log[B]/[BH+],$$

where Ka is the ionization constant of the dissociation constant.

Effect of pH on API solubility and stability is most important for solution formulation development of ionizable compounds, which will guide the selection of formulation pH in the solution dosage form. Salt or co-crystal form is another factor that may also affect the compound solution solubility; salt form screen or *in situ* salt formation should be evaluated to find a salt form that enhances compound solubility.

8.4 TYPES OF PARENTERALS

Parenterals can be officially classified as:

1. *Injection:* Liquid preparations that are drug substances or solutions thereof (e.g., insulin injection, USP)
2. *For injection:* Dry solids that, upon addition of suitable vehicles, yield solutions conforming in all respects to the requirements for injections (e.g., Cefuroxime for injection, USP)

3. *Injectable emulsion*: Liquid preparation of drug substance dissolved or dispersed in a suitable emulsion medium (e.g., Propofol, USP)
4. *Injectable suspension*: Liquid preparation of solid suspended in a suitable liquid medium (e.g., Methylprednisolone acetate suspension, USP)
5. *For injectable suspension*: Dry solids that, upon addition of suitable vehicle, yields preparation conforming in all respects to the requirements for *injectable suspensions* (e.g., imipenem and cilastatin for injectable suspension, USP)

Parenterals can also be classified according to their physical properties as:

1. Solutions
   (a) Aqueous
   (b) Oily
2. Suspensions
3. Sterile powders
4. Implants

The form in which the manufacturer prepares a given parenteral depends on the:

(a) the nature of the drug itself with respect to its physical and chemical characteristics, and (b) on certain therapeutic considerations.

The nature of the product determines the route of administration, e.g., blood-immiscible liquids, such as oleaginous injections and suspensions, can interrupt the normal flow of blood and therefore cannot be administered by the IV route, but can be administered by the IM route.

The desired route also places certain requirements on product, e.g., if the drug has to be administered intravenously than an aqueous solution is desired, thus a water-soluble salt form of the insoluble drug is frequently prepared.

8.5 FORMULATION

Since most parenterals are liquids, the vehicle forms the major component in the formulation. Apart from the drug, additives or added solutes may be present to improve the performance, quality, stability and safety. Typically, the formulation of an injection consists of:

(a) Vehicles
(b) Added solutes

8.5.1 Vehicles

Vehicles are classified as:

1. Aqueous
   (a) Water
   (b) Other aqueous vehicles or IV fluids
2. Non-aqueous
   (a) Water miscible
   (b) Water immiscible

8.5.1.1 Aqueous Vehicles

Water

Most commonly used vehicle since many drugs are soluble in water, apart from being cheap and easily available. The body fluids are mostly composed of water, therefore it is better tolerated by the body. Only water of the highest quality and purity may be used as a vehicle for injections and such water is known as Water for Injection or WFI. Types of water for injection are:

(a) Water for injection
(b) Sterile water for injection
(c) Bacteriostatic water for injection

WFI is water of the highest quality and purity, free of pyrogens purified by distillation or reverse osmosis. It is required to comply with standards in the pharmacopoeia for water for injection. Although water for injection is not required to be sterile, it must be pyrogen-free.

It is intended for use for the manufacture of parenterals whose solvent is water (WFI in bulk), and intended to be terminally sterilized or water that is used to dissolve or dilute substances or preparations for parenteral administration (heat sterilized WFI as vehicle).

Various liquid, gas and solid contaminating substances are adequately separated by distillation and reverse osmosis.

Preparation of WFI

Source water for purification is not fit for direct distillation or reverse osmosis, since it is contaminated by organic and inorganic impurities as well as dissolved gases and needs pretreatment by chemical softening, filtration, deionization, carbon adsorption or reverse osmosis. The pretreated water is then subjected to distillation or reverse osmosis to produce WFI.

Distillation

The features of conventional still are:

1. Boiler (evaporator) containing feed water (distilland).
2. Source of heat to vaporize the water.
3. Headspace above level of distilland with condensing surfaces for refluxing, vapour separator returning nonvolatile impurities to the distilland.
4. A means for eliminating volatile impurities (demister/separation device) before the hot water vapour is condensed; and a condenser.
5. Condenser for removing the heat of vaporization, thereby converting the water vapour to a liquid distillate.

   The specific construction features of the still and the process specifications will affect the quality of the distillate. Only stills designed to produce high-purity water should be used in the production of WFI.

   All surfaces in contact with water or vapour should be made of a non-reactive material such as stainless steel, pure tin, or borosilicate glass.

Types of stills for large-scale production:

(a) Vapour compression stills

(b) Multiple effect stills

Compression Distillation

The vapour-compression still is used for the production of large volumes of high-purity distillate with low consumption of energy and water. Stills are generally made of stainless steel (304 grade). As illustrated in Fig. 8.2, the feed water is heated from an external source in the evaporator to boiling. The vapour produced in the tubes is separated from the entrained distilland in the separator and conveyed to a compressor that compresses the vapour and raises its temperature to approximately 107°C. This superheated steam then flows to the steam chest, where it condenses on the outer surfaces of the tubes containing the distilland. The condensate is drawn off as a distillate, while giving up its heat to bring the distilland in the tubes to the boiling point.

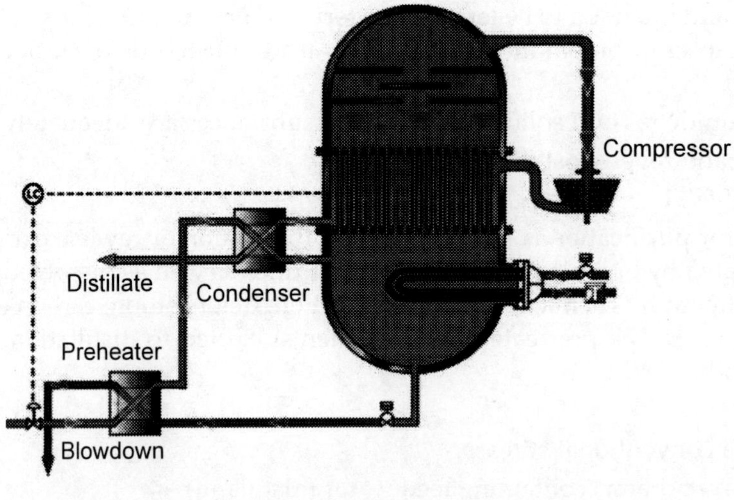

Fig. 8.2. Vapour compression still

Multiple-Effect Stills

The multiple-effect still consists of a series of single-effect stills or columns operating at differing pressures. A series of up to seven effects may be used, with the first effect operated at the highest pressure and the last effect at atmospheric pressure. Figure 8.3 shows a schematic drawing of a multiple-effect still. Steam from an external source is used in the first effect to generate steam under pressure from feed water. The steam produced by the first effect is used as the power source to drive the second effect. The steam used to drive the second effect condenses as it gives up its heat of vaporization and forms a distillate. This process continues until the last effect, when the steam is at atmospheric pressure and must be condensed in a heat exchanger.

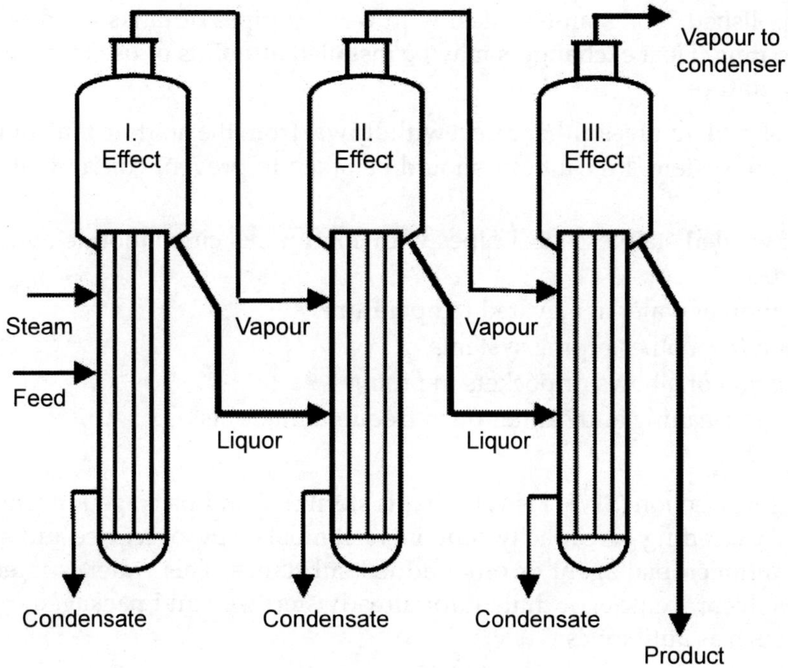

Fig. 8.3. Multiple effect still

Reverse Osmosis

Reverse osmosis is a phenomenon which involves the movement of water in the opposite direction to normal osmosis. Pressures of 200-400 psig are applied to raw water to overcome the osmotic pressure so as to force pure water through a semi-permeable membrane. The membrane may be made of cellulose esters or polyamides which are effective in retaining all macromolecules and 85% of small ions such as sodium chloride. Thus, they are able to remove pyrogens as well as microorganisms. Sometimes two membranes in series may be used for greater efficiency.

Storage and Distribution of WFI

The rate of production of WFI by distillation or reverse osmosis is not sufficient to meet daily production requirements. Therefore, it is the practice in large scale manufacture to collect the WFI in a holding tank (closed system) with a capacity of several thousand gallons. This storage tank will be part of a continuously operating system with piping and is connected to a welded stainless steel distribution loop supplying to various use sites. As per USP, WFI should be stored at 80°C to reduce the risk of microbial growth and therefore production of pyrogens. Generally, these storage tanks have a steam coil at the bottom of the tank for maintaining the required temperature. However, freshly collected WFI can be stored at room temperature, but for a maximum of 24 hours and therefore must be collected in a batch. The system must also have a hydrophobic membrane vent filter to permit changes in pressure. The tank must be constructed from electropolished 316L stainless steel with welded pipes or tanks lined with glass or pure tin coating. Heat exchangers may be installed at points of use to collect water at room temperature.

Distribution of WFI involves either direct withdrawal from the holding tank or through the welded pipe system. Precautions should be taken to prevent contamination such as:

- Use of welded stainless-steel pipes with continuous circulation to avoid water stagnation
- Circulation of water at elevated temperature
- Isolation from other piping systems
- Elimination of elbows or pockets in piping
- Thorough cleaning and sanitation at frequent intervals

Other Types of WFI

Sterile water for injection (SWFI) is WFI that is sterilized and packaged in single dose containers not exceeding 1 L capacity containers. It must be pyrogen-free and must not contain any antimicrobial agent or other added substance. This water is intended to be used as a solvent, vehicle, or diluent for already sterilized and packaged injectable medications such as antibiotics.

Bacteriostatic water for injection (BWFI) is sterile water for injection containing one or more suitable antimicrobial agents. It is packaged in prefilled syringes or in vials containing not more than 30 mL of the water. The container label must state the names and proportions of the antimicrobial agent used. BWFI is used as a sterile vehicle in the preparation of small volumes of injectable preparations. The water must be used only in parenterals that are administered in small volumes because of the presence of antimicrobial agents. Larger volumes would lead to excessive amounts of the antimicrobial agent being administered leading to possible toxic effects. During reconstitution, if more than 5 mL of solvent is required, SWFI is preferred instead of BWFI. Consideration should also be given to the chemical compatibility of the bacteriostatic agent or agents with the intended drug being dissolved.

Purity and Standards of WFI

As per the USP, the chemical and physical standards are as follows: Total organic carbon (TOC), with a limit of 500 ppb (0.5 mg/L). Conductivity, with a limit of 1.3 μS/cm at 25°C or 1.1 μS/cm at 20°C where S stands for Siemens

In the case of biological requirements for WFI, not more than 10 colony-forming units (CFUs)/100 mL and less than 0.25 USP endotoxin units/mL.

Unlike WFI, SWFI must pass the USP sterility test. Since it is a final product, WFI and SWFI may not contain added substances. As with water for injection, SWFI must be pyrogen-free but with an allowable endotoxin level of not more than 0.25 USP EU/mL. SWFI may contain slightly more total solids than water for injection because of the leaching of solids from the glass-lined tanks during sterilization. BWFI may contain one or more suitable antimicrobial agents in containers of 30 mL or less. This restriction is designed to prevent the administration of a large quantity of a bacteriostatic agent that would probably be toxic when large volumes of solution are administered, even though the concentration was low.

8.5.1.2 Other Aqueous Vehicles

Certain large volume parenterals (LVPs) may be used as isotonic vehicles to which the drug is added at the time of administration. Such vehicles include sodium chloride injection, bacteriostatic sodium chloride injection, Ringer's injection, lactated Ringer's injection, dextrose injection, dextrose and sodium chloride injection.

8.5.1.3 Non-aqueous Vehicles

Non-aqueous vehicles are used when:

- Solubility of drug in water is limited
- Drug undergoes hydrolysis in presence of water
- To prolong drug absorption

Requirements of non-aqueous vehicles for use in parenterals are:

- They must be non-toxic, non-irritating, non-sensitizing
- Must be pharmacologically inert
- Compatible with drug and added solutes

The properties of the solvent or vehicle must be considered, evaluated, and determined to be suitable for the task at hand. The solvent's physical and chemical properties to be evaluated are:

(a) Physical and chemical stability at various pH levels
(b) Viscosity and fluidity at a wide temperature range, which may affect syringeability and injectability
(c) Boiling point, sufficiently high to permit heat sterilization
(d) Miscibility with body fluids and polarity
(e) Low vapour pressure to avoid problems during heat sterilization
(f) Constant purity or ease of purification and standardization

Non-aqueous vehicles are of two types:

(a) Water miscible vehicles
(b) Water immiscible vehicles

Water miscible vehicles are used in combination with water to improve drug solubility or to reduce hydrolysis, e.g., ethyl alcohol, polyethylene glycol 400 and 600 and propylene glycol. Dimethyl acetamide and dioxolanes may also be used. Ethyl alcohol is used in the preparation of solutions of cardiac glycosides and the glycols in the solutions of barbiturates, alkaloids and certain antibiotics.

Water immiscible vehicles are the fixed oils (vegetable origin) such as corn oil, cotton seed oil, sesame oil, peanut oil (arachis oil) and esters such as benzyl benzoate, isopropyl myristate, ethyl oleate. The following are the requirements for oils used as vehicles in parenterals:

- Must be of vegetable origin
- Must be easily metabolized. Mineral oil or paraffins cannot be used
- Must be liquid at room temperature
- Must be clear when cooled to 10°C
- Must not become rancid readily
- Limits for degree of unsaturation and free fatty acid content must meet standards, i.e., they must comply with limits for iodine number and saponification number.

The label on the container must state the name of the oil used so the user may be aware in case of known sensitivity or other reactions to it.

8.5.2 Added Solutes

Care must be taken in selecting active pharmaceutical ingredients and excipients to ensure their quality is suitable for parenteral administration. As far as possible, they must be of parenteral grade. They must also be:

- Free of microbial and pyrogenic contamination
- Must be non-toxic in the quantity administered
- Must be compatible with the drug and not interfere with its therapeutic efficacy
- Must not interfere with the specific assay of the drug
- Must be present and active throughout the useful life of the product

The additives used in parenterals include antimicrobial agents, antioxidants, buffers and pH adjusting agents, tonicity adjusting agents, solubilizers, wetting agents, suspending agents, flocculating agents, emulsifiers, protectants and bulking agents.

Antimicrobial Agents (AMA)

According to the pharmacopoeia, antimicrobial agents (AMA) must be added in bacteriostatic or fungistatic concentrations to:

(a) Injectable products in multiple-dose containers
(b) Formulations sterilized by marginal processes
(c) Products prepared by aseptic manufacture

A suitable AMA must be present in adequate concentration at the time of use to prevent the multiplication of microorganisms unintentionally introduced into the preparation while withdrawing a portion of the contents with a hypodermic needle and syringe or during processing in the case of aseptic manufacture. Since AMAs are inherently toxic substances, they must be used only in the concentrations specified. They must be compatible with the drug, excipients and container used and their antimicrobial activity must be evaluated in the total formula. Products packaged in single-dose containers do not require AMA since they remain sterile until opened and expected to be used promptly after opening or discarded. Large volume parenterals (LVPs) are packaged in single-dose containers and may not contain an added antimicrobial preservative. Table 8.1 gives a list of commonly used AMA in parenterals.

Table 8.1: Antimicrobial agents and their recommended concentrations

Name of AMA	Concentration recommended (%)
Benzalkonium chloride	0.01
Benzethonium chloride	0.01
Phenyl mercuric nitrate	0.001
Thiomerosal	0.01
Phenol	0.5
Chlorobutanol	0.5
Methyl paraben	0.18
Propyl paraben	0.02

For oily products, hexylresorcinol (0.5%) and phenylmercuric benzoate (0.1%) may be used.

Antioxidants

Antioxidants are included to protect drugs susceptible to oxidation especially under the accelerated conditions of thermal sterilization. There are four types of antioxidants:

(a) Reducing agents which are preferentially oxidised are gradually used up in the oxidative reaction, e.g., ascorbic acid - 0.02-0.1%, sodium metabisulphite - 0.1%, sodium bisulphite - 0.1%.
(b) Blocking agents which block an oxidative chain reaction in which they are not usually consumed, e.g., butylated hydroxy toluene (BHT), tocopherols.
(c) Synergists which increase the effectiveness of the antioxidants that are blocking agents, e.g.,tartaric acid, phosphoric acid, citric acid.
(d) Chelating agents that chelate metallic ions which act as catalysts that would otherwise accelerate the oxidative reaction, e.g., EDTA salts.

For drugs where oxygen enters into degradative reaction, an antioxidant effect can be produced by displacing the air above the product with an inert gas. After filling, the contents of the container are saturated with nitrogen or carbon dioxide and immediately sealed.

Buffers

Buffers are used to maintain the required pH of a product to stabilize it against chemical degradation, especially for proteins where, aggregation and precipitation might occur at changing pH. Changes in pH may occur during storage for various reasons such as:

(a) Dissolution of glass constituents in the product
(b) Leaching of constituents from rubber closures or plastic containers into the product
(c) Dissolution of gases and vapours from the air space in the container
(d) Diffusion of gases through rubber or plastic components
(e) Reactions between the formulation ingredients

The buffer system selected should have the capacity to maintain the pH of the product against these effects but low enough not to significantly disturb the body's buffering systems when injected. Consideration should be given to their effective range, concentration and chemical effect on the total product. Buffers most frequently used are the citrates, acetates, and phosphates. Amino acid buffers, especially histidine, have been used for controlling solution pH of monoclonal antibody solutions.

Tonicity agents

Tonicity contributors are used in many parenterals to adjust the tonicity of the solution to reduce the pain of injection in areas with nerve endings. Hypotonic injection solutions are made isotonic by the addition of sodium chloride, dextrose or mannitol. Hypertonic injection solutions must be made isotonic by dilution prior to administration, after considering the route of administration and degree of hypertonicity.

It is desirable for every injectable product to be isotonic with physiologic fluids, but is not essential for small volume injectables administered intravenously. Small volumes administered can be quickly diluted by the blood without significant effects. However, the following products administered require to be adjusted to isotonicity:

(a) Large volume parenterals for intravenous use (IV infusions).
(b) Injections into the subcutaneous tissue and muscles to minimize pain and tissue irritation.
(c) Solutions for intrathecal injection.

The tonicity agents most commonly used are electrolytes (sodium chloride, potassium chloride), mono- or disaccharides (dextrose, lactose) and glycerin.

The methods that can be used to calculate the quantity of the tonicity adjusting substance to be added in an aqueous preparation are:

(i) Freezing point depression method
(ii) Based on molecular concentration
(iii) Graphical method using vapour pressure and freezing point determination
(iv) Based on sodium chloride equivalents

The freezing point depression method is most frequently used to determine whether a solution is isotonic. This method is based on the principle that inclusion of ions in a solvent will lower the freezing point of that solvent and the extent of the depression of the freezing point depends on the number of ions in solution (colligative property). Therefore, the freezing point of a solution is a measure of its osmolarity. The freezing point of blood serum/plasma and tears is −0.52 °C. Therefore, an aqueous solution that freezes at −0.52 °C is isotonic. The required amount of adjusting substance required to make a hypotonic solution isotonic is given by the equation:

$$W = (0.52 - a)/b$$

where, W is the concentration in % w/v of adjusting substance in the final solution, a is the freezing point depression of the unadjusted solution (i.e., freezing point depression of 1% solution × strength in % w/v) and b is the freezing point depression of water due to 1% w/v of adjusting substance, usually sodium chloride or glucose. Tables are available which provide the freezing point depressions for various compounds.

Solubilizers

When a solution formulation is desirable, the drug solubility can be increased by the use of solubilizing agents or cosolvents. When using solubilizing agents, the formulator must consider their effect on the safety and stability of the drug. There are three kinds of solubilizers that can be used:

1. Cosolvents or water miscible organic solvents
2. Chemical solubilizers
3. Surfactants

Cosolvents

Solvents that are miscible with water can be used to improve the aqueous solubility of drugs. Apart from solubilization, they also retard the hydrolysis of drugs, e.g., PEG 400, 600, propylene glycol, glycerin and ethyl alcohol.

Chemical Solubilizers

These are single compounds that may be used to solubilize certain drugs when used in combination. For example, solubilization of hydrocortisone with creatinine or niacinamide, caffeine by sodium benzoate in caffeine sodium benzoate injection, theophylline by excess of ethylene diamine in aminophylline injection

Surfactants

Surfactants that are used in injections to improve the solubility of drugs such as oil soluble vitamins and steroids are usually non-ionics, for example, polysorbates (tweens) and polyoxyethylated derivatives (Emulphor-EL 620)

Wetting Agents

Surfactants may be included in a parenteral suspension for wetting powders and to provide acceptable syringability. They help to disperse a water-insoluble drug as a colloidal dispersion by reducing the interfacial tension between the particles and the vehicle. They may also prevent crystal growth, e.g., Polysorbate 80, lecithin, Emulphor EL-620, Pluronic F-68.

Protective hydrocolloids such as sodium carboxymethyl cellulose enhance the effect of surfactants and remove the surface charge of the dispersed particles, water repellency and the tendency to agglomerate.

Suspending Agents, Flocculating Agents and Emulsifiers

Injectable suspensions may require a suspending agent to ensure that the drug can be readily and uniformly resuspended prior to use. The viscosity of the vehicle may be increased to stabilize the suspension by adding hydrocolloids such as acacia, gelatin, sodium carboxymethyl cellulose, hydroxyethyl cellulose, methyl cellulose and polyvinyl pyrrolidone (PVP) or by using polyhydric alcohol such as sorbitol.

To prevent the formation of a dense cake in suspensions, flocculating agents such as Monosodium citrate, benzyl alcohol or phenyl ethanol may be added.

Emulsifiers are added to stabilize parenteral emulsions. Lecithin, a commonly employed emulsifier, is used to stabilize vitamin K emulsion. Likewise with intravenous nutrient emulsions made from cottonseed oil, lecithin may be used as an emulsifier. These emulsions may be further stabilized by the addition of small amounts of gelatin, dextran and methyl cellulose.

Protectants

A protectant is a substance that is added to a formulation to protect against loss of activity caused by some stress that is introduced by the manufacturing process or to prevent loss of active ingredients by adsorption to process equipment or to primary packaging materials. Protectants are used primarily in protein formulations, liposomal formulations, and vaccines. Cryoprotectants and lyoprotectants are used to inhibit loss of integrity of the active substance as a result of freezing and drying, respectively. They stabilize proteins and minimise protein denaturation. Compounds that provide cryoprotection are not necessarily the same as those that provide lyoprotection. Cryoprotectants such as sorbitol, glycerol and lyoprotectants such as glucose and trehalose may be used. Amino acids like glycine, lysine, glutamine; polymers such as liquid polyethylene glycol or dextran; and polyols, such as mannitol can also be used. Human serum albumin (HSA) may be used as a protectant against adsorptive loss of proteins present at low concentrations. For example, insulin is subject to adsorptive loss to hydrophobic materials and can be prevented by the addition of 0.1–1.0% HSA.

8.6 CONTAINERS AND CLOSURES

Containers are in intimate contact with the product. There is no container available that is totally non-reactive with aqueous products. Therefore, the physical characteristics must be considered in the selection of a container.

8.6.1 Glass

Glass is the material of choice for containers of small volume injections. It is composed principally of the silicon dioxide tetrahedron which forms the basic structural network of glass, with varying amounts of other oxides such as of sodium, potassium, calcium, magnesium, aluminium, boron, and iron. Boric oxide will enter into this structure, but most of the other oxides do not. The latter are only loosely bound, are present in the network interstices, and are relatively free to migrate. These migratory oxides may be leached into a solution in contact with the glass, particularly during the increased reactivity of thermal sterilization. Therefore, these migratory oxides lower the chemical resistance of glass. The oxides dissolved may hydrolyze to raise the pH of the solution and catalyze or enter into reactions. Additionally, some glass compounds will be attacked by solutions and, in time, dislodge glass flakes into the solution.

Based on the chemical resistance, there are four types of glass. Their properties and uses are given in Table 8.2.

Table 8.2: Different types of glass and their features

Type of glass	Characteristic features	General use
Type I glass (Borosilicate glass)	Has lower levels of migratory oxides, chemically resistant glass (low leachability) and low thermal coefficient of expansion.	Buffered and unbuffered aqueous solutions, all other uses
Type II or treated soda-lime glass	Higher levels of sodium oxide, lower chemical resistance than Type I glass but higher than Type III glass since inner surfaces are treated with sulphur dioxide under controlled conditions of humidity and temperature, melt at a lower temperature, are easier to mould into various shapes, and have a higher thermal coefficient of expansion.	Buffered aqueous solutions with pH below 7.0. Dry powders, oily solutions
Type III or soda-lime glass	Higher levels of migratory oxides, lower chemical resistance than Types I or II, higher thermal coefficient of expansion, melt at a lower temperature, and are easier to mould into various shapes.	Dry powders, oily solutions
Type IV or NP glass	Soda-lime glass is not suitable for containers for parenterals.	Not for parenterals

The chemical resistance of glass can be evaluated by specific tests that determine the amount of alkaline constituents leached from the glass container under test by highly purified distilled water, under controlled elevated temperature conditions. The USP recommends the powdered glass and the water attack test while the IP (Indian Pharmacopoeia) recommends the hydrolytic resistance of glass test for measuring chemical resistance. The water attack test is used only for Type II glass and is performed on the whole container, due to the dealkalized surface; the former is performed on powdered glass, which exposes internal surfaces of the glass compound. The IP test is to be used for all types of glass. The results of these tests are based on the amount of standardised acid required to neutralize the alkalinity extracted from the container into a sample of high-purity distilled water after an autoclaving cycle.

The desirable properties of glass for the packaging of sterile products are:

1. Must be strong enough to withstand physical shocks and pressure differences as in thermal sterilization.
2. Should withstand thermal shocks from large temperature changes (have low thermal coefficient of expansion).
3. Must be transparent to permit inspection of contents.
4. Containers must have uniform physical dimensions.
5. Must protect light-sensitive products.

8.6.1.1 Types of Glass Containers

Glass containers for sterile products are available in sizes ranging from 0.5 to 1000 mL. The different types of containers are ampoules, vials, cartridges and bottles. Sizes up to 100 mL may be obtained as ampoules and vials, and larger sizes as bottles. All of these may be used as single-dose containers. Smaller sizes are also available as syringes and cartridges. For irrigating solutions, IV fluids or large volume parenterals, bottles of 100-1000 mL are available and are for single use. The size of single-dose containers is limited to 1000 mL by the USP, and multiple-dose containers to 30 mL, unless stated otherwise in a particular monograph. Multiple-dose vials are limited in size to reduce the number of punctures for withdrawing doses and the accompanying risk of contamination of the contents. The contents of single-dose containers are meant to be used immediately on opening the container. The integrity of the container is destroyed when opened, so that the container cannot be closed and reused.

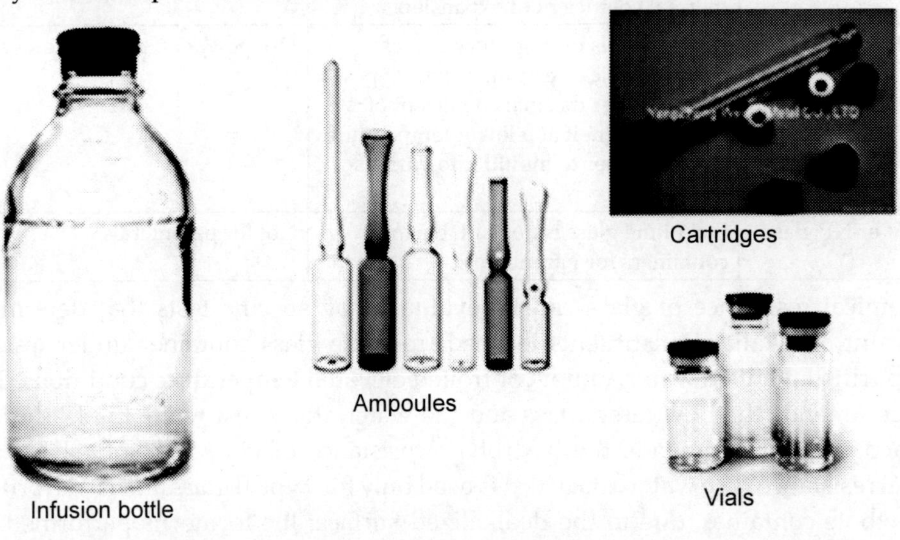

Fig. 8.4. Different types of glass containers

Glass containers may be manufactured by drawing from glass tubing or by blow moulding. Ampoules, cartridges and smaller vials are drawn from tubing, have thinner walls of uniform thickness, are lighter and have better optical clarity. Large vials and bottles are made only by blow moulding and are stronger and heavier.

Advantages

1. Glass containers are mainly used in packaging liquid preparations due to their rigidity and their superior protective qualities.
2. Its high transparency allows easy inspection of its contents.
3. It offers better protection because it is relatively impermeable to air and moisture.
4. It is chemically resistant to most medicinal products.

5. Coloured glass (amber glass and red coloured glass) can protect its content from ultraviolet rays and certain wavelengths.
6. Glass containers can be easily sterilized using heat without adverse effects.

Disadvantages

1. Glass containers are expensive to manufacture.
2. They are fragile and relatively heavy.
3. During heat sterilization, some types of glass containers have the tendency of shedding glass flakes or release alkaline constituents into the formulation that could affect the stability of the product.

8.6.2 Plastic

Thermoplastic polymers have been used as packaging materials for sterile preparations, such as large-volume parenterals, ophthalmic solutions, and recently for small-volume parenterals. The principal ingredient in these plastics is the thermoplastic polymer such as low-density polyethylene (LDPE). High-density polyethylene (HDPE), polypropylene, polyvinyl chloride (PVC) flexible and rigid, polycarbonate, polyamide (nylon), polystyrene, and polytetrafluoroethylene (Teflon). Additives that may be present include plasticizers, fillers, anti-static agents, antioxidants, etc. These compounds are not chemically bound, but free to migrate.

There are three principal problems when these materials are used:

1. Permeation of vapours and other molecules in either direction through the wall of the plastic container.
2. Leaching of constituents from the plastic into the product.
3. Sorption (absorption and/or adsorption) of drug molecules or ions on the plastic material.

Permeation is the most extensive problem when the plastic container allows migration of volatile constituents, water, or specific drug molecules through the wall of the container to the outside and, thereby, be lost. This problem can be minimised by the use of an overwrap in the packaging of IV solutions in PVC bags to prevent loss of water during storage. Reverse permeation in which oxygen or other molecules may penetrate the inside of the container and cause oxidative or other degradation of susceptible constituents may also occur. Polystyrene has the highest level of permeation.

Leaching may be a problem when the additives in the plastic formulation, such as plasticizers or antioxidants, migrate into the product. Thus, the plastic container should be formulated with as few additives as possible, which is possible for most plastics used for parenteral packaging.

Sorption occurs only with few plastics, that is, sorption of a certain drug molecules occurs on specific polymers. For example, sorption of insulin and other proteins, vitamin A acetate, and warfarin sodium has been shown to occur on PVC bags and tubing, when these drugs are present as additives in IV admixtures.

Many of the thermoplastic materials soften or melt under the conditions of thermal sterilization. But most types of thermoplastic polymers can withstand autoclaving (although they soften at such temperatures) with the exception of LDPE and polystyrene. Careful selection of the plastic used and control of the autoclave cycle has made thermal sterilization of some products possible, especially large-volume injectables. In some cases, ethylene oxide or radiation sterilization may be employed for the empty container with subsequent aseptic filling.

Nowadays, polypropylene and the copolymer polyethylene-polypropylene are increasingly being used for packaging of IV fluids and even some small-volume parenterals such as ampoules by blow-fill-seal (BFS) technology. Polypropylene is most widely used and is a linear polymer, highly crystalline with a high tensile strength. It has a high melting point of 165°C and a low permeability to gases and vapour. It is also translucent, abrasion resistant with high surface gloss and can withstand normal autoclaving temperatures.

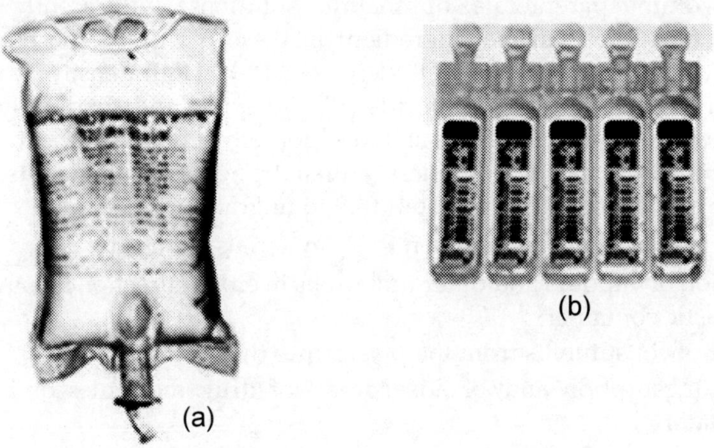

Fig. 8.5. (a) Infusion bag made from PVC
(b) Plastic ampoules made by BFS technology

Advantages

1. Plastic containers are not breakable.
2. They are light weight.
3. In the case of the flexible bags of polyvinyl chloride used for large-volume intravenous fluids, no air interchange is required; the flexible wall simply collapses as the solution flows out of the bag.
4. Usually formulated to be low in additives and low reactivity.
5. They are non-toxic.

Disadvantages

1. Possible problems of permeation, leaching and sorption and affecting the composition and stability of the product as described earlier.
2. They lack the clarity of glass, making inspection of contents difficult.
3. They melt when heated, therefore cannot be sterilized by dry heat.

8.6.3 Rubber Closures

Rubber closures are used to seal the mouths of cartridges, vials and bottles and kept in place by aluminium caps. Rubber is a material that is soft and elastic enough to permit the entry and withdrawal of a hypodermic needle without loss of integrity of the sealed container.

Rubber closures are principally made from natural rubber (latex) and/or a synthetic butyl or halobutyl rubber or polymer; a vulcanizing agent such as sulphur; an accelerator such as 2-mercaptobenzothiazole; an activator, usually zinc oxide; fillers such as carbon black or limestone; and a number of other ingredients such as antioxidants and lubricants. These multiple ingredients are plasticized into a homogeneous mass using a roller mill. The fluid mass is placed in moulds and vulcanized (cured) under high temperature and pressure. During vulcanization the polymer strands are cross-linked by the vulcanizing agent, along with the accelerator and activator to produce the elastic, solid moulded closure. Ingredients not involved in the cross-linking reactions remain dispersed within the compound and are capable of being leached out into the aqueous product.

Desirable physical properties of rubber closures

The physical properties considered in the selection of a particular formulation include elasticity, hardness, porosity, tendency to fragment, and permeability to vapour transfer.

1. Rubber closures must be sufficiently elastic to provide a snug fit between the closure and the neck of the glass container.
2. The elasticity should be sufficient to allow the rubber closure to spring back and reseal the hole produced by the needle, immediately after withdrawing the needle.
3. Closure must not be so hard or produce excessive resistance to the insertion of a needle and in the process produce minimal number of rubber fragments as the hollow needle cuts through the closure.
4. Although porous, rubber closures should not permit the easy transfer of water vapour and gases in either direction.

Closures should be completely non-reactive with the products with which they are in contact. In practice, this is not the case and the ingredients, dispersed throughout the rubber compound, are capable of leaching into the product contacting the closure. Therefore, rubber closures should be tested for compatibility with the intended product. There are two compatibility problems with rubber closures.

(i) Leaching of additives from the closure and reaction with the product.

(ii) Removal of ingredients by sorption from the product by the rubber compound or by vapour transfer through the closure.

Rubber closures may be given a plastic or lacquer coating on the surfaces that will be in contact with the product to minimise vapour transfer, sorption and leaching.

8.6.3.1 Types of Rubber Closures

The common flanged rubber closures have a lip and a protruding flange that extends into the neck of the vial or bottle. Disk closures pre-assembled with aluminium caps are being used now, particularly in the high-speed packaging of antibiotics. Slotted closures are used on freeze-dried products to permit the escape of water vapour, since they are inserted only partly into the neck of the vial until completion of the drying phase of the cycle. Plunger type of rubber closures are used to seal the ends of syringes or cartridges. Closures for intravenous infusion bottles have permanent holes for adapters of administration sets. These closures are shown in Fig. 8.6.

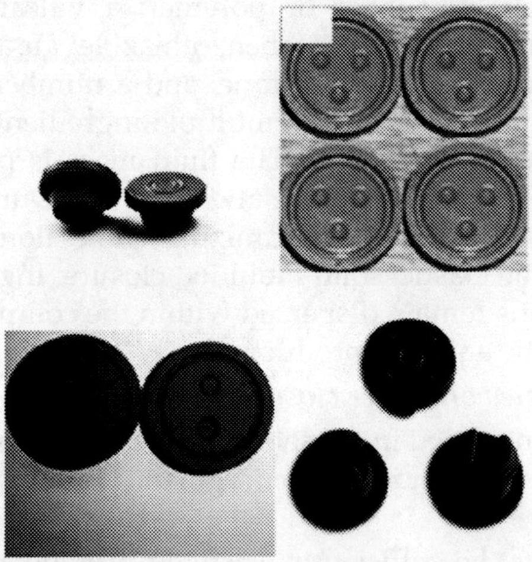

Fig. 8.6: Types of rubber closures. A- Common flanged rubber closure, B-Disk closures, C-Punctured rubber closures for infusion bottles, D- Slotted rubber closure

8.7 PARENTERAL DOSAGE FORMS

Parenteral dosage forms can be classified as:

1. Solutions
2. Suspensions
3. Emulsions
4. Dry powders
5. Subdermal implants

8.7.1 Solutions

Most injectable products are solutions. Solutions of drugs suitable for parenteral administration are referred to as injections. Although usually aqueous, they may be mixtures of water with glycols, alcohol, or other non-aqueous solvents. Many injectable solutions are manufactured by dissolving the drug and any excipients, adjusting the pH, sterile filtering the resultant solution through a 0.22 µm membrane filter and, when possible, autoclaving the final product. Most solutions have a viscosity and surface tension very similar to water. For some injections, thickeners may be added to increase the viscosity of the solution such as methyl cellulose, sodium carboxymethyl cellulose and polyvinyl pyrrolidone (PVP). Parenteral solutions are filtered through 0.22 µm membrane filters to achieve sterility and remove particulate matter. Large-volume parenterals (LVPs) and small-volume parenterals (SVPs) containing no antimicrobial agent should be terminally sterilized. It is common practice to include an antimicrobial agent in SVPs that cannot be terminally sterilized or are intended for multiple dose use, e.g., ascorbic acid injection, I.P. Injections and infusion fluids must be manufactured in a manner that will minimize or eliminate extraneous particulate matter. LVPs include IV fluids, irrigation solutions and dialysis solutions.

Intravenous fluids: Intravenous fluids or IV fluids are large volume parenterals (LVPs) that are sterile, pyrogen-free aqueous solutions intended to be administered by intravenous infusion. They are single-dose injections administered in volumes of 100 mL or more. They are packaged in containers of capacity of 100–1000 mL. IV fluids are solutions of simple chemicals such as sugars, electrolytes or amino acids that can be easily carried into the blood and assimilated. They are prepared in water for injection. Some examples of IV fluids are; dextrose injection (2.5–50%), dextrose and sodium chloride injection (varying concentrations of dextrose, 5–20% with varying concentrations of sodium chloride, 0.22–0.9%), sodium chloride injection (0.9%). The following are the requirements for LVPs or IV fluids:

1. Must be sterile and pyrogen free.
2. Must be free of particulate matter.
3. Must not contain any added solutes such as antimicrobial agents.
4. Must be isotonic.

IV fluids are used for the following purposes:

1. Correction of disturbances in electrolyte balance.
2. Correction of disturbances in body fluids.
3. As a means of providing basic nutrition.
4. The basis for the practice of total parenteral nutrition.
5. As vehicles for drug substances.

Oil solutions: Oil solutions of drugs may be prepared for intramuscular injection. They produce prolonged drug effects, due to the slow absorption of the therapeutic agent from the site of injection. Such long-acting injectable formulations are known as 'repository' or 'depot' injections. The drugs are dissolved in fixed oils of vegetable origin such as sesame oil, cottonseed oil, arachis oil, olive oil, almond oil, maize or corn oil, e.g., fluphenazine enanthate in sesame oil.

8.7.2 Suspensions

When a drug is not soluble, aqueous or oil suspensions may be prepared. They are the most difficult to formulate and require a delicate balance of variables to formulate a product that should be easy to fill, not cake or settle easily, is easily resuspended and can be ejected through an 18 to 21-gauge needle throughout its shelf life and usage. To achieve these properties, it is necessary to select and carefully maintain particle size distribution, zeta potential, and rheological properties, as well as the formulation and manufacture to control wettability and surface tension. The solids content range between 0.5 and 5% and as high as 30% in case of some antibiotics. When suspensions are administered by I.M. or S.C. routes, they provide a longer duration of action than solutions and hence can be classified as depot or repository injections.

8.7.2.1 Properties of Suspensions

(a) Rheological properties

Rheological properties are important for syringeability and injectability. The flow properties of parenteral suspensions are usually characterized on the basis of syringeability or injectability. The term syringeability refers to the handling characteristics of a suspension while drawing it into and manipulating it in a syringe. Syringeability is the ease of withdrawal of the product from the container into the syringe and can affect accuracy of dose measurement. The term injectability refers to the ease with which the suspension can be injected. The syringeability and injectability characteristics of a suspension are closely related to viscosity and to particle characteristics. The amount of solids present and the nature of the vehicle determine the viscosity. The property of thixotropy is sometimes used to improve the stability of the suspension. For example, with oleaginous suspensions, thixotropic properties can be obtained by the use of suspending agents such as aluminium monostearate. Such suspensions have the sedimentation stability of a gelled preparation during storage and syringeability of a fluid for administration.

(b) Small and uniform particle size

Particle size is a critical parameter for injectable suspensions. Small, uniform particle size of the suspended solids is required for slow uniform rates of sedimentation, adequate dissolution and drug release. Uniform particle size reduces the tendency for crystal growth during storage. Particle size growth can cause caking, difficulty in syringeability and affect dissolution and drug release rates. Size reduction of the solids to be dispersed can be achieved by various milling methods. For example, dry or wet ball milling, micropulverization, fluid energy milling, ultrasonication of shock cooled saturated solutions, spray drying, etc.

(c) Stability of suspension

Stability is important for ensuring content uniformity of a suspension. To minimise settling and caking, surfactants can be added to reduce interfacial tension between particles and the vehicle, e.g., Polysorbate 80, lecithin, Emulphor EL-620, Pluronic F-68. The use of hydrocolloids can enhance the effect of the surfactant and reduce agglomeration, e.g., sodium CMC, gelatin, methyl cellulose, and PVP. Suspensions can be further stabilized by thickening agents in the form of protective colloids or compounds such as sorbitol.

Flocculating agents may be included to bring about controlled flocculation which could prevent the formation of a dense cake, e.g., monosodium citrate.

8.7.2.2 Formulation and Manufacture

A formula for an injectable suspension might consist of the active ingredient suspended in an aqueous vehicle containing an antimicrobial preservative, a surfactant for wetting, a dispersing or suspending agent, and perhaps a buffer or salt.

Parenteral suspensions are usually processed by aseptic manufacture by one of the following methods:

(a) Sterile vehicle and powder combined aseptically

(b) Aseptic crystallization (sterile solutions combined and crystals formed *in situ*)

Sterile vehicle and powder combined aseptically

The aqueous vehicle containing the soluble components (surfactants, AMA, buffers, etc) is clarified by filtration through 0.22 μ membrane filter. This solution is heat sterilized and transferred into a presterilized mixing-filling tank. The sterile powdered drug previously prepared by freeze drying, aseptic crystallization or spray drying is gradually added to the sterile solution in a mixing tank aseptically, with continuous mixing. After tests, the suspension is aseptically filled into final containers and sealed. Procaine penicillin suspension is prepared by this method.

Aseptic crystallization (sterile solutions combined and crystals formed in situ)

The vehicle containing soluble additives is prepared and sterilized by filtration. The selected vehicle must be a non-solvent for drug. The drug is dissolved in the desired solvent and sterilized by filtration. The sterile drug solution is aseptically added to the sterile vehicle causing the drug to crystallize. The resulting suspension is diluted further with the sterile vehicle, mixed and the crystals are allowed to settle; and the supernatant solution is siphoned out. This washing is repeated several times until the solvent (organic) is completely removed. The suspension diluted to volume and transferred to the filling line, e.g., testosterone suspension.

8.7.3 Emulsions

The main problem in the formulation and manufacture of parenteral emulsions is the attainment and maintenance of very small oil droplets of uniform size of 1-4 μ in the dispersed phase. There is also limited selection of stabilizers and emulsifiers, mainly due to the difficulties arising from autoclave sterilization and parenteral injection. In addition, there may be unwanted physiological effects (e.g., pyrogenic reaction and haemolysis) that have further limited the use of intravenous emulsions. Nevertheless, a few emulsions have been formulated for parenteral use.

There are three types of parenteral emulsions.

1. Water-in-oil emulsions of allergenic extracts (subcutaneous)
2. Oil-in-water emulsions of nutrients (intravenous)
3. Oil-in-water sustained release depot preparations (intramuscular)

Lecithin is frequently used as an emulsifier for the formulation of nutrient parenteral emulsions., e.g., vitamin K emulsion and cottonseed oil emulsion.

Small amounts of gelatin, methyl cellulose and dextran have been used to stabilize these emulsions.

Total body nutrition is often administered as an IV emulsion to enable co-administration of both water-soluble and water-insoluble nutrients. IV fat emulsion usually contains 10% oil. Fat emulsions yield triglycerides that provide essential fatty acids and calories during total parenteral nutrition of patients who are unable to absorb nutrients through the GI tract. IV lipid emulsions are usually administered in combination with dextrose and amino acids in the aqueous phase. Glycerol is commonly added to make the product isotonic.

Multiple emulsions have been formulated as depot injections in the administration of anticancer drugs such as methotrexate and vinblastine.

8.7.4 Dry Powders (Sterile Solids)

There are many drugs that cannot be formulated as a solution, suspension, or emulsion because they are too unstable in an aqueous medium. The drug is then formulated as a dry powder that is reconstituted by addition of water before administration. The reconstituted product is usually an aqueous solution; however, occasionally it may be an aqueous suspension, e.g., ampicillin trihydrate and spectinomycin hydrochloride are prepared as sterile powders for suspension.

The methods for the preparation of sterile powders are:

1. Freeze drying
2. Aseptic crystallization
3. Spray drying

8.7.4.1 Freeze Drying

Freeze drying, also known as lyophillization, is a drying process where the solvent/water is first frozen and removed by sublimation in a vacuum environment. Freeze-drying takes place below the triple point of water, at which solid, liquid, and vapour all coexist in equilibrium. The product to be dried is first frozen in the range of -35 to about -45°C, then the pressure in the freeze-dry chamber is reduced to a pressure less than the vapour pressure of ice at the temperature of the product. Heat is applied to the product by increasing the temperature of the circulating fluid in the drying chamber. Under these conditions, water is removed by sublimation of ice, or a phase change from the solid state directly to the vapour state without the appearance of an intermediate liquid phase.

Advantages

1. Since water can be removed at low temperatures, damage to heat-sensitive materials can be avoided.
2. Biologicals and pharmaceuticals unstable in aqueous solution and thermolabile can be dried so that shelf life is prolonged (elevated temperatures not used).
3. Freeze-dried product has high specific surface area which facilitates rapid and complete rehydration and rapid solubility during reconstitution.
4. Dispersions are stabilized throughout shelf life.
5. Enhances stability of products subject to degradation by oxidation since process is carried out under vacuum.
6. Allow product to be filled as liquid into vials which ensures better content uniformity due to greater accuracy of filling than solids.
7. Since drug is filled as a solution, there is minimal contamination by air-borne particles and cross-contamination which is a problem with dry powder filling can be avoided.

8. Biologicals, tissue sections and viable microorganisms can be preserved, e.g., multiple vitamin combinations, antibiotics, hormones, etc.

Disadvantages

1. Biological preparations such as proteins, liposomal systems, and vaccines may be damaged by freezing, freeze-drying or both. This problem can be minimized to a certain extent by using protectants.
2. Expensive operation, hence process is limited to drying of products whose stability is enhanced in dry state.
3. Stability of a drug in solid state depends on its physical state, i.e., crystalline or amorphous.
4. Volatile compounds or drugs may be removed by the high vacuum.

A freeze dryer consists of the following components:

1. Drying chamber with temperature controlled shelves.
2. Compressor for circulating refrigerant (freon, ammonia or ethylene glycol) through pipes in the drying chamber.
3. Heating coil or element.
4. Condenser chamber interconnected to the drying chamber.
5. Vacuum pump.
6. Additional compressor for condenser chamber.

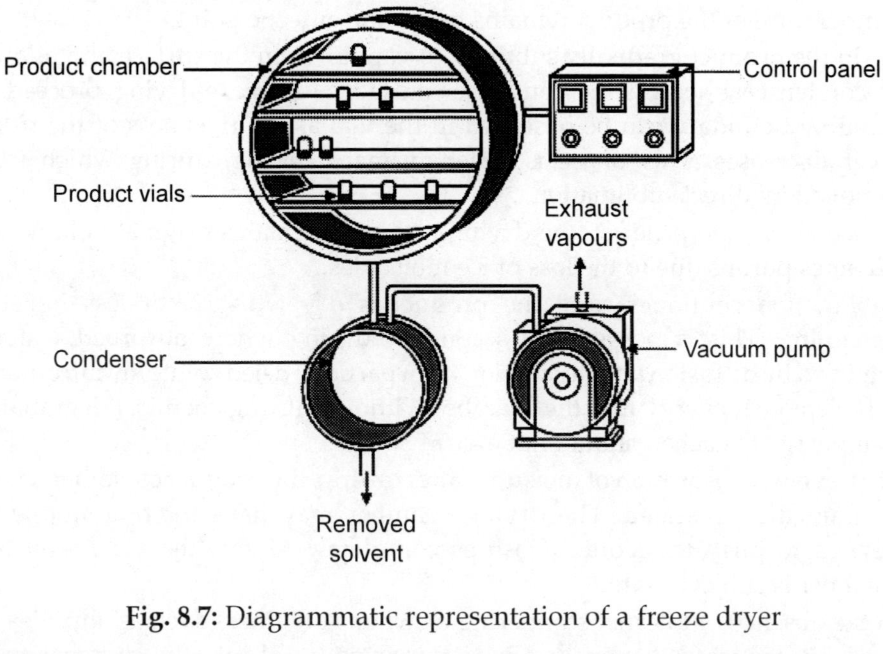

Fig. 8.7: Diagrammatic representation of a freeze dryer

Process:

The product to be freeze-dried is prepared and handled as an aqueous solution or suspension in the same manner as discussed earlier. Aqueous solutions may be sterilized by filtration, while suspensions and emulsions are prepared by aseptic manufacture. The product is filled into vials and slotted rubber closures are partially inserted into the necks (to allow for water vapour to escape during drying. The trays of filled vials are transferred to the freeze dryer.

Since the filled product containers are kept partially open, the batch must be protected from contamination during transfer from the filling area to the freeze-drying chamber (HEPA filtered LAF) and during freeze drying until the containers are fully sealed.

The important steps during this operation are described below and the stages are depicted in Fig. 8.8.

(a) Trays of vials filled with product are loaded onto the shelves in the drying chamber. Temperature of the chamber is lowered to –50°C or below the eutectic temperature of the product by the circulating refrigerant. The aqueous product is rapidly frozen (mixture of ice and solid solute).

(b) When the product is completely frozen, the chamber and the condenser are sealed and evacuated by the vacuum pump. The condenser should have been previously chilled by the circulating refrigerant to –60°C. The pressure of evacuation is about 100 μm of Hg.

(c) Heat is introduced into the shelves to supply the latent heat of vaporization to initiate sublimation. Heating must be carefully controlled so that the temperature of the product remains below the eutectic point.

(d) Ice in the product gradually sublimes to vapour from the surface and allowed to condense as ice on the condenser surface. As freeze-drying proceeds, a receding boundary can be observed in the vial as the thickness of the frozen layer decreases. This phase is called primary drying, during which ice is removed by direct sublimation.

(e) As ice leaves the product, the drying residue maintains original volume and becomes porous due to the loss of ice molecules.

(f) Sublimation continues until the product is dry with 1% or less moisture remaining. This is possible by secondary drying where adsorbed water is removed by diffusion and desorption from partially dried solute, by introducing sufficient heat energy into the chamber without causing chemical degradation (temperature reached should not exceed 30°C).

(g) To prevent reabsorption of moisture, after drying, the product container should be immediately sealed. The drying chamber may have internal stoppering devices to push the slotted closures completely to seal the vials while the chamber is still evacuated.

(h) In the absence of internal stoppering or when containers such as ampules are used, then filtered dry air or nitrogen is introduced into the chamber to re-establish atmospheric pressure. Under controlled low humidity conditions, the containers are removed and transferred to the sealing line under the protection of HEPA filtered LAF.

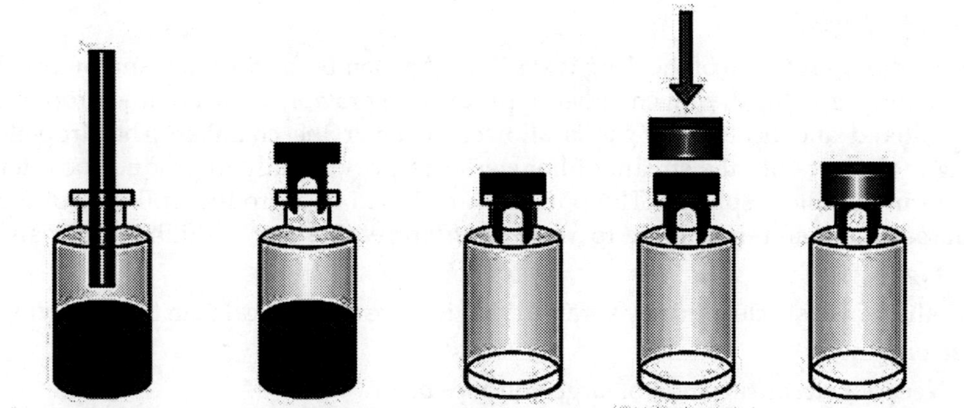

Fig. 8.8: Stages of lyophilization of product packaged in vials

8.7.4.2 Aseptic Crystallization and Dry Powder Filling

Manufacture of sterile solids by aseptic crystallization consists of the following steps:

(a) The drug is dissolved in a suitable solvent (organic) and the solution sterilized by filtration through an appropriate membrane filter.

(b) A second solvent (non-solvent for the drug), sterilized by filtration, is added at a controlled rate to the above solution, causing crystallization and precipitation of the drug.

(c) The crystals are collected on a funnel, washed if necessary, and dried by vacuum-drying.

(d) After drying, the drug crystals may be milled to reduce size and blended with additives.

(e) The powder is then transferred to dry powder filling equipment and filled into vials.

Advantages

1. Large variety of organic solvents can be used.
2. Better control over physical form of crystallized drug by choice of solvent.
3. Inexpensive.

Disadvantages

1. Batch-to-batch variability in crystal habit and crystal size give rise to variability in physical properties, leading to inconsistent product quality.
2. Maintenance of asepsis between sterile crystallization and powder filling is difficult resulting in decreased sterility assurance.
3. Since the drug is filled into vials as a powder, accuracy of filling will be difficult to control leading to greater chances of non-uniformity of drug content.

8.7.4.3 Spray Drying

In this method, a solution of the drug is sterilized by membrane filtration and pumped into an atomizer in the drying chamber to produce a spray or aerosol of fine droplets. Sterile filtered and heated air/gas is allowed to enter the chamber. The droplets coming in contact with the stream of hot sterile gas, dry rapidly to produce powder in the form of hollow spheres. The powder is collected in a product collector of the cyclone separator and transferred to a powder filling equipment, for filling into vials.

Advantage

The production of sterile solids by spray-drying is more economical than freeze-drying

Disadvantages

1. Need for sterile filtration of large volumes of air.
2. Construction and maintenance of a spray dryer that can be readily sterilized.
3. Difficulties of aseptic transfer of sterile powder from spray dryer to powder filling line.
4. Need for precise control of drying conditions to prevent overheating of the drug powder while providing adequate drying.
5. Difficulties in ensuring content uniformity due to less accuracy of filling powders.

Because of the many disadvantages, this method is not widely used in the production of sterile solids.

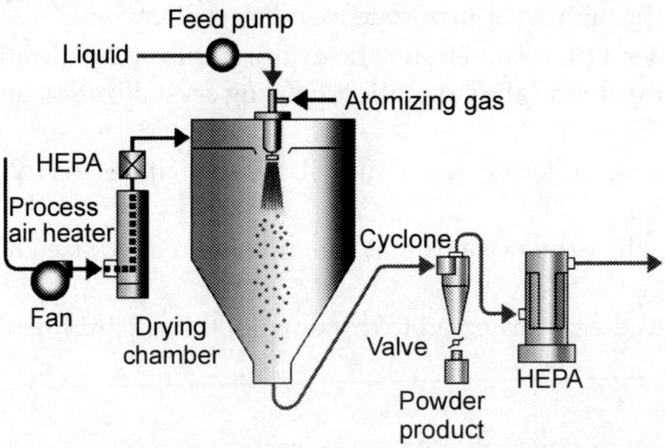

Fig. 8.9: Schematic drawing of a spray dryer

8.7.5 Subdermal Implants

Subdermal implants are also known as implantable drug delivery systems and are categorized as parenteral controlled release drug delivery systems. They are defined as sterile solid objects/devices intended to be implanted subcutaneously for the purpose of providing continuous release of drug over prolonged periods. After implantation, the drug is released, and slowly dissolves into the subcutaneous tissues. The slow absorption of the drug into the systemic circulation, produces sustained drug levels in the blood and prolonged effects.

For implantation, a surgical incision is required. The first subdermal implants made were cylindrical pellets prepared by compression of drug crystals with/without small fraction of pharmaceutical excipients. The newer implants provide a better control over drug release by utilizing rate controlling polymers or technologies using physical/chemical/biochemical processes to activate and control drug release, e.g., osmotic pressure. The Alzet osmotic pump and the Norplant are examples of two such devices.

8.8 PYROGENS AND THEIR SIGNIFICANCE IN PARENTERAL DOSAGE FORMS

Pyrogens or endotoxins are products of metabolism of microorganisms. The most potent pyrogenic substances are produced by Gram-negative bacteria (e.g., *Seudomonas* sp, *Salmonella* sp., *Escherichia coli*). Gram-positive bacteria and fungi also produce pyrogens but of lower potency and of different chemical nature. Chemically, endotoxins are lipopolysaccharides that exist in high molecular weight aggregate forms. The lipid portion of the molecule is responsible for the biological activity.

When present in parenteral drug products and injected into patients, within 1 hour of administration, pyrogens can cause fever, chills, pain in the back and legs, and malaise. Although pyrogenic reactions are rarely fatal, they can cause serious discomfort and, in the seriously ill patient, shock-like symptoms that can be fatal. The intensity of the pyrogenic response and its degree of hazard depend on factors such as the medical condition of the patient, the potency of the pyrogen, the amount of the pyrogen, and the route of administration (intrathaecal is most hazardous followed by intravenous, intramuscular, and subcutaneous).

8.8.1 Source of Pyrogens and their Control

Pyrogens are aqueous soluble, non-volatile, pass through most filters and cannot be destroyed at autoclaving temperatures. Therefore, it is impractical, if not impossible, to remove pyrogens, once present, without adversely affecting the drug product. Hence, the emphasis should be on preventing the introduction or development of pyrogens in all aspects of the compounding and processing of the product. Pyrogens can enter a product by any means that introduce microorganisms or the products of their growth. To control the entry of pyrogens into parenteral dosage forms, it is important to identify the sources of pyrogens which may then be controlled. The common sources of pyrogens are:

(a) Water
(b) Added solutes
(c) Containers and equipment

Water

Water is the biggest source of pyrogens, since all microorganisms require water for their growth. Therefore, raw water can be expected to be pyrogenic and must be appropriately treated to render it free from pyrogens. Such water is WFI which can be obtained by appropriate purification of potable water by distillation or reverse osmosis. As described earlier, it is also important that the prepared WFI is collected and stored in a sterile condition.

Added Solutes

Solutes to be used in the formulation of parenteral dosage forms must be pyrogen free. Additives and drugs may be sources of pyrogens, since the manufacturing of bulk chemicals involves the use of pyrogenic water for process steps, such as crystallization, precipitation, or washing. Bulk drug substances derived from cell culture fermentation will also be heavily pyrogenic. Therefore, all lots of solutes used to prepare parenteral products should be tested to ensure that their endotoxin levels do not exceed valid limits.

Only parenteral grade additives should be used, that has been prepared from vehicles free of pyrogens and stored in a manner to prevent subsequent contamination. Production lots or batches should be designed to use the entire contents of the packages of chemicals whenever possible, to minimise contamination on opening them.

Containers and Equipment

Pyrogenic materials adhere strongly to glass and other surfaces, especially rubber closures. Residues of solutions used in equipment can become bacterial cultures, with subsequent pyrogenic contamination. Since drying does not destroy pyrogens, they may remain in the equipment for long . Adequate washing reduces contamination, and subsequent dry heat treatment can make contaminated equipment suitable for use. Since pyrogens can be destroyed by heating at high temperatures, depyrogenation of glassware and equipment is possible by maintaining a dry heat temperature of 250°C for 45 minutes. Exposure of 650°C for 1 minute or 180°C for 4 hours, will also destroy pyrogens. Other techniques for removing pyrogens from containers and equipment are:

(a) Heating with strong alkali or oxidizing solutions.

(b) Washing with detergent and thorough rinsing with pyrogen-free water will make glassware pyrogen free.

(c) Rubber stoppers cannot withstand pyrogen-destructive temperatures, so they must be washed thoroughly, finally rinsed with WFI and immediately sterilized by autoclaving. Treated closures must be stored appropriately to prevent contamination. Plastic containers and devices must be protected from pyrogenic contamination during manufacture and storage, since all known ways of destroying pyrogens affect the plastic adversely.

Solutions can be made pyrogen free by adsorption on adsorptive agents. However, it is possible that the drug may also be removed in the process, and therefore this method has limited applications. Other in-process methods for the removal of pyrogens from solutions are selective extraction procedures and careful heating with dilute alkali, dilute acid, or mild oxidizing agents.

8.9 PRODUCTION FACILITIES

Facilities should be designed for control of cleanliness in every step. The production facilities and procedures for processing the product must meet cGMP standards. Prevention of contamination must be the primary objective of the design of these facilities.

8.9.1 Design of Production Area

To achieve the goal of a manufactured sterile product of exceptionally high quality, many functional production areas are involved: warehousing or procurement; compounding (formulation); materials (containers, closures, equipment) preparation; filtration and sterile receiving; aseptic filling; stoppering; lyophilization (if required); and packaging, labelling, and quarantine. All these areas must be designed and constructed for ease of cleaning, appropriate environment control, efficient operation and personnel comfort. Near-perfect cleanliness must be achieved in aseptic filling areas. The extra requirements for the aseptic area are designed to provide an environment where a sterile product is briefly exposed during the filling process without being contaminated. The surrounding areas should provide buffer area in which the standards of cleanliness may not be as stringent.

The design and control of the aseptic area is to ensure reduction in contaminants such as dust, lint, microorganisms so that they are not a hazard to aseptic processing. Areas are adjacent to each other for efficient flow of components.

Barriers must be placed between areas to minimise entry of contaminants into aseptic area. These barriers may be in the form of sealed walls, manual or automatic doors, air lock pass - throughs, ports of various types or plastic curtains. Glass is often used in partitions to permit supervisory view of the operation. Such partitions also provide more pleasant, better lighted, and less confining surroundings for operators. Adjacent support areas are the equipment wash rooms, capping, inspection, etc.

8.9.2 Flow Plan

The formula ingredients, container components, processing equipment released for use from stock room or storage areas to the compounding area. The containers and equipment are washed in the clean-up area or materials support area and sent for sterilization and depyrogenation. In the compounding area, ingredients are compounded according to the master formula. The product goes for filling in aseptic filling areas. If the product is a solution, then filtration is followed by filling and sealing in final containers in aseptic area. The product then passes into the quarantine area where it is held until all tests are performed.

If product is to be sterilized in its final container (terminal sterilization), there may be a change in flow pattern. After filling and sealing in the aseptic area, the product goes for sterilization. When the results from all tests are known, and the product has been found to comply with its release specifications, it passes to the finishing area for final release for shipment.

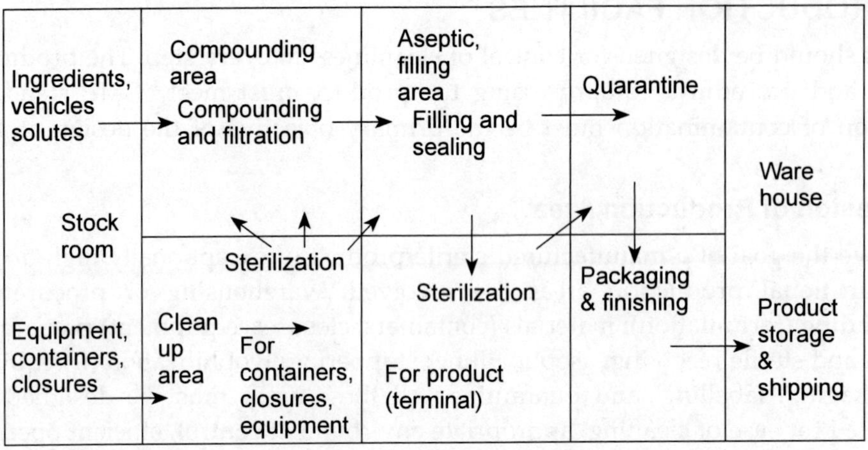

Fig. 8.10: Process flow diagram showing the movement of materials during manufacture of sterile dosage forms

Facilities in the different functional areas are described below.

Materials Support Area

Materials support area is where equipment, container and closures are washed before they are used for the formulation and further processing. This area is constructed to withstand moisture, steam and detergents. The ceiling, walls and flooring are constructed of impervious materials so that moisture will run off and not be held. On the ceiling and walls, a 'spray-on-tile' finish can be produced by using a ceramic epoxy or vinyl paint applied as sealing coat to seal off holes or crevices. For flooring, ceramic plastic cement is applied as a thick coat to provide continuous smooth, sealed surface. All such surfaces can be washed at regular intervals to keep them thoroughly clean. Adequate exhaust facilities must be provided to remove heat and humidity for the comfort of personnel. Precautions should be taken to prevent accumulation of dirt and microorganisms. There should be adequate sink and counter space. This area need not be aseptic but must be cleanable and kept clean at all times. The microbial load must be monitored and precautions taken to prevent deposit of particles or other contaminants on clean containers and equipment until boxed or wrapped for sterilization and depyrogenation.

Compounding Area

The formulation is compounded here. This area need not be aseptic (except in the case of aseptic manufacture) – control of microorganisms and particulate matter should be more stringent than in the materials support area or clean up area. The dust generated from the weighing and compounding operations must be controlled. The ceiling, walls and flooring are constructed similar to that of the materials support area. Cabinets and counters are to be constructed of stainless steel. They should fit snugly to the walls and there must be no catch areas for dirt to accumulate.

Aseptic Area

The aseptic area is considered to be a critical area and requires constructional features designed for maximum microbial and particulate control. The ceiling, walls and flooring should be sealed in the similar way as the materials support area. All surfaces must be washed and sanitized with disinfectant at regular intervals. Counters should be constructed of stainless steel and hung from the walls. There must be no legs to accumulate dirt. All light fixtures, utility service lines, ventilation fixtures are to be recessed in the walls or ceiling to eliminate ledges, joints, etc., where dirt can collect. All equipment and supplies introduced into the aseptic filling area must be sterile, preferably coming directly from sterilization. As far as possible, tanks containing compounded product must remain outside the aseptic filling area and fed through hose lines. Mechanical equipment located in this area must be housed as completely as possible within stainless steel cabinets which prevent operating parts coming directly in contact with the aseptic environment. All such equipment parts should be located below the filling line. Mechanical parts in contact with product must be demountable so that they can be sterilized after use. Entry of personnel into the aseptic area must be only through an air lock after proper gowning and movements within the aseptic area must be restricted.

All Other Areas

The construction and maintenance of ceilings, walls and flooring are the same as described under 'materials support area'. The level of cleanliness need not be as stringent as the aseptic area, but the microbial load must be monitored.

Environmental Control

The need for sterility, freedom from pyrogens and particulate matter in parenteral dosage forms necessitates effective environmental control during production. Both physical and biological control is essential. The levels achieved depend on the characteristics of facilities and consideration should also be given to variations in control associated with seasonal changes. The standards of environmental control depend on the area involved and the type of product to be manufactured, e.g., for products prepared by aseptic manufacture without terminal sterilization, the entire area for preparation must be under the most rigid biological control. For products requiring terminal sterilization, less degree of biological control may be achieved.

The measures for environmental control are:

1. Air control
2. Isolation (barrier) technology
3. Personnel control
4. Traffic control
5. Housekeeping and maintenance
6. Surface disinfection and UV radiation

Air Control

Air is the greatest source of contamination; therefore, the incoming air must be made free of dirt, microorganisms and other contaminants. The air is subjected to a series of treatments:

(i) First air is passed through prefilters made of glass wool, cloth or shredded plastic to remove large particles. More than one prefilter may be used in series, starting with the largest pore size and ending with the smallest pore size.

(ii) Next, the air is passed through an electrostatic precipitator which unit induces an electrical charge on particles in the air and removes them by attraction to oppositely charged plates.

(iii) The air then passes through the most efficient cleaning device, a HEPA (high efficiency particulate air) filter which makes it virtually free from foreign matter.

A HEPA filter is defined as a filter is at least 99.97% efficient in removing particles of 0.3 μ in size and larger and is made of glass fibres and fillers or electrostatic precipitators. For personnel comfort air conditioning and humidity control should be included in the system.

Another air cleaning device is the Kathabar system which washes the air with disinfectant solution and removes dirt and microbes while simultaneously controlling humidity.

Clean aseptic air flows into the maximum-security areas (e.g., aseptic filling area) at the greatest volume flow rate, thus producing positive pressure in these areas. This prevents unclean air from rushing into the aseptic area through cracks, open doors and other openings.

Laminar Air Flow (LAF) systems: For greater environmental control in aseptic areas, an air control system based on laminar air flow principles is utilized. The entire body of air moves with uniform velocity of 100 ± 20 feet/minute along parallel lines originating through a HEPA filter occupying an entire side of the confined space and exhausted from the opposite side. This system provides a total sweep of the confined space, bathing it with clean air and sweeping away contaminants. A confined space can be an entire room or work bench or part of a room sectioned off by plastic curtains.

The direction of the airflow maybe vertical or horizontal. Any contamination introduced upstream by an equipment, operator or leaks in the filter will be blown downstream.

In horizontal LAF, the HEPA filters are mounted on the back of work bench or entire wall of a room. In such an arrangement, the risk of blowing any introduced contaminants downstream into a critical working area is more, resulting in greater chances of cross-contamination. Horizontal LAF is more suitable for work benches as shown in Fig. 8.11.

In vertical LAF, HEPA filters are mounted on the ceiling used or placed in the top of a work bench. By this arrangement, there is less risk of introducing contamination and is suitable for protecting critical operations in processing lines. Vertical LAF is also recommended for sterility testing procedures.

Clean Room Classified Areas

HEPA filtered LAF is the only means for achieving a Class 100 clean room which is defined as a room/environment in which the particle count in the air is not more than 100 particles/cubic foot of 0.5 μ in size and larger.

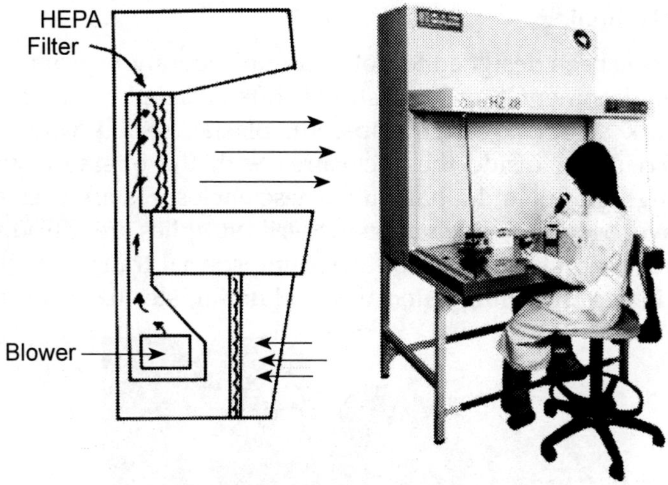

Fig. 8.11: Horizontal laminar airflow workbench

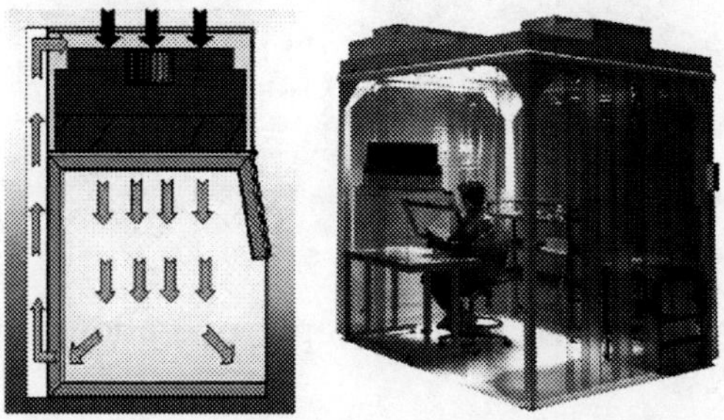

(a) (b)

Fig. 8.12: (a) Direction of airflow in vertical LAF (b) Enclosure with vertical LAF

Critical areas of processing where the product is briefly exposed to environment, such as the aseptic areas should meet Class 100 clean room standards. Achieving such levels requires effective maintenance and monitoring of Class 100 environment which is expensive. Not all operations associated with parenteral manufacture require such standards. Other classes of clean rooms can also be defined.

Class 10,000 room is one in which particles of size 0.5 μ and larger do not exceed 10,000/cubic foot. Such standards of cleanliness are suitable for buffer areas around aseptic areas, e.g., material support areas, process filtration, aseptic gowning, etc.

Class 1,00,000 clean room is suitable for laboratories, stock rooms, finishing and packaging areas. Clean room design, traditionally, has Class 100 rooms adjacent to Class 1,00,000 rooms. Due to concerns about this significant change in air quality from critical to controlled areas, it is now preferable to have an area classified from Class 1,000 to Class 10,000 in a buffer area between a Class 100 and Class 100,000 area.

Isolation (Barrier) Technology

Isolation systems have been designed to isolate aseptic operations from personnel and the surrounding environment. Sterility testing is often carried out in isolators which are enclosures/work stations with transparent, plastic, sealed walls. The aseptic operations are carried out inside the enclosures with the operator sitting outside and working through gloves and a half suit. These enclosures are presterilized with peracetic acid or hydrogen peroxide vapours. Sterile supplies are introduced into the sterilized enclosures from sterilizing modules using special transfer ports or directly from attached sterilizers, including autoclaves and hot-air sterilizing tunnels.

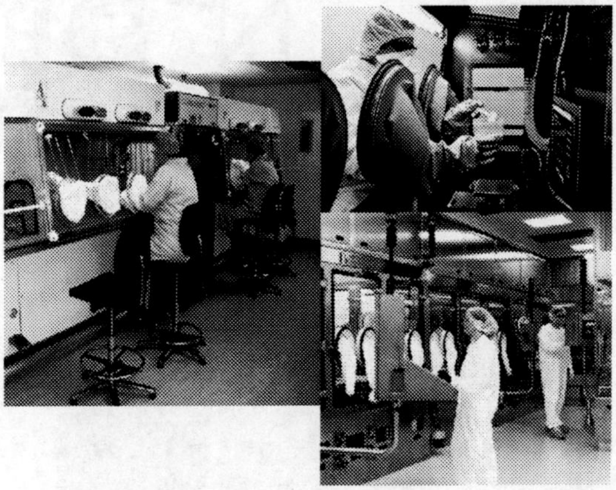

Fig. 8.13: Personnel carrying out aseptic operations in isolators

Personnel Control

Personnel working on the preparation of parenteral products must be neat, orderly, reliable, and alert with the required skills. They must be aware of the vital role that every movement they make in determining final quality and safety of the finished product. They should be in good health and free from dermatological diseases. They also must be subjected to periodic health check-ups. They must be responsible enough to report the development of a cold, sore throat or other infections and should not be permitted to work in the critical areas.

Even healthy persons may shed large number of viable and non-viable particles from their body surfaces. Therefore, uniforms/overalls are worn to control this emission to a certain extent. In addition, personnel assigned to work in clean rooms are given effective training and proper gowning to reduce the problem of particle shedding.

Operators in aseptic areas should be given training in the principles of aseptic processing and techniques. Their acquired knowledge and skills must be evaluated to determine their effectiveness. If found effective, such personnel may then be allowed to work in critical areas. Personnel entering aseptic areas need to follow the preparatory procedure as given below:

(i) Removing outside clothing.

(ii) Scrubbing hands and arms thoroughly with disinfectant. For biological product processing, a full body water and soap shower is required before entering or leaving.

(iii) Sterile gowning. Operators are required to wear sterile overalls made of synthetic fiber (e.g., Dacron), hoods/caps to cover hair, face masks, foot covers or plastic boots, gloves and goggles.

Fresh, sterile uniforms should be used after every break period or whenever the individual returns to the aseptic area. In some plants, this is not required, if the product is to be sterilized in its final container. After gowning, an air shower may be directed at the gowned person to blow away loose lint. In addition, vibrating foot mats/tacky mats or disinfectant foot baths maybe used to reduce the transfer of contamination. Personnel working in equipment washrooms, sterilizing and packaging rooms are required to wear freshly laundered uniforms daily and do not need to follow special procedures or aseptic gowning.

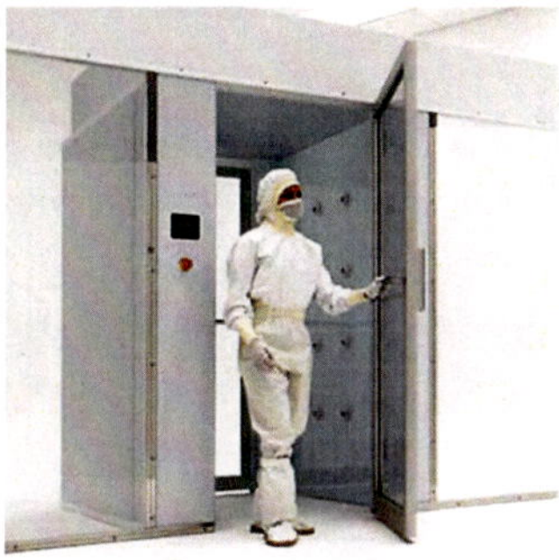

Fig. 8.14: Personnel stepping out of an airlock after sterile gowning

Traffic control

Traffic is the movement of personnel and supplies from area to area. Environmental control would be easy to achieve if it were not necessary for traffic during manufacture. Therefore, facilities should be designed to control and minimize traffic in production area, especially in and out of the aseptic area.

Floor plan in Fig. 8.15 shows that the only access directly from the outside is to personnel wash- rooms, equipment washrooms and the non-sterile manufacturing area and the packaging area. Access by personnel to the aseptic corridor and the aseptic compounding and filling rooms are only through air locks. Supplies should be introduced into the aseptic areas in a manner without disturbing the aseptic state. Pass-through openings and double ended sterilizers are provided to allow for the controlled passage of supplies from non-aseptic to aseptic areas. All equipment and supplies introduced into the aseptic area should be sterile, having come directly from the sterilization process. Or packages, hose lines from equipment and supplies are passed through ports of minimal size that can be reclosed promptly under aseptic conditions.

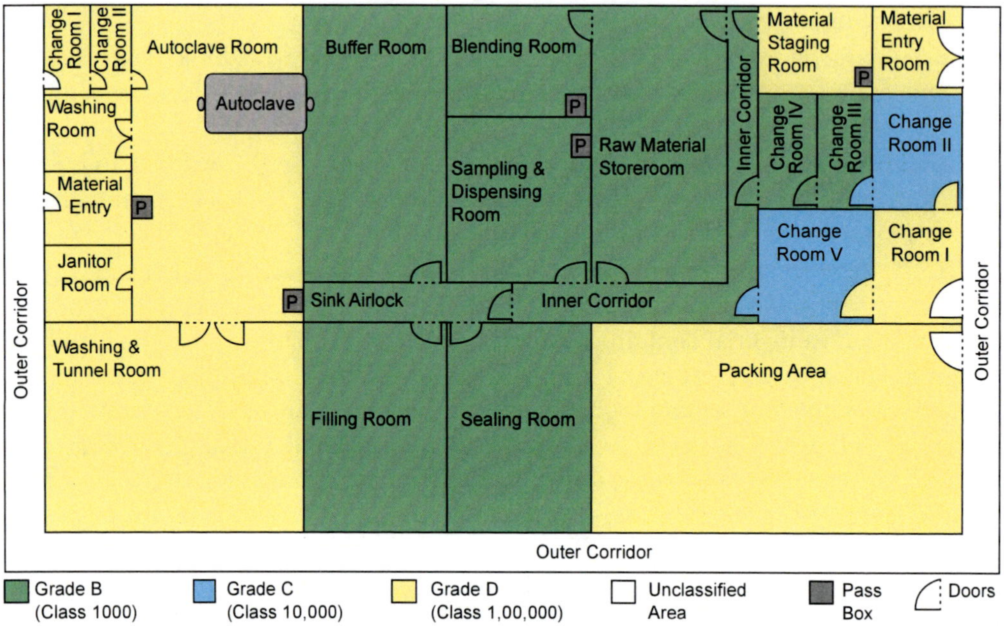

Fig. 8.15: Floor plan for sterile products production areas

Figure 8.16 shows the aseptic transfer of the compounded product through hose lines into the aseptic filling area. Outer wrappings of packages are loosened and contents received by the personnel in aseptic filling area, by grasping them by the inner wrapping. When double wrapping is not possible, outer surfaces of boxes, packages or equipment wiped with disinfectant as they are transferred. Personnel should be permitted to enter into the aseptic area only after following strictly the prescribed preparatory procedures for sterile gowning. Once inside, in and out movements without re-gowning should not be permitted. Personnel assigned to cleaning and packaging should be restricted to those areas.

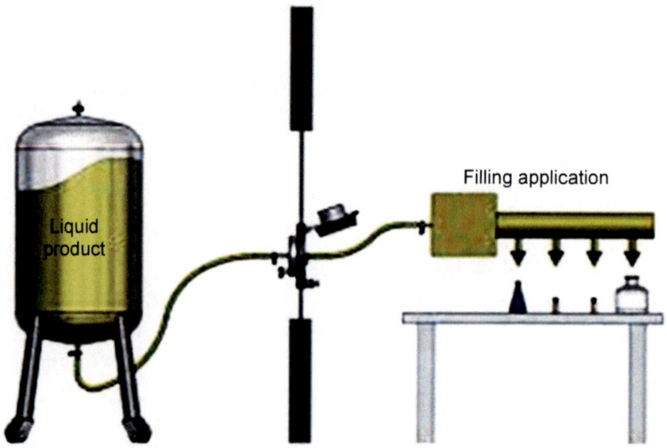

Fig. 8.16: Aseptic transfer of compounded product through transfer port

Housekeeping and Maintenance

Housekeeping and maintenance should be done by crews given special instructions and working under the supervision of trained personnel. These tasks should be done after the completion of the day's work. It is important that a carefully planned cleaning schedule should be developed, ranging from daily to monthly, depending on the location and its relation to the most critical Class 100 areas. Cleaning personnel should have the attitude that not even one remaining particle of debris is acceptable. They must also be aware during cleaning that most contaminating particles are subvisual in size. All equipment and surrounding work area must be cleaned thoroughly to remove contaminating residues of the completed operation. The ceiling, walls, flooring and other surfaces must be cleaned and sanitized according to the schedule and the prescribed procedures. Cleaning and maintenance equipment should be selected for effectiveness and freedom from lint producing tendencies. Cleaning equipment for aseptic areas should be restricted for use in these areas only.

Surface disinfection and Ultraviolet (UV) radiation

After thorough cleaning all surfaces are to be disinfected especially the aseptic areas. An effective liquid disinfectant, e.g., 2% solution of phenolic germicide, 0.01% solution of quaternary ammonium salts, isopropyl alcohol, or glutaraldehyde. The germicide must be sprayed or wiped on the surfaces.

The most effective means of surface disinfection is UV radiation from ultraviolet lamps. UV rays have antibacterial action and disinfect directly irradiated surfaces and thereby reduce the bacterial count on irradiated surfaces. Since UV rays cannot penetrate most materials, only a surface effect is produced.

UV rays travel in straight lines, therefore objects in the path of the beam can cast shadows with a lack of irradiation in these areas. UV rays are irritating to the skin and eyes, hence personnel in area of irradiation should be protected from direct exposure. Preferably, direct irradiation should be done when personnel is absent. UV rays are useful to irradiate inside exposed surfaces of processing tanks, surfaces under hoods, surfaces of conveyor belts, etc. They are not suitable for inside pipe connections, underside of conveyors, inside of containers which cannot be exposed to UV radiation.

The best source of UV radiation is the cold cathode mercury vapour lamp, which emits radiation at 253.7 nm wavelength. These lamps must be kept clean, since dust and grease reduce the effective emission drastically. With prolonged usage, there may be a change in the glass structure as well. The irradiation intensity for effective antibacterial activity of irradiated surfaces is 20 $\mu w/cm^2$.

8.10 PRODUCTION

The processes required for preparing sterile products start with the procurement of approved raw materials (drugs, excipients, vehicles, etc.) and primary packaging components (containers, closures, etc.) and ending with the sterile product sealed in its dispensing package. Each step in the process must be controlled very carefully, so the product has its required quality. For this, each process should be validated to ensure it is accomplishing what it is intended to do. The various steps involved in the manufacture of parenteral products are as follows:

1. Cleaning containers, closures and equipment
2. Compounding
3. Filtration
4. Filling
5. Sealing
6. Sterilization
7. Quality control
8. Packaging and labelling

8.10.1 Cleaning Containers, Closures and Equipment

Containers and equipment come in intimate contact with the product and therefore must be perfectly clean.

8.10.1.1 Cleaning of Containers

Dust, fibres, chemical films contaminate new unused containers which can be easily removed by rinsing alone and do not require detergents. Use of detergents should be avoided for new containers so as to prevent the risk of leaving detergent residue.

During the cleaning process, containers are subjected to a cycle of high-pressure rinsing treatments which is an alternate use of hot water or steam with cold treatment. Final rinse should be done with filtered WFI. For containers with constricted openings (ampoules), the final treatment is a blast of clean air to blow out the remaining water.

A variety of machines are available for cleaning new containers for parenteral products. These vary in complexity from a small, hand loaded, rotary rinsers to large, automatic washers capable of processing several thousand containers per hour, e.g., rotary rinsers, rack loading rinsers, conveyor rinser, etc. The selection of the particular type is determined largely by the physical type of containers, the type of contamination, and the number to be processed in a given period of time. In all these machines, the cycles of rinsing treatments are delivered through jet tubes over which containers are inverted.

Irrespective of the type of washing machine, certain fundamental characteristics are required as follows:

- The liquid treatment must be introduced from the jet tubes in such a manner that it strikes the bottom of the inside of the inverted container spreads in all directions and smoothly flows down. The pressure of the jet stream should be such that there is minimal splashing and turbulence inside.
- Containers must receive a simultaneous rinse on the outside
- All parts of the machine coming in contact with the treatments must be non-corrosive to prevent deposition of metallic contaminants on glassware.

As per cGMP all cleaning procedures must be properly validated.

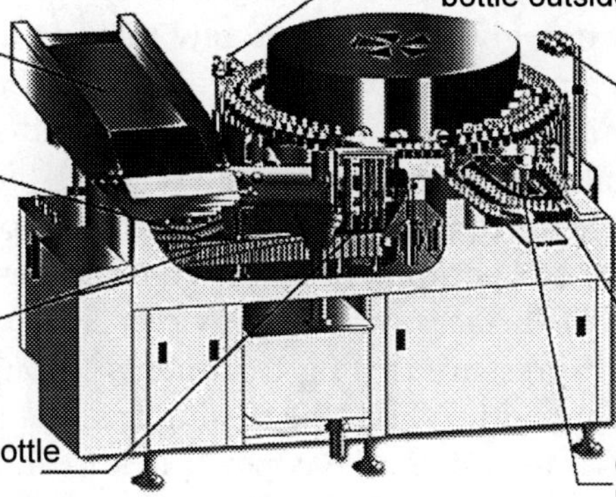

Fig. 8.17: Rotary ampoule/vial washing machine

Handling of Washed Containers

The wet, clean containers must be handled in such a way that contamination is not reintroduced. A wet surface will attract contaminants much more readily than a dry surface will and also encourage the growth of microorganisms. Therefore, wet, rinsed containers must be handled under the protection of HEPA filtered LAF and dry-heat sterilized, as soon as possible after washing. Washed containers are removed from the rinsers and placed in clean stainless steel boxes for sterilization. Doubling the heating period is required to destroy pyrogens; for example, increasing the dwell time at 250° from 1 to 2 hours.

The development of continuous, automated line processing has the advantage of requiring a minimum of individual handling while providing adequate cleaning of containers. In this process, the clean, wet containers are protected by filtered, laminar-flow air from the rinser, through the tunnel, and until they are delivered to the filling line.

8.10.1.2 Cleaning of Rubber Closures

Rubber closures may be coated with a lubricant from the moulding operation, debris, dust held on the surface by electrostatic attraction, all of which need to be removed by adequate washing. Closures are washed by gentle agitation in a tank of hot detergent solution or water softener (0.5% sodium pyrophosphate). They are then rinsed several times with water and finally rinsed with filtered WFI. Wet closures are immediately sterilized by autoclaving and stored in closed boxes until use. The equipment used for washing large number of closures is usually an agitator or horizontal basket-type automatic washing machine.

8.10.1.3 Cleaning of Equipment

All equipment should be disassembled as much as possible to provide access to internal structures for cleaning. Surfaces are scrubbed thoroughly using stiff brush and detergent, with extra attention given to joints, screw threads, crevices where dirt can collect. Streams of live steam are used to dislodge debris from areas not easily accessible. After thorough cleaning, the equipment is then rinsed several times with water and finally with WFI followed by sterilization. For large tanks, pipelines and large equipment which are difficult to clean manually, the concept of clean-in-place (CIP) may be used. For this purpose, equipment made from stainless steel is designed to have smooth rounded internal surfaces without crevices. An automatic, computer controlled system delivers high pressure rinsing treatments through nozzles within the equipment, and a final rinsing with WFI. If the rinsing treatments are followed by steam sanitization within the same system, the concept is known as sterilization-in-place (SIP).

8.10.2 Compounding

The product should be compounded under clean environmental conditions. Aseptic conditions are not required, with the exception of products requiring aseptic manufacture. However, the equipment and as far as possible, the ingredients used must be sterile.

The product must be prepared as per the batch formula which is developed from the master formula on file. The accuracy of compounding must meet rigid standards accepted in pharmaceutical procedures. All measurements of quantities must be made as accurately as possible and checked by a second qualified person.

Liquid formulations should be prepared by weight instead of by volume, since weighing is more accurate and is unaffected by changes in temperature. Care must be taken that the equipment is not wet enough to significantly dilute the product or cause physical incompatibility in case of anhydrous products. The order of mixing ingredients is important and significant especially for large batches where attaining homogeneity requires considerable mixing time. For example, in the adjustment of pH, the addition of acid though diluted, may cause excessive local reduction in pH so that adverse effects (degradation of drug) may be produced before the acid can be uniformly dispersed through the entire batch.

Parenteral dispersions such as colloids, emulsions and suspensions also produce problem such as:

- Difficulty in achieving and maintaining proper reduction in particle size under aseptic conditions.
- Dispersions must be kept in uniform state of dispersion throughout preparation, transfer and filling operations.

Biopharmaceuticals are extremely sensitive to many environmental and processing conditions exposed to during production, such as temperature, mixing time and speed, order of addition of formulation components, pH adjustment and control, and contact time with various surfaces, such as filters and tubing. Therefore, the effect of manufacturing conditions on the stability of proteins must be thoroughly evaluated during the product development stage.

8.10.3 Filtration

Products that are solutions must be filtered after compounding. The primary objectives of filtration are clarification or sterilization. A high degree of clarification is known as 'polishing' the solution when particulate matter down to 2-3 μ in size are removed. Solutions with a high degree of polish convey the impression of high quality and purity. The removal of particles down to 0.2 μ in size eliminates microorganisms and their spores as well and would accomplishes 'cold sterilization'.

The filters used for the purpose of clarification include seitz filters, sintered glass filters of suitable grade and membrane filters. Membrane filters are used exclusively for parenteral solutions, due to their particle-retention effectiveness, non-shedding property, non-reactivity, and disposable characteristics. These filters may be made from cellulose esters, nylon, Polysulfone, Polycarbonate, PVDF, or Polytetrafluoroethylene (Teflon). They are available as flat membranes or pleated to increase surface area and therefore, the flow rate.

Each filter in its holder must be tested for effectiveness before it is used especially if it is being used to eliminate microorganisms. The test frequently used is the 'bubble point' test or the 'diffusion or forward flow' test. This test is commonly used on smaller filters.

Bubble point test is used to detect any tear, opening or large pore in the membrane by increasing air pressure on the upstream side of a water wet filter. The pressure at which bubbles first appear on the downstream side is the bubble point pressure. These pressures are characteristic for each pore size of a filter and are provided by the filter manufacturer. The measured pressure should not be lower than the pressure provided by the filter manufacturers.

Although membrane filters are disposable, the filter holders must be cleaned thoroughly between uses. Clean, sterile, pretested, disposable assemblies for small, as well as large, volumes of solutions are available commercially.

After filtration, the filtrate must be protected from environmental contamination until sealed in the final containers by collecting within a closed system and fed directly to the filling machine.

8.10.4 Filling

Filling is the subdivision of the liquid/solid product from the bulk container into individual final containers. The most stringent measures are taken to prevent contamination during filling especially if the product has already been sterilized by filtration and will not be sterilized in the final container. The latter process is known as *aseptic filling*. The process of filling exposes the sterile product briefly to the environment, equipment and manipulation of the operator until sealed. Therefore, filling should be done as quickly as possible, even though the process is carried out under the protection of HEPA-filtered laminar-flow air within the aseptic area.

8.10.4.1 Filling of Liquids

Liquids are easier to fill than solids and mobile liquids are much easier to transfer and subdivide than viscous, sticky liquids, which require heavy-duty machinery for rapid production filling.

The filling of a small number of containers, can be done by using a hypodermic syringe and needle, the liquid drawn into the syringe and forced through the needle into the container. Faster filling by hand can be achieved by using a Cornwall pipette which has a two-way valve between syringe and the needle for setting the stroke of the syringe to deliver the same volume. On a large scale, semi-automatic machines are used. Although there are several types of machines that can be used for the filling of liquids into containers, certain features are fundamental to them all.

(i) A means of repetitively forcing a measured volume of liquid through the orifice of a delivery tube which is introduced into the container.
(ii) The size of the delivery tube required depends on the physical characteristics of fluid, desired filling speed, and the inside diameter of the neck of the container. The delivery tube diameter may range from a 20-gauge hypodermic needle to a tube of 1/2 in or more in diameter.
(iii) The tube must enter the neck and deliver the liquid well into the neck to eliminate spillage, with sufficient clearance to allow air to leave the container as the liquid enters.
(iv) The delivery tube should be as large in diameter as possible to reduce resistance and decrease velocity of flow of the liquid.
(v) After delivery, the drop of liquid that hangs at the tip of the tube may wet the narrow neck of containers such as ampoules, during the withdrawal of the delivery tube. Therefore, filling machines should have a retraction mechanism by which this drop can be drawn back into the lumen of the tube.
(vi) All parts of machine in contact with product should be non-reactive and demountable for cleaning and sterilization.

For small volume parenterals (SVPs), accuracy of filling is important, hence the filling machines should be designed for high delivery volume precision. Delivery of the liquid is by the stroke of a plunger in the syringe which can be repeated precisely. With every stroke of the syringe, the liquid is forced through a two-way valve, allowing alternate filling of syringe and delivery of mobile liquids. For heavy, viscous liquids, such as emulsions and suspensions, specially designed equipment using a sliding piston valve with stainless steel syringes are required. They can handle high pressures of filling to improve the flow rate.

Large volume injections which normally are solutions of low potency, do not require the accuracy of filling needed by SVPs. The bottles are filled by gravity, pressure or vacuum filling devices. The quantity delivered is measured in the container by the level of fill in the container. The force required to transfer the liquid is provided by gravity, pressure or vacuum.

The USP requires that each container be filled with a sufficient volume in excess of the labelled volume to ensure withdrawal of the labelled volume and provides a table of suggested fill volumes.

8.10.4.2 Filling of Solids

Sterile solids are more difficult to subdivide accurately and precisely into individual dose containers than liquids. The rate of flow of solids is slow and irregular although containers have larger openings. It is difficult to introduce the solid particles into the container, and there is always the risk of spillage. The accuracy of filling cannot be controlled well and therefore larger tolerances are permitted for the content in each container.

Some sterile solids can be subdivided by individual weighing using a scoop that holds a volume approximately equal to the weight required. But the quantity filled into the container is finally weighed on a balance. This is a slow process.

If the solids are granular in nature, they have better flow properties. Then machines can be used for filling such solids into the final containers. The use of such machines involves measurement and delivery of a volume of solid granular material, calibrated in terms of the weight desired as is the case with the Accofil machine. In this machine, there is an adjustable cavity in the rim of the filling wheel filled by vacuum as the wheel passes under the hopper as shown in Fig. 8.18. The contents are held by vacuum until the cavity is inverted over the container, then a jet of sterile air discharges the solids the contents into the container beneath.

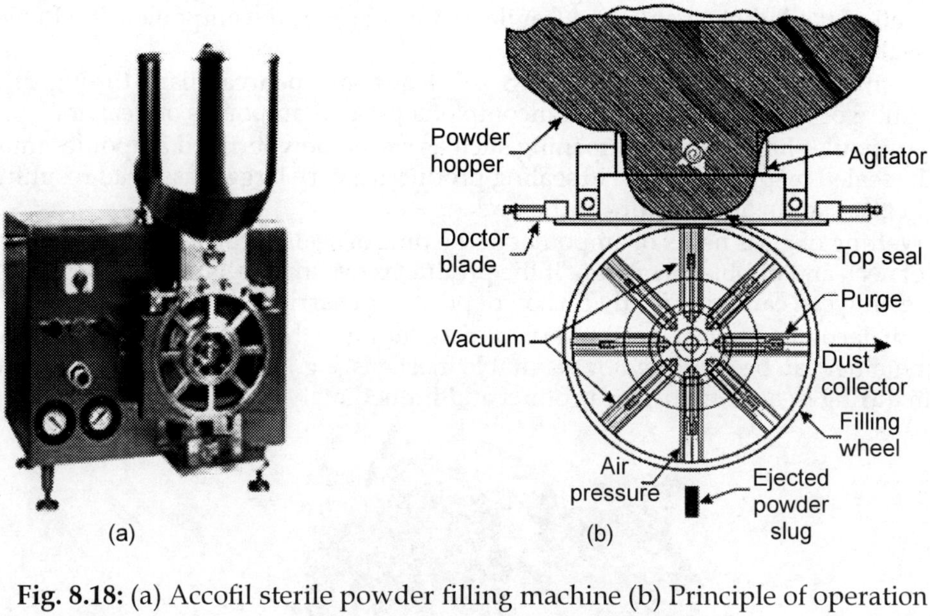

Fig. 8.18: (a) Accofil sterile powder filling machine (b) Principle of operation

8.10.5 Sealing

Filled containers should be sealed immediately after filling to prevent the contents from being contaminated by the environment. The sealing is carried out in the aseptic area usually by machines that carry out filling and sealing in the same equipment. Figure 8.19 is a photograph of an ampoule filling and sealing machine.

8.10.5.1 Ampoules

Ampoules are sealed by melting a portion of the glass neck to close the opening. Two types of seals are employed normally: tip seals (bead seals) or pull seals.

Tip sealing (Bead sealing)

Tip seals are made by melting enough glass at the tip of the neck of an ampoule to form a bead and close the opening. These can be made rapidly in a high-temperature gas-oxygen flame. To produce a uniform bead, the ampoule neck must be heated evenly on all sides, such as by burners on opposite sides of stationary ampoules or by rotating the ampoule in a single flame.

Pull Sealing

Pull seals are made by heating the neck of the ampoule below the tip, leaving enough of the tip for grasping with forceps or other mechanical devices. The ampoule is rotated in the flame from a single burner. When the glass has softened, the tip is grasped firmly and pulled quickly away from the body of the ampoule, which continues to rotate. The small capillary tube, thus, formed is twisted closed. Pull sealing is slower, but the seals are more secure than tip sealing.

Problems with ampoule sealing

(a) With tip sealing excessive heating results in 'bubble' formation. Expansion of gases within ampoule neck against soft bead seal causes bubble formation. The wall of the bubble is thin and fragile and if it bursts, the ampoule is no longer sealed.

(b) In tip sealing, insufficient heating will leave an open capillary through the centre of the bead, resulting in incompletely sealed ampoules or 'leakers'

(c) Ampoules having a wide opening such as sterile powderfilled ampoules must be sealed by pull sealing. Tip sealing produces a very large glass bead resulting in glass strain and fracture of the neck.

(d) Wetting of glass necks of ampoules at the time of sealing can also cause fracture of neck and bubble formation. If the product is organic, wet necks at the time of sealing can cause unsightly carbon deposits or charring.

To prevent decomposition of oxidizable products, the air in the space above the product in the container can be displaced by a suitable inert gas, e.g., nitrogen is introduced as a stream during or after filling the product and immediately sealed.

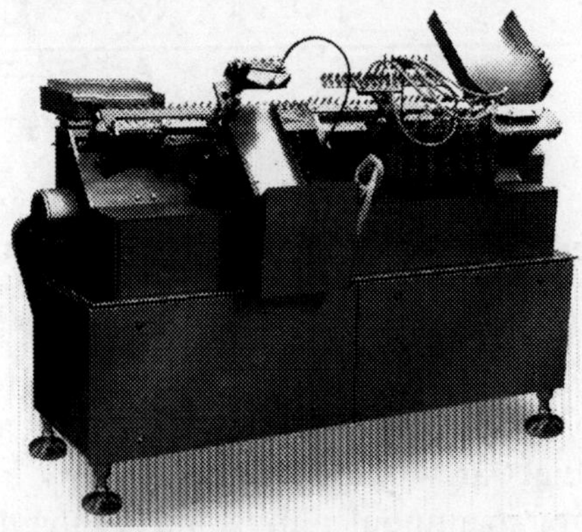

Fig. 8.19: Ampoule filling and sealing machine

8.10.5.2 Vials and Bottles

Vials and bottles are sealed by closing the openings with rubber closures. The closure must fit the mouth of the container snugly so that elasticity will produce a seal but at the same time it must not be difficult to introduce in the mouth.

With small lots of vials or bottles, manual stoppering can be done where the pre-sterilized stoppers are inserted into the mouths of the containers with sterile forceps.

With large lots, machines are used, which insert the closures mechanically, using an automated process, especially with high-speed processing. The closure surfaces are halogenated or treated with silicone to reduce friction as they slide from the vibrating drum to the bottom of the chute where it is positioned over the mouth of the container for insertion by a plunger.

Aluminium caps hold rubber closures in place and are crimped under the lip of the vial/bottle and serves as a tamper-proof feature. Thus, an intact cap is proof that the aluminium cap has not been removed intentionally or otherwise. Single, double and triple layered aluminium caps are available. The aluminium caps are designed so the outer layer of double layered caps, or the centre of single layered caps, can be removed to expose the centre of the rubber closure, without disturbing the band that holds the closure in the container. Triple layered caps are used for infusion bottles with rubber closures that have a permanent hole.

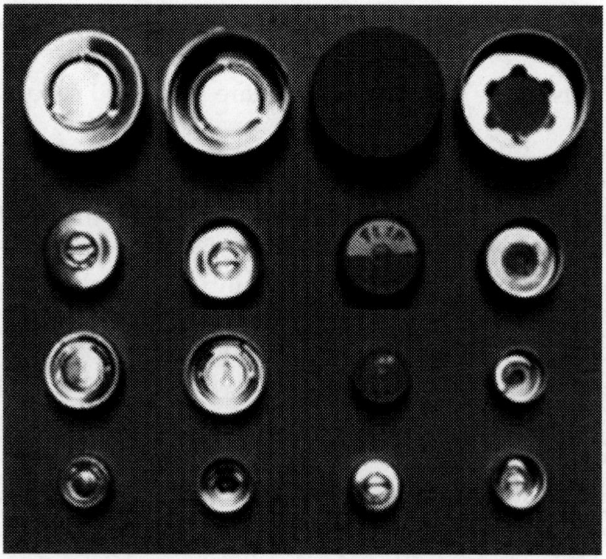

Fig. 8.20: Different types of aluminium caps to be used with rubber closures

8.10.6 Sterilization

Whenever possible, the product should be sterilized after being sealed in its final container (terminal sterilization) and quickly after filling and sealing are completed. Since this usually involves a thermal process, consideration should be given to the effect of elevated temperature upon the stability of the product.

Heat labile products must be sterilized by a non-thermal method such as filtration through a bacteria-retentive filter. When filtration is used for sterilization, all operations must be carried out under stringent aseptic conditions to prevent the contamination of the filtrate.

Colloids, suspensions, oily solutions and emulsion that are thermolabile require a process in which each component is sterilized separately and the product is formulated and processed under aseptic conditions. Such a process is referred to as aseptic manufacture.

Dry heat sterilization may be suitable for anhydrous or dry solids not adversely affected by high temperatures. Autoclaving can be used for the sterilization of aqueous liquids, and substances that are penetrated by steam. The effectiveness of any sterilization technique must be proved (validated), before it is employed in practice.

8.10.7 Quality Assurance and Control

Every component and step of the manufacturing process must be evaluated to be confident that quality is attained in the finished product. The responsibility for achieving this quality is divided appropriately in concept and practice into quality assurance (QA) and quality control (QC). QA relates to the studies made and the plans developed for ensuring quality of a product prospectively, with a final confirmation of achievement. QC is responsible for carrying out these plans during production and includes all the tests and evaluations performed to ensure quality of a specific batch of the product.

Quality control tests of the finished product are discussed separately in the next section.

8.10.8 Packaging and Labelling

Package is an important part of the product, since it presents the product to the user. The final packaged product must be dignified, neat and attractive in appearance to convey the impression of quality, purity and reliability. The packaging should provide ample protection against physical damage from shipping, handling and storage. It should also provide adequate protection from UV light if necessary. The package must also provide complete and accurate information with instructions necessary for the safe and proper use of the product. Such information should be placed clearly on the label or accompanying leaflets, inserts, etc.

The USP specifies the following requirements for the packaging and storage of injections:

1. Volume of injections in single-dose containers should not exceed 1 litre.
2. Parenterals for intra-cisternal, intraspinal and peridural administration should be packaged in single dose containers only (to prevent use of added solutes such as AMA to which nerves are sensitive).
3. Volume of injection in multiple dose containers should not exceed 30 mL (to prevent withdrawal of more doses which can increase the potential for contamination).

4. Injections packaged for use as irrigation solutions, haemofiltration, dialysis or for parenteral nutrition are exempt from the above requirements relating to packaging and may contain a volume in excess of 1 litre.
5. Injections intended for veterinary use are exempt from the limitation to single-dose containers and to the volume of multiple-dose containers.

8.10.8.1 Labelling Requirements

The labelling of an injection must provide the physician or other user with all information needed to ensure the safe and proper use of the product. Since all this information cannot be placed on the immediate container and be legible, it may be provided on accompanying printed matter.

The label on the immediate container should be so arranged, that sufficient area is uncovered to permit inspection of contents. The details required are:

1. Name of the preparation.
2. Composition, percentage content of active ingredient.
    - For single-dose injections of large volume (LVP), the strength is expressed as % w/v or gm/litre and for electrolytes as mmoles/litre.
    - For single-dose injections of small volume, the strength is expressed as the amount of drug in a nominal volume (e.g., 1mL) or the volume that the user expects to remove, e.g., mg/mL, μg/mL
    - For multiple dose injections, the strength is expressed as the amount of drug in a suitable dose volume, e.g., mg/2mL, if 2 mL is one dose.
3. Name of the vehicle, composition of non-aqueous vehicles. In case of sterile powders, the name and volume of the sterile solvent to be added to prepare injection or suspension.
4. Name and strength of any bactericide used.
5. Name and strength of any stabilizer, antioxidant used.
6. Intended route of administration
7. Storage conditions
8. Batch/lot number
9. Date of manufacture, expiry date, name and address of the manufacturer
10. Special instructions, e.g., for dilution, warnings, etc.

8.10.9 Quality Control

There are three general areas of quality control

1. Incoming stock (raw material control): Raw materials used in the formulation and packaging of parenteral dosage form are subjected to various tests such as routine tests on all ingredients and special evaluation tests such as pyrogen test on WFI, glass tests on containers, tests on rubber closures, etc. Tests on the microbial load to determine the number and types of microorganisms present in the environment are also included.
2. Process or manufacture control (in-process testing): Process control includes all the tests, observations and readings made throughout the manufacture of

the product.For example, conductivity measurement of WFI during distillation, confirmation of volume of fill, recording cycle time and temperature of autoclaving., etc.

3. Finished product testing: Evaluation of the finished parenteral product consists of a number of tests, the most important being:
   - (i) Leaker test (container/closure integrity test)
   - (ii) Particulate evaluation (clarity) test
   - (iii) Pyrogen test
     - (a) Rabbit test (in vivo)
     - (b) LAL test or bacterial endotoxin test (in vitro)
   - (iv) Sterility test
   - (v) Safety test

8.10.9.1 Leaker Test (Container/Closure Integrity Test)

Ampoules are intended to provide hermetically sealed containers for single doses of the product and thereby preventing any interchange between the contents and the environment. It is possible that in a batch, there may be incompletely sealed ampoules or leakers, due to capillary pores or tiny cracks around the seal or base of the container. The significance of the presence of leakers is:

- Microorganisms and contaminants may enter the container from the outside.
- Contents may leak to the outside and spoil the package and the label.
- Changes in temperature during storage may cause expansion or contraction of the ampule/content, worsening the leak if present.

Therefore, ampoules that have been sealed by fusion must be subjected to a test to determine whether or not a passageway remains to the outside.

Objective: To detect incompletely sealed ampoules (leakers) so that they may be discarded from a batch.

Method

The ampoules under test are immersed in a bath of dye solution (0.5-1% methylene blue) in a vacuum chamber and a vacuum (27 inches of Hg) is applied for 30 minutes. A negative pressure will be produced only within the incompletely sealed ampoules. The vacuum is released sharply, consequently the atmospheric pressure causes the dye to penetrate openings in the leakers. The ampoules are washed externally to remove any adhering dye and the contents are inspected. Ampoules with coloured contents are discarded.

Other Methods

Leaker testing is considered to be more effective when autoclaving ampoules in a bath of dye solution. The advantage is that both sterilization and leak detection can be accomplished in one operation. Alternatively, the ampoules can be removed from the autoclave while hot and quickly submerged in a bath of cold dye solution. The ampoules are further treated and inspected as explained earlier.

Vials and bottles are not subjected to the container/closure integrity test since the rubber closure is not rigid and the results would therefore, be meaningless. However, if the bottles were filled by vacuum filling, the presence of a vacuum can be detected by striking the base of the bottle/vial with the palm of the hand or with a rubber mallet, when a sharp 'click' sound heard or 'water hammer' sound is heard.

8.10.9.2 Particulate Evaluation (Clarity) Test

The presence of particulate matter in parenteral solutions is unacceptable for 2 reasons:

- Produces an impression of poor quality to the user. High degree of clarity (polish) is an important requisite for parenteral solutions.
- Harmful harticles can produce emboli in vital organs in man and animals. Presence of particulate matter in infusion fluids is also known to cause infusion phlebitis.

Objective: To detect and discard individual containers of product from a batch containing visible particulate matter.

Methods

1. ***Human visual inspection:*** The USP specifies that it is a good manufacturing practice that every product unit or container in a batch be subjected individually to visual inspection by human inspectors so that those containers with particles can be discarded. This 100% inspection of a batch prevents distribution and use of parenterals which contain particulate matter. For the inspection, all product units (externally clean) from a production line, are individually examined under a good light, baffled against reflection, viewed against black and white background with the contents set in motion by a swirling action and inverted as final step. The latter actions are necessary since moving particles are easier to detect than stationary.

   Advantage: This is the only test that can be done on 100% of the batch without destroying the integrity of the sealed product container and is suitable for in-line detection.

Limitations:

- The smallest particle size detected by the unaided human eye is 50 μ, therefore smaller particles may be undetected.
- Reduction in efficiency of the test due to eye strain, fatigue, distractions, emotional disturbances, etc.

2. ***USP tests for particulate matter in injections:*** The USP prescribes two tests for the detection of particulate matter in injections:
   (a) Light obscuration test
   (b) Microscopic count test

   Since the human inspection test cannot identify sub-visual particles, i.e., particles of size less than 50 μ, the USP identifies these additional tests for LVPs and SVPs. The tests used, however, are destructive of container units. Therefore, they are performed on appropriately selected samples of products. In addition, these methods require very stringent, ultraclean preparation techniques to ensure accuracy in the counting and sizing of particles only in the product, without interference from those particles that have been introduced accidentally during the sample preparation or the testing procedure.

The light obscuration test uses an electronic instrument designed to count and measure the size of particles by means of a shadow cast by the particle as it passes through a high-intensity light beam. If the injection formulation is not a clear, colourless solution (e.g., an emulsion) or it exceeds the limits specified for the light obscuration test, it is to be subjected to the microscopic count test.

In the microscopic count test, a measured sample of solution is filtered through a membrane filter under ultraclean conditions to retain particles. The particles on the surface of the filter are counted using oblique light under a microscope at both 40x and 100x magnification.

The USP limits for the microscopic test are as follows:

For LVPs: Not more than 50 particles/mL of size 10 μ and larger and not more than 5 particles/mL of size 25 μ and larger.

For SVPs: Not more than 10,000 particles/container of size 10 μ and larger and not more than 1000 particles/container of size 25 μ and larger.

8.10.9.3 Pyrogen Test

Pyrogens are considered impurities and should not be present in parenteral dosage forms. The test for the presence of pyrogens must be performed on all sterile vehicles intended to be used for injections and sterile products that do not interfere with the test. The Indian Pharmacopoeia (I.P.) prescribes two methods for evaluating the presence of pyrogens in parenteral preparations:

1. *In vivo* test in rabbits
2. Limulus Ameobocyte Lysate (LAL) test or bacterial endotoxin test (*In vitro* test)

1. *In Vivo* Test in rabbits

The pyrogen test in rabbits is a qualitative biological test based on the fever response in rabbits. Rabbits are used because they show a physiological response to pyrogens similar to humans.

Objective: To measure the rise in body temperature of rabbits following the IV injection of a sterile solution under test.

The test is used for products tolerated by test rabbits in doses not exceeding 10 mL/kg body weight when administered IV within the period not exceeding 10 minutes.

Method

Three healthy adult rabbits male/female of body weight not less than 1.5 kg, are fed on a complete and balanced diet. All glassware, syringes, needles, etc., to be used for the test must be washed with WFI and heated in a hot air oven at 250°C for 30 minutes or 200°C for 1 hour. The body temperature is measured by a rectal thermometer or thermocouple. Rabbits showing a body temperature higher than 39.8° C are not used.

Those rabbits with a temperature variation greater than 0.2°C between two successive readings for initial (normal) body temperature before product is administered are also not used.

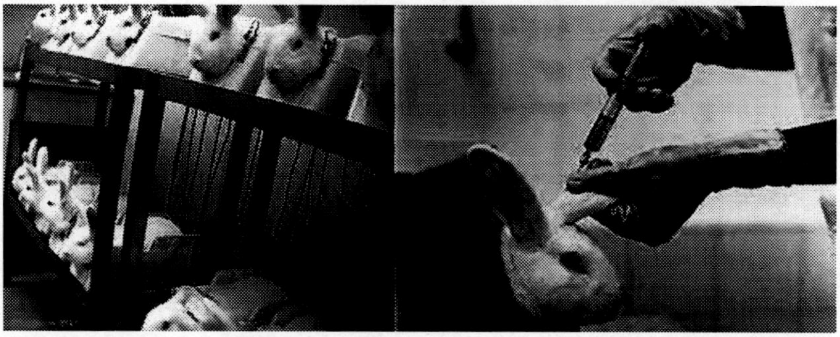

Fig. 8.21: Pyrogen test in rabbits

Preliminary test (Sham Test)

First, a preliminary test or sham test is conducted for rabbits used for the first time or not used during the previous 2 weeks (for conditioning them). Pyrogen-free isotonic saline (warmed to 38.5°C) is injected through the marginal ear vein of these rabbits. Animals showing a body temperature rise of more than 0.6°C are discarded.

Actual Test

The test preparation is dissolved or diluted in pyrogen-free saline and warmed to 38.5°C. Two normal readings, 90 minutes before injection are taken at half-hour intervals for each rabbit. The mean of these readings is taken as the initial temperature of the rabbit. The sterile test solution is injected slowly through the marginal ear vein in a dose volume of 0.5 - 10 mL/kg of body weight. The body temperature of each rabbit is recorded at intervals of 30 minutes for 3 hours after injection. The difference between the initial and maximum temperature is taken as the response.

Interpretation of results

The test sample passes if the sum of responses of the 3 rabbits does not exceed 1.4°C and if the response of an individual rabbit is less than 0.6°C.

If the response of any rabbit is 0.6°C or more or the sum of responses exceeds 1.4°C, then the test is continued with 5 other rabbits (5+3 = 8). The test sample passes the test, if the sum of responses of the 8 rabbits does not exceed 3.7°C and the individual response of not more than 3 rabbits is 0.6°C or more.

2. Limulus Ameobocyte Lysate (LAL) Test or Bacterial Endotoxin Test

The bacterial endotoxins test (BET) is an *in vitro* test based on the formation of a gel or the development of colour in the presence of bacterial endotoxins and the lysate of the amebocytes of the horseshoe crab (*Limulus polyphemus*). The Limulus Amebocyte Lysate (LAL) test is a biochemical test performed in a test tube and is simpler, more rapid, and of greater sensitivity than the rabbit test. This test however, detects only pyrogens of Gram-negative bacteria.

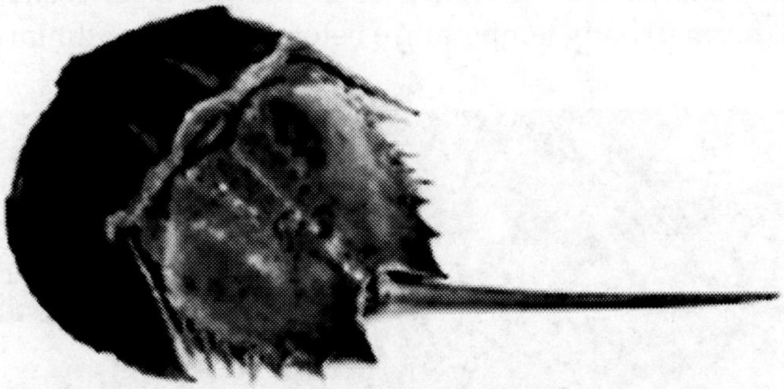

Fig. 8.22: The horseshoe crab, *Limulus polyphemus*

Principle: The addition of a solution containing endotoxins to a solution of lysate (derived from the amoebocytes of the horseshoe crab, *Limulus polyphemus*) produces turbidity, precipitation or gelation of the mixture. The rate of the reaction depends on the concentration of the endotoxin, pH and temperature of the mixture.

Method

Glassware and apparatus used for the test should be made free of pyrogens/endotoxins by the method specified under the *in vivo* test in rabbits. The sample under test is mixed with lysate of the amoebocytes and incubated at 37ºC for 60 minutes. A firm gel is formed if pyrogens are present.

Advantages over the rabbit test

- The LAL test is simpler and 5-10 times more sensitive than the rabbit test.
- Can be a semi-quantitative test by use of serial dilutions of the lysate.

For the standardization of the semi-quantitative test, a suitable reference standard is required against which all lots of lysate should be standardized. In the I.P., the Endotoxin Reference Standard is the freeze-dried purified endotoxin of *Escherichia coli* calibrated in endotoxin units by comparison with the international standards. The sensitivity of the lysate is expressed in terms of endotoxin units (EU), e.g., for WFI- not more than 0.25 EU/mL. The LAL test is also used in in-process testing.

8.10.9.4 Sterility Test

All products labelled, 'sterile' must be subjected to the sterility test. This test is carried out strictly under aseptic conditions of a Class 100 environment.

Principle: When microorganisms are placed in a media containing nutrients and water and under conditions required for growth, they will grow and their presence is detected in the form of turbidity in the media.

Objective: To detect the presence of all forms of viable microorganims in products meant to be sterile.

The test is done on sufficient number of samples of units or containers from a batch based on the assumption that the samples are representative of the batch/lot from which they are taken.

Methods as per the I.P.

1. Method A: Membrane filtration method
2. Method B: Direct inoculation method

1. Membrane Filtration Method

The membrane filtration method is preferred for an oil or oily preparation, liquid products of volume 100 mL or more or soluble powder or liquid with bacteriostatic and fungistatic properties.

Procedure

The test sample is filtered through a membrane filter of porosity of not more than 0.45µ and a diameter of 50 mm. The membrane is aseptically removed from the holder and cut into two halves. One half is transferred to 100 mL sterile fluid Thioglycollate medium (for anaerobic bacteria) and incubated at 30-35ºC for 7 days. The other half is transferred to 100 mL of sterile soyabean-casein digest medium (for fungi and aerobic bacteria). The media are incubated at 20-25ºC for 7 days. At the end of this period, the media are observed for turbidity or growth.

2. Direct Inoculation Method

Procedure

The test sample is drawn aseptically from the container (quantity used depends on the volume in the container) and inoculated or transferred to tubes of culture media (sterile fluid thioglycollate and soyabean casein broth). The contents are mixed and incubated for 14 days at 30-35ºC and 20-25ºC respectively. At the end of this period, the broth tubes are observed for growth or turbidity.

Observation and interpretation of results (applies for methods A and B)

- No growth or turbidity- Preparation passes.
- There is growth - Preparation fails, isolate and identify microorganisms microscopically.
- Do not repeat test unless it is clearly shown that the test was invalid due to reasons not related to preparation under test. The test is considered invalid only if microbial growth was found in the negative controls or testing procedure is faulty or contamination has taken place during testing. Also, if on identifying the microorganisms isolated from the preparation showing growth, it is clear that it is due to materials or faulty technique.
- If test is invalid, repeat test with same number of samples and media.
- After retest, if there is no growth - Preparation passes.
- Growth is present - Isolate and identify the microorganism. If they are similar to the first test, then preparation fails.

8.10.9.5 Safety Test for Freedom from Abnormal Toxicity

Most pharmaceutical preparations are now required to be tested for safety. Because it is entirely possible for a parenteral product to pass the routine sterility test, pyrogen test, and chemical analyses, and still cause unfavourable reactions when injected.

Therefore, a safety test in animals is essential, particularly for biological products, to provide additional assurance that the product does not have unexpected toxic properties.

The safety test prescribed in the I.P. is indicated for biological preparations. The animals used for the test are 5 healthy mice and 2 healthy guinea pigs.

General Test

Method

The test preperation is dissolved or diluted in 0.5 mL WFI or sterile normal saline. A dose of 0.5 mL is injected intravenously into mice. The test preparation passes if no death occurs in 24 hours or within the time specified in the monograph. If more than one animal dies, the preparation fails. If only one animal dies, the test is repeated. The sample passes if no animal in the second group dies within the time specified.

For vaccines and antisera

A dose of 1.0 mL is injected intra-peritoneally into each of the 5 mice and not more than 5 mL into each guinea pig intra-peritoneally. The preparation passes if no animal dies or shows signs of ill health in 7 days. The preparation fails, if more than one animal dies. If one animal dies or shows ill health, the test is repeated. If no animal in the second group dies or shows signs of ill health in the time interval specified, the preparation passes.

REVIEW QUESTIONS

Long Essays

1. Explain the formulation of parenterals.
2. Describe the facilities required for the manufacture of sterile dosage forms.
3. What is the significance of environmental control in the manufacture of sterile dosage forms? Explain the measures used to control the environment and the facilities required for the same.
4. Describe the steps involved in the manufacture of parenterals. Explain.
5. What are the packaging materials used for injections? Elaborate on various materials for containers, closures, their advantages, disadvantages and pharmacopoeial tests for their evaluation.
6. Discuss the various quality control tests for parenterals.

Short Essays

1. Define parenterals. Classify and list out advantages and disadvantages.
2. Briefly describe the various routes of injection. Which routes are most commonly used and why?
3. What are pyrogens? What is their significance in the use of parenterals? How can they be controlled during the formulation and manufacture of parenterals?
4. What is "water for injection"? Discuss its preparation, standards, storage and distribution.
5. Write a brief note on various types of WFI and their significance as vehicles in the preparation of injections.

6. Classify and describe various vehicles used in the manufacture of parenterals.
7. Explain the significance of the use of antimicrobials or preservatives in parenterals.
8. What are the various types of glass permitted for use in parenterals? Give the advantages, disadvantages, types of glass containers and pharmacopoeial standards.
9. Write briefly on the characteristics of plastic containers, advantages, disadvantages and types of containers used in parenterals.
10. Write a short note on rubber closures used in the packaging of parenterals.
11. Explain the design or layout of the manufacturing unit for parenterals.
12. What is the significance of air control on the quality, purity and safety of parenterals? Briefly explain the various measures that can be taken to control air quality.
13. Discuss the conduct and requirements for personnel working in a parenteral manufacturing unit.
14. List out and briefly explain various types of parenteral products with examples.
15. What is the significance of administration of paratonic injections? Which methods are used in the adjustment of injections to isotonicity?
16. How are sterile powders manufactured?
17. Briefly explain the formulation design and manufacture of sterile suspensions.
18. Define pyrogens and explain the pyrogen tests.
19. What are the objectives of the sterility test? Explain the procedures, standards and interpretation of results of the official sterility test for parenterals.
20. Explain the leaker test and particulate evaluation test for injections.

9

OPHTHALMIC DOSAGE FORMS

Learning Objectives

After going through this chapter, you would be able to:

1. Describe the structural features of the human eye.
2. Classify ophthalmic drug delivery systems.
3. Enumerate and explain characteristics of different ophthalmic dosage forms.
4. Explain the important requirements of ophthalmic dosage forms.
5. Describe the formulation and preparation of eye drops and eye ointments.
6. Explain the packaging and labelling requirements of ophthalmic preparations.

9.1 INTRODUCTION

Ophthalmic dosage forms are sterile topical preparations, free from foreign particles meant to be instilled onto the external surface or into the *cul-de-sac* of the eye for therapeutic or diagnostic purposes and include solutions, suspensions, ointments, gels and solid inserts.

They may also be administered inside the eye (intraocular) or adjacent to it or used in conjunction with an ophthalmic device such as solutions used in the maintenance of contact lenses.

Pharmaceutical preparations are applied topically to the eye to treat surface or intraocular conditions, including bacterial, fungal, and viral infections of the eye or eyelids; allergic or infectious conjunctivitis or inflammation; elevated intraocular pressure and glaucoma; and dry eye due to inadequate production of fluids bathing the eye.

Ophthalmic preparations are similar to parenteral dosage forms in their requirement for sterility as well as considerations for osmotic pressure (tonicity), preservation, tissue compatibility, the avoidance of pyrogens in intraocular dosage forms, particulate matter, and suitable packaging. However, it was not until 1953 that there was a legal requirement by the US Food and Drug Administration (FDA) that all manufactured ophthalmic solutions be sterile. This is because the ocular tissues are highly sensitive to contaminants and easily prone to infection that may be serious enough to cause loss of eyesight.

9.2 ANATOMY AND PHYSIOLOGY OF THE HUMAN EYE

The eyeball consists of a wall made of three concentric layers: the outer fibrous layer, middle vascular layer and the neural retina (Fig. 9.1).

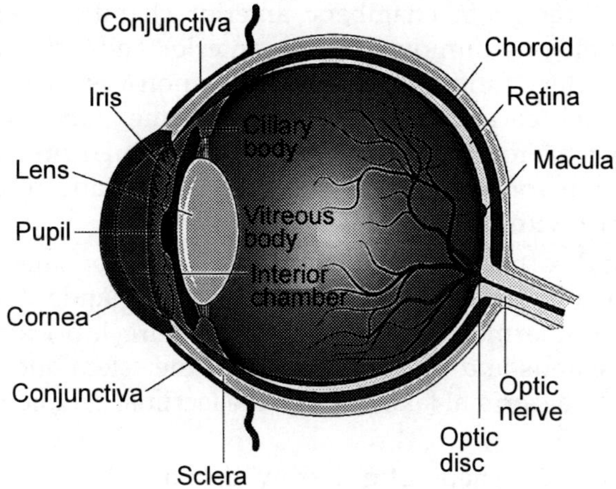

Fig. 9.1: A cross section of the eyeball showing the various structures inside

The outer fibrous layer is tough and pliable but only slightly elastic. It consists of the sclera and cornea, which are continuous with each other. Their main functions are to provide shape to the eye and support the deeper structures. The most anterior portion of this layer forms the cornea, which is transparent, free of blood vessels and positioned centrally at the front of the eye. Light entering the eye is refracted by the cornea.

Over the remaining two-thirds of the globe, the fibrous collagen-rich coat is opaque (the white of the eye) and is called the sclera. It contains the microcirculation, which nourishes the tissues of the anterior segment. The conjunctiva is a thin, transparent mucous membrane that covers the visible part of the sclera and extends to the inside of the eyelids.

The middle vascular layer, or uvea, provides nourishment to the eye and consists (from the back of the eye to the front) of the choroid, the ciliary body, and the iris.

The choroid consists of a pigmented vascular layer, coloured by melanocytes and traversed by blood vessels that nourish the neural retina. The ciliary body contains muscles that control the extension of the lens and the ciliary processes that secrete the aqueous humor into the posterior chamber to maintain the intraocular pressure (IOP) that, in turn, keeps the eyeball fully expanded. The pigmented iris is a ring of muscular tissue around the pupil, which is a round central hole or aperture to control pupil diameter.

The inner layer of the eye is the retina, which is a complex network of neurons that process light. The layer of the retina surrounding the vitreous cavity is the neural retina. The neural cells of the retina are arranged in several parallel layers and consist mostly of the photoreceptors (the rods and cones that are responsible or the conversion of light into an electrical signal through the presence of pigments.

The lens of the eye is located anteriorly, between the vitreous humour and the pupil. The shape of the lens is altered by the ciliary body, altering its refractive power.

The eye contains three main chambers: anterior chamber, posterior chamber and vitreous cavity. Aqueous humour fills the anterior and posterior chambers. It is a clear, colourless, watery fluid that nourishes the non-vascularized tissue of the anterior chamber, lens and corneal endothelium. It fills the globe anterior to the lens and is primarily responsible for maintaining correct intraocular pressure. The gel-like vitreous humour accounts for most of the weight of the eye and resides posterior to the lens, in direct contact with the retina.

The conjunctival and corneal surfaces are covered and lubricated by a precorneal tear film, a fluid secreted by the conjunctival and lacrimal glands. The inner surfaces of the eyelids and the outermost surfaces of the eye are lubricated by the tears, produced by lacrimal glands and specialized cells of the sclera and the conjunctiva. Tears are drained from the lacrimal lake through the lacrimal canaliculi into the upper nasolacrimal duct.

The antechamber has the shape of a narrow cleft directly over the front of the eyeball, with pocket-like extensions upward and downward. The pockets are called the superior and inferior fornices (vaults), and the entire space is known as the conjunctival 'cul-de-sac'.

9.3 SITE OF APPLICATION FOR TOPICAL OPHTHALMIC DOSAGE FORMS

Most topical formulations are applied or instilled into the conjunctival sac or *cul-de-sac* of the eye. The application of medication to the eye or conjunctival sac affects the surface of the eye and underlying tissues as the drug penetrates. The cornea is the main route through which ocular topically administered drugs reach the aqueous humour. The cornea functions as a bilayer barrier, with the hydrophobic epithelium as the primary barrier to hydrophilic molecules and the hydrophilic stroma as the primary barrier to hydrophobic molecules. Therefore, drugs should have the necessary hydrophilic-lipophilic balance for optimum permeation through the cornea.

For drugs that are poorly absorbed by the cornea, the conjunctiva and sclera provide an alternate route.

9.4 OPTIMUM VOLUMES OF ADMINISTRATION FOR TOPICAL PREPARATIONS

The normal volume of tear fluid in the *cul-de-sac* of the human eye is about 7 to 8 μL. The unblinking eye can accommodate a maximum of about 30 μL of fluid, but, when blinked, can retain only about 10 μL. Because the capacity of the eye to retain liquid and semisolid preparations is limited, topical applications are administered in small amounts, liquids dropwise, and ointments as a thin ribbon applied to the margin of the eyelid. Larger volumes of liquid preparations may be used to flush or bathe the eye. Excessive liquids, both normally produced and externally delivered, rapidly drain from the eye. A single drop of an ophthalmic solution or suspension measures about 50 μL (based on 20 drops/mL), so much of an administered drop may be lost. The optimal volume to administer, based on eye capacity, is 5 to 10 μL. The eye droppers commonly used are not calibrated in terms of microlitres. Hence, there is a loss of instilled medication using standard eye droppers, since the average dropper delivers about 25 to 50 μL/drop.

9.5 TYPES OF OPHTHALMIC DOSAGE FORMS

Based on their physical properties, topical ophthalmic dosage forms can be classified as:

1. Ophthalmic solutions
2. Ophthalmic suspensions
3. Ophthalmic emulsions
4. Ophthalmic ointments and gels
5. Ocular inserts

9.5.1 Ophthalmic Solutions

These are the most common dosage forms for delivering drugs to the eye. They are simple to manufacture and scale up. Ophthalmic solutions are also desirable where a rapid onset of action is required as the drug is already in the dissolved form. Since the ingredients are completely soluble, dose uniformity is not an issue, and there is little physical interference with vision. However, their main disadvantage is the relatively brief contact time of the drug with the absorbing corneal membrane. Contact time can be increased by the inclusion of viscosity imparting agents; provided that the resulting viscosity of the solution is low enough to allow dispensing of the eye drop from the container or eye dropper and on application, not cause excessive blurring of vision.

Aqueous soluble salt forms of the drug are used in formulation. The selection of the appropriate salt form of the drug depends on its solubility, therapeutic concentrations required, ocular toxicity, the effect of pH, tonicity, and buffer capacity, its compatibility with the total formulation, and the intensity of eye sting or burning sensations (i.e., discomfort reactions). The most common salt forms used are the hydrochloride, sulphate, nitrate, and phosphate. Salicylate, hydrobromide, and bitartrate salts are also used. For drugs that are acidic, such as the sulfonamides, sodium and diethanolamine salts are used.

Ophthalmic solutions are prepared sterile and may be buffered or pH adjusted with the addition of additives such as preservatives, antioxidants and tonicity contributors. They are used as eye drops, eye lotions or intra-ocular solutions.

9.5.2 Ophthalmic Gel Forming Solutions

These are solutions that are liquid in the container and thus can be instilled as eye drops but gel on contact with the tear fluid. Thus, they provide increased contact time with the possibility of improved ocular absorption and increased duration of therapeutic effect. The liquid-to-gel phase transition can be triggered by a change in temperature, pH, ionic strength, or presence of tear proteins, depending on the particular polymer system employed. For example, eye drops of timolol maleate, which is used to reduce elevated intraocular pressure (IOP) in the management of glaucoma. Thermally sensitive systems, which are transformed to a gel phase at body temperature and pH-sensitive systems are the most commonly investigated.

9.5.3 Ophthalmic Suspensions

Ophthalmic suspensions are dispersions of finely divided, relatively insoluble drug substances in an aqueous vehicle containing suitable suspending and dispersing agent. This approach has been used to administer drugs which are sparingly soluble in water, e.g., steroids, or to prolong drug release. The particles tend to be retained in the cul-de-sac, hence, the contact time and duration of action of a suspension could exceed that of a solution. The ophthalmic suspensions are prepared from steroid anti-inflammatory agents such as: prednisolone acetate, dexamethasone, fluorometholone, and rimexolone.

Characteristics to be kept in mind are particle size, storage stability, dosage uniformity, intrinsic solubility and dissolution rate.

Size of the dispersed particles can affect irritation potential, ocular contact time and stability of the suspension. To minimise irritation to the sensitive ocular tissues, 95% or more of the particles must have a diameter of 10 μm or less. This is to ensure that the particles do not cause irritation of the sensitive ocular tissues which can cause excessive tearing and rapid drainage and loss of the instilled dose.

The vehicle is considered to be a saturated solution of the drug substance. Only the dissolved drug is absorbed from the solution, and the solution concentration is replenished from retained particles. Dissolution of the particles will increase with smaller particle size while the retention of particles in the cul-de-sac is favoured by larger size. Hence, it is important that an optimum particle size is achieved during formulation of the suspension.

The particles of a suspension need to be readily dispersible on shaking by the patient to ensure uniform dose administration. Label should clearly indicate that the suspension should be shaken well before use. Fluctuations in storage temperature can give rise to polymorphic changes of the crystal structure of the drug. This can lead to changes in drug solubility and dissolution with increased or decreased bioavailability. Storage at freezing temperatures should be avoided and indicated accordingly in the label to prevent particle agglomeration.

9.5.4 Ophthalmic Emulsions

Poorly water-soluble drugs can be delivered in a solubilized form by formulating them as emulsions. The drug is dissolved in a nonaqueous vehicle, such as castor oil, and emulsified with water, using a non-ionic surfactant and an emulsion stabilizer. An emulsion with water as the external phase can be less irritating and better tolerated by the patient than use of a purely nonaqueous vehicle, e.g., Cyclosporine has been formulated as an emulsion for the topical treatment of chronic dry eye conditions. Ocular submicron emulsions with a droplet size of less than 0.1 μm have the ability of prolonging drug release and achieving significantly higher drug concentrations in the cornea and aqueous humour compared to suspensions.

Ophthalmic solutions may be dispensed as eye drops or eye lotions, whereas ophthalmic suspensions and emulsions as eye drops only. For the benefit of the reader, a brief discussion on eye drops and eye lotions is given in the following paragraphs.

Eye drops

Eye drops are sterile ophthalmic solutions, suspensions or emulsions instilled as drops, using a dropper into the conjunctival sac or cul-de-sac of the eye, to produce topical effects or affect the structures in the anterior segment of the eye such as the cornea, conjunctiva and anterior uvea. They may be used for therapeutic or diagnostic purposes and are sterile, isotonic, buffered with added viscosity enhancers, preservatives or antioxidants. They usually contain antibiotics, antibacterial/fungal, antiviral, corticosteroids, NSAIDS, cycloplegics, miotics, local anaesthetics, diagnostic stains, antihistamines, antiglaucoma drugs, etc. The two major physical forms of eye drops are aqueous solutions and suspensions. Nearly all the major ophthalmic therapeutic agents are water soluble or can be formulated as water-soluble salts.

To help improve the accuracy and consistency of dosage and to prevent contamination, it is important that certain precautions are followed. The hands of the user or patient must be clean and he must be instructed to not touch the dropper tip to the eye, surrounding tissue, or any surface, refrain from blinking; and to place the drop in the conjunctival sac, not on the globe; and to close the lids for several moments after instillation.

The disadvantage of eye drops is the difficulty in administering the exact volume or weight leading to inaccuracy of dosage. The volume of a drop depends on the physiochemical properties of the formulation, such as surface tension; the design and geometry of the dispensing office; and the angle at which the dispenser is held during instillation. One drop is approximately 30-50 µL and since the blinking eye can retain only 10 µL of the administered liquid, much of the administered volume is lost. Hence, the eye drops may require to be administered frequently (3-4 times a day) for adequate efficacy.

Eye lotions

Eye lotions are sterile, isotonic, pH adjusted or buffered aqueous solutions meant to irrigate the eye for the purpose of removing foreign particles, secretions, irritants, etc., from the surface of the eye. Eye lotions are simple solutions and are iso-osmotic with tears because they cause much greater dilution of the lachrymal fluid or tears and hence are more likely to cause discomfort if not adjusted. They are generally used in large volumes to bathe the eye. For example, sodium chloride eye lotion and sodium bicarbonate eye lotion are commonly used to remove foreign substance from the eye. Eye lotions may be packaged for single or for multiple use.

9.5.5 Ophthalmic Ointments and Gels

These are soft sterile semisolids in which drug/s may be solubilized, dispersed or emulsified in a suitable ointment or gel base generally meant for topical application in the eye. Compared with ophthalmic solutions, ophthalmic ointments and gels provide extended residence time on the surface of the eye, increasing the duration of their surface effects and bioavailability for absorption into the ocular tissues but with slower onset and time to peak absorption.

Ophthalmic ointments: Ointments formulated for ocular application are mostly anhydrous and contain mineral oil and white petrolatum as the base ingredients, the proportions of which can be varied to adjust consistency and the melting temperature. They are applied as narrow bands along the margin of eyelids. Ointments have the advantage of longer contact time and greater total drug bioavailability, but with slower onset and time to peak absorption. Although ointments provide prolonged effects of the drug, they can cause blurring of vision as the base melts on application and spreads across the lens, therefore their use is usually limited to bedtime instillation. The anhydrous nature of the base enables its use as a carrier for moisture-sensitive drugs. The petrolatum base can be made more miscible with aqueous components by the addition of lanolin or wool fat which acts as an absorption base. The ointment base selected for an ophthalmic ointment must not be irritating to the eye and must permit the diffusion of the medicinal substance throughout the secretions bathing the eye. Ointment bases used for ophthalmic use should have a softening point close to body temperature, both for comfort and for drug release. Usually, mixtures of white petrolatum and liquid petrolatum (mineral oil) are used as the base in medicated and unmedicated (lubricating) ointments.

Ophthalmic gels: These are aqueous transparent or translucent semisolids and are administered to the eye for soothing, lubricating or medicating purposes. They are more suitable for water-soluble drugs, e.g., Timolol maleate. They have the potential to prolong residence of the drug at the corneal surface. They are mainly applied as tear substitutes in the treatment of dry eye because they present numerous drawbacks, which limit their use for the administration of ophthalmic drugs. Gel eye drops do not allow accurate and reproducible drug administration and can produce crusting on the eyelids, and tearing. Although they contain a large proportion of water, they can still cause blurring of vision. Gel-forming polymers used are cellulose derivatives, such as carboxymethylcellulose, hydroxypropyl methylcellulose, carbomer (Carbopol), or hyaluronic acid. They are packaged and administered the same as ointments. Many of these polymers display bioadhesion, further improving the bioavailability of the active agent. The viscous gels have significantly increased topical residence time and can increase drug bioavailability and decrease dosage frequency, compared to solutions.

9.5.6 Ocular Inserts

Ocular inserts are sterile solid devices meant to be inserted into the cul-de-sac of the eye and have been designed to release the drug at a near-constant known rate by diffusion. They minimize side effects by avoiding excessive absorption peaks and provide prolonged drug effects thereby avoiding the need for frequent administration as is the case with eye drops. An example of an ocular insert is the Ocusert which is a non-erodible insert designed to be placed in the lower cul-de-sac to provide a weekly dose of pilocarpine, after which it needs to be removed and replaced by a new one. This device produces a zero-order release rate.

Ocular inserts that gradually erode in the tear fluid have also been developed and have the advantage of not requiring removal at the end of the therapeutic cycle, which would provide more precise unit dosing, e.g., Lacrisert

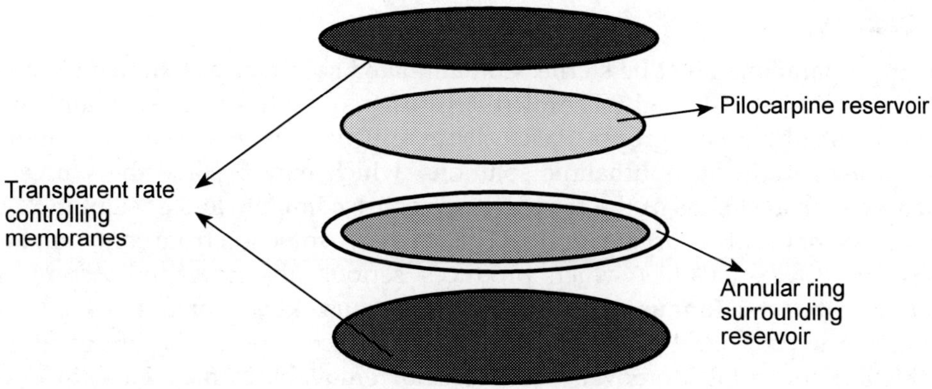

Fig. 9.2: Components of the Ocusert

9.5.7 Intraocular Dosage Forms

Intraocular dosage forms are specialized dosage forms introduced into the anterior chamber or vitreous chamber of the eye during ocular surgery. They are considered parenteral-type products requiring both sterility and non-pyrogenicity and their manufacture requires strict control of particulate matter. Therefore, they require additional pharmaceutical considerations in their formulation, packaging, and manufacture. In some cases, when used during eye surgery, sterility of the exterior of the primary package is required. They are also designed and packaged as preservative-free single-use products, since the commonly used preservatives in topical ophthalmic dosage forms can be toxic to sensitive intraocular tissues, such as the corneal endothelium. These formulations include irrigating solutions, intraocular injections, intravitreal injections/implants, juxta scleral injections, intracameral injections, iontophoresis, subconjunctival injections, retrobulbar injections, iontophoresis, packs, etc.

9.6 REQUIREMENTS OF OPHTHALMIC DOSAGE FORMS

Ophthalmic dosage forms should be designed and formulated with the following characteristics in mind:

1. Sterility
2. Use of antimicrobial agent
3. Clarity
4. Viscosity
5. Stability
   (a) pH and buffer
   (b) Antioxidants
   (c) Chelating agents
6. Tonicity
7. Particle size
8. Sterility

9.6.1 Sterility

All ocular preparations must be sterile. Contaminated solutions are known to cause corneal ulcers and loss of eyesight. The microbes most frequently found as contaminants are from the staphylococci group. *Pseudomonas aeruginosa* is less commonly found but also grows readily in ophthalmic solutions, which may become the source of extremely serious infections of the cornea. It can cause complete loss of sight in 24 to 48 hours. Some of the other organisms that can cause eye infection from contaminated solutions are *Bacillus subtilus* which produces serious abscesses and *Aspergillus fumigatus*, a pathogenic fungus and viruses that can cause keratoconjunctivitis. Virus contamination is particularly difficult to control, because none of the preservatives now available is virucidal. Moreover, viruses are not removable by filtration. However, they are destroyed by autoclaving.

Methods of Sterilization

The USP recognizes 6 methods of sterilization for ophthalmic preparations:

(a) Steam sterilization (autoclaving)
(b) Dry heat sterilization
(c)Gas sterilization
(d) Sterilization by ionizing radiation
(e) Sterilization by filtration

Thermal sterilization: As far as possible ophthalmic dosage forms should be sterilized in their final container. A thermal method would then be required such as steam sterilization or dry heat sterilization. In steam sterilization or autoclaving at 121°C (250°F) for 15 minutes, it is important that the drug solution or suspensions must be sufficiently heat resistant to survive the procedure. If sterilization is carried out in the final container, the container also must be able to withstand heat and pressure.

Dry heat sterilization would be preferred for non-aqueous solutions and suspensions that are stable at temperatures of 160°C, e.g., liquid paraffin eye drops

Most ophthalmic products, however, cannot be heat sterilized. In most cases, the drug is not stable to heat, either physically or chemically. High molecular weight polymers used to impart viscosity in aqueous products are also affected adversely by heat. For such preparations, a non-thermal method of sterilization such as filtration may be used.

Filtration: According to the USP, sterile membrane filtration under aseptic conditions is the preferred method of sterilization of ophthalmic solutions. In case of suspensions, the vehicle may be sterile filtered before dispersing the sterile solids. The advantage of membrane filtration is that the sterilization can be done at room temperature without adversely affecting the product. This method involves the transfer of the finished sterile product into previously sterilized containers, using aseptic techniques. The membrane filtration equipment itself is sterilized as an assembly by autoclaving.

Gaseous sterilization: This method is suitable for the sterilization of heat-sensitive materials by exposure to ethylene oxide (EtO) gas in the presence of moisture using gas autoclaves. EtO sterilization requires careful consideration of conditions required to effect sterility such as exposure time, EtO concentration, and moisture. EtO sterilization is suitable for some drug solids and the preferred method for plastic containers, caps and droppers.

Sterilization by ionizing radiation

This method may be used for the sterilization of the total product, such as certain ophthalmic ointments and oily suspensions formulated with heat labile drugs. Gamma sterilization is currently the method used in place of EtO for sterilizing most of the packaging components. Radioisotopes such as ^{60}Co (a source for gamma irradiation), are utilized in linear electron accelerators for sterilization. Sometimes, sterilization by radiation may produce untoward effects, such as chemical changes in product components as well as changes in colour or physical characteristics of package components.

9.6.2 Use of Preservatives or Antimicrobial Agents (AMA)

A sterile ophthalmic solution in a multiple-dose container, such as eye drops can be contaminated in a number of ways unless precautions are taken. Therefore, the pharmacopoeia specifies that one or more antimicrobial agents to prevent growth of, or destroy, microorganisms accidentally introduced during use must be added to ophthalmic preparations that are packaged in multiple dose containers, regardless of the method of sterilization employed, unless otherwise directed in the individual monograph, or unless the formula itself is bacteriostatic. Preservatives should not be used in intraocular solutions and single dose ophthalmic solutions or eye drops meant for eye surgery (packaged for single use).

Preservatives/AMA to be used in ophthalmic preparations should:

1. have broad spectrum of activity against Gram +ve, Gram –ve and rapid bactericidal activity against *pseudomonas aeruginosa*,
2. be stable over a wide range of conditions, autoclaving temperatures, pH range during storage,
3. be compatible with other components and package, and
4. be non-toxic, non-irritant.

Some of the commonly used AMAs are quarternary ammonium compounds such as Benzalkonium chloride (0.013%) and Benzethonium chloride (0.01%); Organic mercurials such as phenyl mercuric nitrate/acetate (0.002-0.004%) and Thiomerosal (0.01%); Parahydroxybenzoic acid esters such as methyl paraben (0.1-0.2%) and propyl paraben (0.04%) and substituted alcohols and phenols such as Chlorobutanol (0.5%) and Chlorhexidine acetate (0.01%).

Preservative mixtures of benzalkonium chloride (0.01%) and either polymyxin B sulphate (1,000 USP U/mL) or disodium ethylenediaminetetraacetate (0.01% to 0.1%) are effective against most strains of *Pseudomonas*. The latter agent, which is commonly employed as a chelating agent for metals, renders strains of *P. aeruginosa* more sensitive to benzalkonium chloride.

9.6.3 Clarity

Ophthalmic solutions are required to be free of undissolved ingredients and are essentially free from foreign particles. Clarity is an important requirement which reflects quality and purity and influences consumer acceptability. In addition, ocular solutions must be free from foreign particles to avoid irritation to the eye.

The clarity of solutions can be improved by filtration. The filtration equipment must not contribute to particulate contamination and must be clean and well rinsed before use. All filtration operations must be performed in clean surroundings with the use of laminar-flow hoods and controlled environment. The operators are required to wear proper non-shedding garments to prevent contribution of foreign particles in the final product. Filtration can be used to achieve both clarity and sterility depending on the choice of the pore size of the membrane filters used. Containers and closures must be clean, sterile and free of particulate matter.

9.6.4 Viscosity

Ophthalmic solution and suspension eye drops may contain viscosity imparting polymers to thicken the tear film and increase corneal contact time (i.e., reduce the rate of tear fluid drainage). The increase in viscosity of aqueous formulations improves therapeutic response due to better absorption and activity. For suspensions, the increased viscosity also retards the settling of particles between uses and at the same time maintains their suspension for uniform dosing.

Requirements of thickeners for aqueous solutions and suspensions are:

(a) Ease of filtration especially if the solution is to be sterilized by filtration.

(b) Should not deteriorate or be affected by heat at temperatures of thermal sterilization, e.g., precipitation of gums at autoclaving temperatures.

(c) Should produce solutions that have the requisite refractive index and clarity.

(d) Should be chemically stable and compatible with other components of the formulation.

(e) Should be resistant to microbial growth.

Thickeners, commonly used in aqueous ophthalmic solutions or suspensions, are given below:

Substituted cellulose ethers such as methyl cellulose, hydroxyethyl cellulose (HEC), hydroxypropyl cellulose (HPC), Carboxymethyl cellulose (CMC).

Methyl cellulose (4000 cps viscosity grade) was one of the first thickeners used usually in concentrations of 0.5 - 2%. Solutions of methyl cellulose are neutral, odourless, tasteless and stable in the pH range tolerated by the eye. Solutions of methyl cellulose do not support bacterial or fungal growth and are unaffected by light or aging.

Today, methyl cellulose is largely replaced by hypromellose or hydroxypropyl methyl cellulose which has better solubility and produces mucilages with better clarity and are unaffected by salts. Hypromellose of 4500 cps grade in a concentration of 0.3% w/v is used as Hypromellose Eye Drops BPC or artificial tears in reducing dryness of eyes in keratoconjunctivitis sicca.

Other thickeners

Polyvinyl alcohol (PVA) is used in a concentration of 1.4% w/v and is a good thickening and wetting agent. It provides better contact time than methyl cellulose even at low viscosity of its solutions. Also PEG, polyvinyl pyrrolidone (PVP) or dextran may be used.

Natural gums such as acacia, tragacanth and gelatin are never used because of their high refractive indices, chemical instability and susceptibility to microbial growth.

Thickeners are not included in intraocular solutions used in eye surgery.

9.6.5 Stability

The stability of ophthalmic products depends on the chemical nature of the drug, product pH, method of preparation, additives used and the type of packaging. Stability refers to the total product stability and not just the chemical stability of a single product component. The characteristics that determine stability are:

(a) pH of the solution or buffer used
(b) Antioxidants
(c)Chelating agents

(a) pH and buffer

The pH of an ophthalmic solution may be adjusted for 3 reasons, namely:

(i) To reduce eye discomfort
(ii) To maintain chemical stability
(iii) To improve therapeutic response

To reduce eye discomfort

Ideally, ophthalmic preparations should be formulated at a pH equivalent to the tear fluid value of 7.4. Instilled solutions outside this pH can cause pain and irritation which produce excessive tearing and the washout of the drug. Adjustment of instilled solutions to the lachrymal or tear pH is not practical, since most ophthalmic drugs are salts of weak bases and are most stable at acidic pH. However, most eye drop medicaments have low buffer capacity and their pH can be quickly adjusted by the tears. Tears have some buffer capacity and are able to adjust or neutralize pH of unbuffered instilled solution, provided that the quantity of the solution is not excessive and does not have a large buffer capacity and strong resistance to neutralization. Further the pH is from neutral, longer will be the adjustment and the faster the adjustment, lesser will be the ocular irritation or eye sting.

When concentrated solutions of very acid drugs, e.g., adrenaline bitartrate, pilocarpine hydrochloride are used, then buffers will be required. Buffers used should be of low capacity; since strongly buffered solutions can be very painful (e.g., phosphate buffer pH 5) as they resist buffering action of tears.

To maintain chemical stability

The majority of eye medicaments are salts of weak organic bases and strong acids and are most stable at low pH (3 - 5). For examle, pilocarpine and physostigmine are active and comfortable in the eye at pH 6.8, but at this pH the chemical stability is reduced to a few days or months or 1 year. On the other hand, at pH 5, the solutions are stable for several years. The attainment of optimum stability may impose several compromises on the formulator. The optimum pH for stability may be lower than that preferred for eye comfort. Therefore, the pH values of solutions should be adjusted to a range where acceptable shelf-life stability of at least 2 years can be achieved or buffered within the required range.

Ophthalmic solutions usually are lightly buffered. Buffers selected should have a capacity adequate to maintain pH within stability range for the duration of product shelf life but minimal enough not to interfere with tears buffer capacity for better eye comfort.

To improve therapeutic response

Absorption of drugs through the cornea is facilitated if most of the instilled drug is in unionized form, since the latter is more lipid soluble and readily diffuses through the corneal membrane. The majority of the ophthalmic drugs are strong acid-weak base salts and produces the unionized free base form at alkaline pH. Therefore, the therapeutic activity of these salts can be increased if their solutions are adjusted to neutral or alkaline pH, but this adjustment can greatly reduce their chemical stability and shelf life. However, due to buffer capacity of tears, any instilled acidic unbuffered solution can be quickly adjusted to near neutrality, making the free base available. Alternatively, buffers of low capacity can be used, for example:

pH adjusting agents: Sodium bicarbonate, boric acid

Vehicles of adjusted pH: Boric acid vehicle (pH 4.7), special boric acid vehicle

Buffered vehicle: Isotonic phosphate vehicle

Table 9.1: Buffers used in ophthalmic solutions

Buffer	Components	pH range
Borate buffer	Boric acid/borax	6.8 - 9.1
Phosphate buffer	Sodium acid phosphate	4.5 – 8.5
Citrate buffer	Citric acid/sodium citrate	2.5 – 6.5

(b) Antioxidants

Several drugs on exposure to air, oxidize with loss of potency, e.g., adrenaline, phenylephrine, physostigmine. Plastic packaging such as low density polyethylene (LDPE) permits oxygen permeation resulting in oxidative decomposition of certain drugs.

In such cases inclusion of an antioxidant is recommended for enhancing stability and prolonging the shelf life of the product, e.g., sodium metabisulphite (0.1 – 0.3%) for acidic preparations and sodium sulphite for alkaline preparations. Sodium thiosulphate (0.1 – 0.2%), ascorbic acid and acetyl cysteine are other examples of anti-oxidants that may be used.

In the case of eye drops of certain drugs such as adrenaline (epinephrine) and sulphacetamide, the air in bottle can be replaced by an inert gas such as nitrogen to improve stability. Development of an epinephrine solution with 2 to 3 years' stability in a plastic package requires the use of a pH of about 3.0 for protection from oxidation, whereas an epinephrine borate solution formulated at a pH of about 7.0, which is more comfortable to the patient, requires an antioxidant system and the use of glass packaging.

(c) Chelating agents

Chelating agents remove traces of heavy metals by complexation that otherwise catalyse breakdown of some drugs. For example., Disodium edetate (0.01 - 0.3%) is soluble in water, stable to autoclaving, compatible with common eye medicaments and enhances the antibacterial activity of some bactericides such as benzalkonium chloride. It is often used together with antioxidants.

9.6.6 Tonicity

Tonicity refers to osmotic pressure exerted by salts in aqueous solution. An ophthalmic solution is considered isotonic when its tonicity is same as that of 0.9% sodium chloride solution. Earlier, the common practice was to adjust tonicity of eye drops for the sake of eye comfort, today more importance is given to sterility, stability and the need for AMAs.

The eye can tolerate solutions having isotonicity range equivalent to that of 0.6 - 2.0% sodium chloride solutions, and a range of 0.5 - 1.5% is acceptable in most persons.

Eye tolerates hypertonic solutions better than hypotonic solutions. Very hypotonic solutions cause temporary oedema of cornea with impaired vision and highly hypertonic solutions cause discomfort. Hypotonic solutions can be adjusted to isotonicity with tonicity contributors such as sodium chloride, potassium chloride, dextrose, glycerin, and propylene glycol. Buffer salts added to maintain desired pH also contribute to tonicity.

Isotonicity is a must for intraocular solutions and eye lotions. Ophthalmic solutions can be adjusted to isotonicity by using one of the three methods such as freezing point depression, determination of sodium chloride equivalents and on the basis of molecular concentrations.

9.6.7 Particle Size

Particle size of dispersed drug solids in suspensions and ointments is an important characteristic to be considered that can influence eye comfort and the retention ability of the drug in the cul-de-sac of the eye. Particle size can also affect stability of the product and uniformity of dosage.

In suspensions, microfine particles are required, and 95% or more particles should have a size less than 10 μ.

9.6.8 Use of Surfactants

The use of surfactants is restricted in ophthalmic solutions. Topical eye products sometimes incorporate surfactants to disperse insoluble ingredients or to aid in solubilization. Formulators use them in the smallest concentration possible to achieve the desired function, because they can be irritating to sensitive ocular tissues. Nonionic surfactants are preferable, because they are less irritating than ionic surfactants, e.g., polysorbate 80, tyloxapol and polyoxyl 40 stearate. Formulators often add surfactants to stabilize hydrophobic drugs. They are also used in suspensions such as of steroids as wetting and dispersing agents. Non-ionic surfactants may be used as cosolvents/ solubilizers, e.g., to solubilize chloramphenicol to prepare 0.5% W/V solution.

9.7 FORMULATION AND PREPARATION OF EYE DROPS

9.7.1 Formulation

Vehicles

Vehicles used in the formulation of eye drops may be aqueous or oily. Most eye drop formulations are aqueous fluids using purified water USP as the solvent. Water for injection is not required as it is in parenterals. Purified water meeting USP standards may be obtained by distillation, deionization, or reverse osmosis.

The formulation of intraocular preparations requires the use of water for injection (WFI), sterile water injection, or bacteriostatic water for injection as a pharmaceutical aid or vehicle.

Oils have been used as vehicles for several topical eye drop products that are extremely sensitive to moisture. Tetracycline HCl is an antibiotic that is stable for only a few days in aqueous solution. It is supplied as a 1% sterile suspension with Plastibase 50 W and light liquid petrolatum. Vegetable oils must be used carefully, since rancidity can be a problem, e.g., parenteral grades of olive oil, castor oil, sesame oil.

Additives

The adjuvants or additives used in eye drops should have the following requirements:

1. Physically, chemically and therapeutically compatible with active ingredients and other adjuvants.
2. Compatible with the container.
3. Unaffected by method of sterilization used.
4. Non-toxic and non-irritant to the tissues.
5. Effective over the shelf life of the product in the concentrations used.

The additives used in eye drops are as follows:

- Antimicrobial agents
- Tonicity modifiers
- Viscosity modifiers
- pH adjusting agents and buffers
- Stabilizers - antioxidants
- Chelating agents
- Wetting agents

A detailed description of these additives has been given earlier 'in Section 9.6'.

9.7.2 Manufacture of Ophthalmic Solutions and Suspensions (Eye Drops, Eye Lotions and Intaocular Solutions)

Due to sterile nature of ophthalmic dosage forms, facilities for manufacture, measures for environment control similar to that of parenterals. Strict adherence to aseptic technique and proper sterilization procedures are crucial in the preparation of ophthalmic products.

Laminar air flow (LAF) with Class 100 environment is required in aseptic manufacture or filling areas. Only personnel who are properly gowned with sterile, non-shedding garments, trained and proficient in the techniques and procedures for aseptic manufacturing should prepare ophthalmic products.

Quality-assurance principles for compounding sterile products should be followed, and methods should be established to validate all procedures and processes related to sterile product preparation.

Production under clean conditions followed by sterilization by autoclaving

The active ingredient and all or a portion of the excipients is dissolved into all or a portion of the water and the sterilization of this solution by using moist-heat sterilization (assuming the drug is chemically stabile under these conditions). This sterile solution is then mixed with the other sterile components, such as previously sterilized solutions of viscosity imparting agents, preservatives, and so on, and the batch is brought to final volume with additional sterile water.

Production under clean or aseptic conditions followed by aseptic sterilization by filtration

If the drug is thermolabile, thermal sterilization should be avoided. The production of ocular solutions is then performed by initially manufacturing the dosage form under clean or aseptic conditions. Clarification of the solution is performed by filtration through sintered glass filters or membrane filters (pore size: 0.45 – 1.2 μm). The filtrate is collected in a closed vessel protected from contamination. The solution is further subjected to sterilization by membrane filtration (0.22 μ filter) and packaging under strict aseptic conditions (Class 100 environment).

Production under aseptic conditions (aseptic manufacture)

Ophthalmic suspensions cannot be sterilized by filtration and those containing thermolabile drugs cannot be sterilized by thermal methods. In such situations, the ophthalmic suspensions may be prepared by aseptic manufacture which usually involves the dispersion of the sterile therapeutic agent into the sterile vehicle (with added excipients) and subsequent packaging, both under aseptic conditions. The solids to be suspended are previously sterilized by heat, by exposure to ethylene oxide or ionizing radiation (gamma or electrons), or by dissolution in an appropriate solvent, sterile filtration, and aseptic crystallization. The sterile solid is then added to the sterile vehicle, either directly or by first dispersing the solid in a small portion of the batch. After adequate dispersion, the batch is brought to final volume with sterile water. The control of particle size of the final suspended material is very important, not only for comfort of the product but also for improving physical stability and re-suspendability of the suspension throughout the shelf life and usage by patients.

9.8 FORMULATION AND PREPARATION OF EYE OINTMENTS

9.8.1 Formulation

Ointment bases: Ointment base used must be non-irritating to the eye and permit diffusion of drug throughout secretions bathing the eye. The selected base must have melting point close to body temperature, to ensure adequate release of the drug.

The various types of ointment bases that can be used in ocular administration are as follows.

Hydrocarbon bases: Hydrocarbon bases are widely used in ophthalmic ointments and are composed of a mixture of paraffins (to achieve the correct viscosity) such as liquid and soft paraffins. In the formulation of these systems, yellow soft paraffin is preferred to white soft paraffin. White soft paraffin is a bleached form of yellow soft paraffin, therefore traces of bleaching agent in the former can be a source of ocular irritancy.

Non-emulsified absorption bases: These bases are composed of one or more paraffins (e.g., liquid and yellow soft paraffin) and a sterol containing emulsifying agent (e.g., lanolin derivatives). An example of such a composition is of liquid paraffin, wool fat and yellow soft paraffin in the ratio of 1:1:8 (Simple Eye Ointment B.P.) These bases are less greasy than those prepared using hydrocarbons alone and in addition, aqueous solutions of drug may be incorporated into non-emulsified absorption bases. In tropical/subtropical climates, varying proportions of hard paraffin are included to raise the melting point of the base. Aliphatic alcohols, e.g., cetyl and stearyl alcohols or fats/waxes such as cholesterol, beeswax may be included to facilitate incorporation of water.

Water-soluble bases/aqueous gels: Water-soluble bases are associated with a lower incidence of blurred vision due to their watermiscibility. These bases are primarily formulated using polyethylene glycols.

In ophthalmic gels, gelling agents such as poly(acrylic acid) or carbomers are commonly used. Drug-free poly(acrylic acid) gels have also been used for the treatment of keratoconjunctivitis sicca (dry-eye syndrome).

Adjuvants: The type of excipients used in ophthalmic ointments depends on the nature of the ointment base used in the formulation. Hydrocarbon based ointment bases that are either devoid of or contain lower concentrations of water require no further excipients.

Eye ointments are less likely to be contaminated than eye drops but still require AMAs as a precautionary measure since they are for multiple use. Examples of preservatives used in eye ointments are chlorobutanol, methyl and propyl parabens, phenethyl alcohol.

The inclusion of non-aqueous antioxidants, e.g., butylated hydroxytoluene, butylated hydroxyanisole, may be required if the therapeutic agent is prone to degradation by oxidation. When aqueous liquids are be incorporated in the ointment, and if its pH is outside the limits tolerated by the eye, then buffers or pH adjusting agents may be included, e.g. pH of aqueous phase of sulphacetamide eye ointment BP is very alkaline.

Water based semisolids such as poly(acrylic acid) gels which may contain 95% w/w water), require the same types of excipients that are commonly used in aqueous solutions, e.g., preservatives, buffers and water-soluble antioxidants.

9.8.2 Manufacture of Ophthalmic Ointments

Ointments can be more difficult to manufacture in sterile form than eye drops. Due to their high viscosity, terminal sterilization of ointments is difficult and can be done only at elevated temperatures. Therefore, ointments are typically manufactured from sterile components and packaged in an aseptic environment. This is known as aseptic manufacture.

Vehicles, drugs, additives and packaging components must be made separately sterile before compounding. The ointment base is sterilized by heat and filtered while molten to remove foreign particulate matter. It is then placed into a sterile steam jacketed kettle to maintain the ointment in a molten state under aseptic conditions, and the previously sterilized active ingredient(s) and excipients are added aseptically. If an aqueous fluid is to be incorporated, such as a drug solution, then it can be sterilized by heat, filtration, or ionizing radiation before addition. While hot, the contents in the kettle may be agitated until homogeneous and the entire ointment may be passed through a previously sterilized colloid mill for adequate dispersion of the insoluble components. Filling of the sterile ointment is performed under aseptic conditions into previously sterilized containers. Packaging components may be sterilized by thermal methods, ethylene oxide gas, and ^{60}Co (gamma) irradiation.

Most ophthalmic pharmaceutical products are aseptically manufactured and filled into previously sterilized containers in aseptic environments using aseptic filling and capping techniques. This is the case for ophthalmic solutions, suspensions, and ointments, and specialized technology is involved in their manufacture.

9.9 PACKAGING AND LABELLING OF OPHTHALMIC DOSAGE FORMS

Ophthalmic products should be packaged such that they are easily administered and their sterility maintained. When selecting the packaging material, it must be determined that the container:

(a) Does not adversely affect chemical stability of drug and adjuvants
(b) Extracts nothing from contents
(c) Yields nothing to contents
(d) Provides protection from light if necessary
(e) Is able to withstand sterilization by heating if necessary (autoclaving or heating with bactericide)

(f) Should preserve sterility of contents

(g) Should be convenient to use (patient friendly)

The type of container selected would depend on the product and mode of administration.

Packaging by Blow-fill-seal (BFS) technology

Also known as form/fill/seal method. BFS technology is widely used in the manufacture of preservative-free ophthalmic products, especially for artificial tear products. It is considered to be the superior form of aseptic processing by various medicine regulatory agencies including the U.S. Food and Drug Administration (FDA). In this process, the container is blow-moulded, filled and sealed in one continuous operation by the same equipment under sterile conditions without operator intervention. The first step is to extrude polyethelene resin at high temperature and pressure and to form the container by blowing the resin into a mould with compressed air. Then the product is filled, as air is vented out, and finally the container is sealed on the top. This process provides a high level of quality assurance. The steps involved in the formation of the container followed by filling and sealing is displayed in Fig. 9.3. BFS technology is most suitable for the packaging of aqueous solutions that contain heat labile components and cannot be subjected to terminal sterilization.

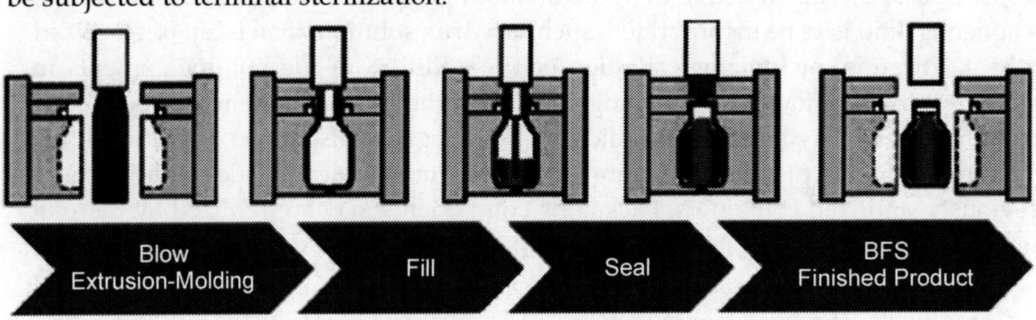

Fig. 9.3: Packaging of eye drops by BFS technology

9.9.1 Containers for Eye Drops

Eye drops may be packaged in single or multiple dose containers of glass or plastic.

Single-dose Containers

Eye drops that are devoid of preservatives or AMAs may be packaged in single-use containers. Such preparations are preferred by consumers who may be sensitive to the AMA or preservative used. The single-dose containers ensure that the eye drops don't get contaminated with pathogens between uses.

Single-use dropper ampoules

The BFS technology is especially suited for the packaging of single-dose eye drops that will be preservative free. Single doses will be packaged in a block of five or ten ampoules and are made from low density polyethylene (LDPE). Filling volumes may be up to 0.5 mL.

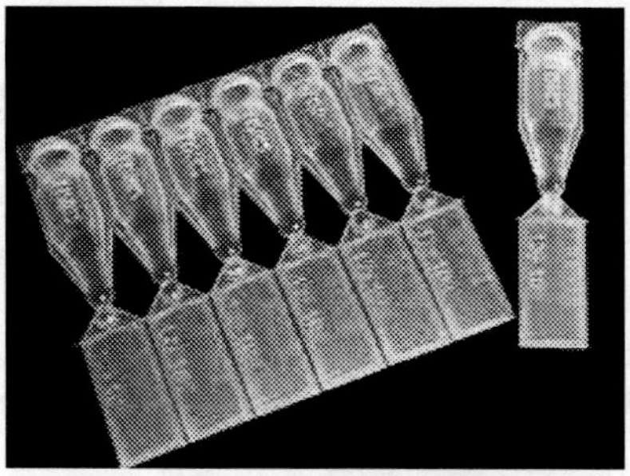

Fig. 9.4: Single-use dropper ampoules fabricated by BFS technology

Minims unit

An older form of the single-dose container is the Minims unit. It is still manufactured today and is available in select countries.

It consists of disposable, pliable tube-like applicator made from polypropylene by ultrasonic sealing and has a nozzle protected by a cap. Until used it is enclosed in a heat-sealed envelope, fronted by transparent polypropylene sheet and backed with paper that can be peeled off to remove the tube. The entire pack can be sterilized by autoclaving. The tube may be marked with a code that indicates nature and concentration of the drug.

For use, the backing paper is peeled off, the applicator removed, the cap is twisted off and the tube is gently squeezed to expel the drops into the eye.

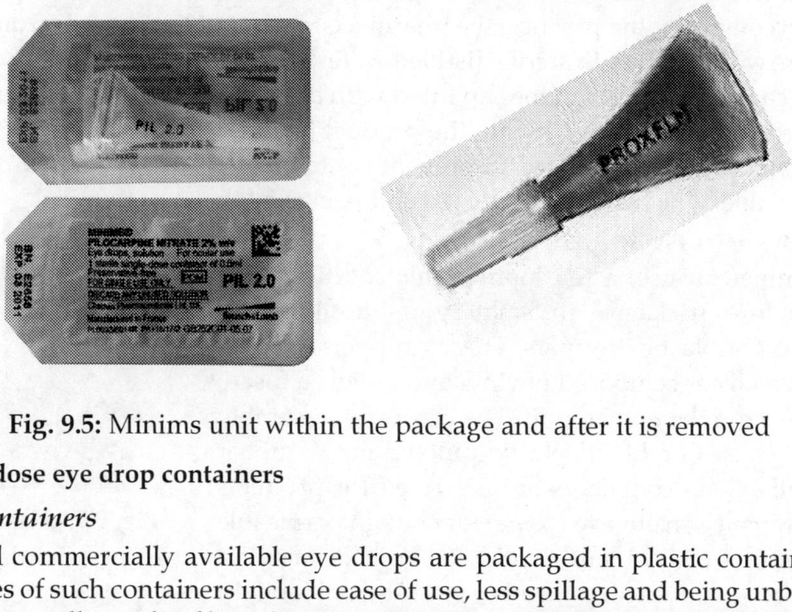

Fig. 9.5: Minims unit within the package and after it is removed

Multiple-dose eye drop containers

Plastic containers

Almost all commercially available eye drops are packaged in plastic containers. The advantages of such containers include ease of use, less spillage and being unbreakable. They are generally made of low-density polyethylene (LDPE) resin, either without any colourants or with opacifying agents or other colorants for light protection. When held in the inverted position at the time of administration, the LDPE gives the necessary flexibility for squeezing the walls of the bottle to expel the drops. These bottles have an inbuilt dropper tip or plug type dropper tip, also made of LDPE and protected by an outer polystyrene or polypropylene outer screw cap. The LDPE resins used are compatible with a wide range of drugs and formulation components. However, they have the disadvantage of allowing sorption and permeation of the actives or excipients from the contents of the container. Volatile ingredients such as the preservatives chlorobutanol and phenylethyl alcohol can migrate into the plastic and permeate through the walls of the container.

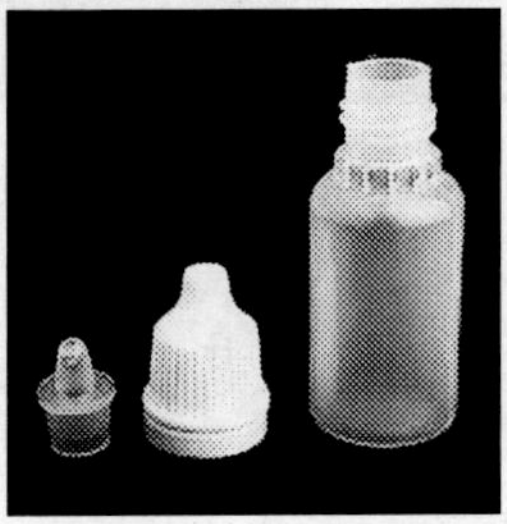

Fig. 9.6: LDPE eye dropper bottle with plug type dropper tip and polypropylene cap

BFS technology is also used in the packaging of eye drops for multiple use with filling volumes ranging from 5-10 mL. These bottles have dropper tips that are specially designed to prevent bacterial entry into the ophthalmic solution.

Glass containers

Glass containers are usually used in the extemporaneous preparation of ophthalmic solutions. In compounding practice, the pharmacist uses containers made from Type 1 glass that are well rinsed with sterile distilled water, and sterilized by autoclaving. The glass bottle carries a dropper in the cap fitted with a teat. The pharmacist should place the dropper assembly aseptically into the product before dispensing and instruct the patient on precautions to be used to prevent contamination. Pre-sterilized droppers are also available, which are pre-sterilized and packaged in a convenient blister pack.

For commercial use, a few ophthalmic solutions and suspensions are packaged in small glass bottles with separate glass or plastic droppers. These droppers are gas-sterilized in a blister composed of vinyl and Tyvek, a fused, porous polypropylene material. The dropper assembly is made of a glass or LDPE plastic pipette and a rubber dropper bulb. Glass containers are preferred for products that are extremely sensitive to oxygen or contain permeable components that are not sufficiently stable in plastic. For drugs that are sensitive to light, amber glass is used for light resistance and is superior to green glass.

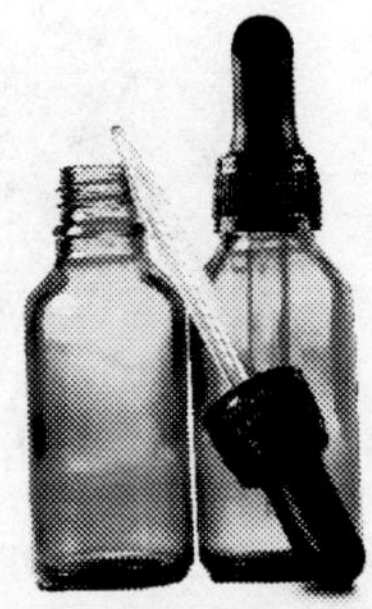

Fig. 9.7: Glass eye dropper bottle with dropper in the screw cap

Powders for reconstitution also use Type 1 glass containers, owing to their heat transfer characteristics, which are necessary during the freeze-drying process. The glass container is made sterile by dry heat or steam autoclave sterilization.

9.9.2 Containers for Eye Lotions and Intraocular Solutions

Ophthalmic solutions used as eyewashes or eye lotions are usually packaged in glass bottles with screw caps containing rubber, plastic or other impervious liner. These bottles may be supplied with an eye cup, which should be cleaned and dried thoroughly before and after each use.

Intraocular solutions of 250 and 500 mL have been packaged in glass, sealed with rubber closures and aluminium caps. Even these parenteral-type products are now packaged in specially fabricated polyethylene/polypropylene containers or flexible bags. Type 1 glass vials with appropriate stoppers are used for intraocular ophthalmic products administered by injection. These packaging components should meet the same requirements as parenteral products.

9.9.3 Containers for Eye Ointments/Gels

Single application containers

For preservative-free single use, ophthalmic ointments of certain drugs such as antibiotics may be packaged in soft gelatin capsules. They help to prevent contamination during use, e.g., Chloramphenicol eye ointment (Chloromycetin Applicap 50's by Pfizer).

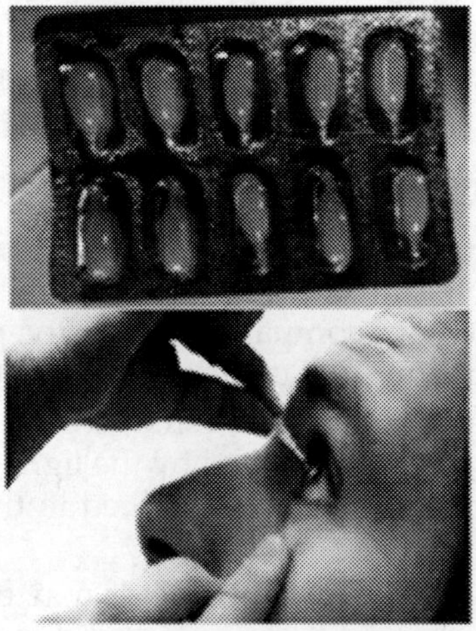

Fig. 9.8: Ophthalmic ointment in soft gelatin capsules (applicaps)

Multiple application containers

Ophthalmic ointments are packaged in small collapsible tin tubes, usually holding 3.5 g to a maximum of 5 g of the product with plastic screw caps of polyethylene or polypropylene. Metallic tubes made of aluminium or tin alloy may also be used and have an inner lining of epoxy or vinyl plastic to prevent any possibility of product incompatibility. These tubes have narrow nozzle tips which help to expel narrow bands of ointment for applying along the margin of the eyelid. Plastic tubes made from flexible LDPE resins have also been considered an alternative material, but they do not collapse and tend to suck back the ointment.

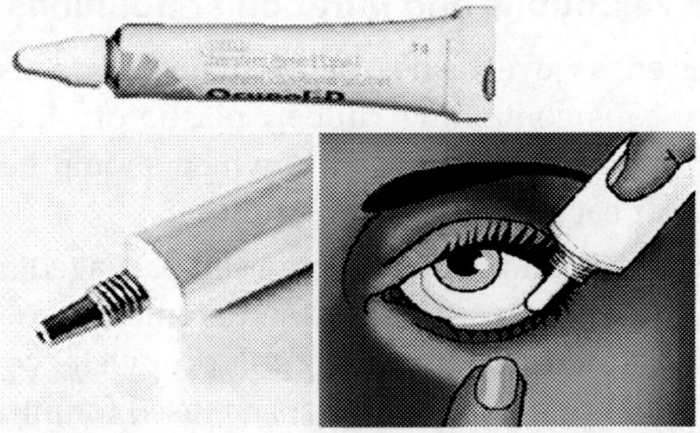

Fig. 9.9: Eye ointment tube showing narrow nozzle and application to the eye

9.9.4 Tamper Proof Feature

Irrespective of the type of packaging used for ophthalmic products, some form of tamper-proof feature should be included for consumer protection. The common tamper-evident feature used on most ophthalmic preparations is the moisture- or heat-sensitive shrink band. In case of ophthalmic solutions and suspensions, a cellulosic or metal band around the cap and bottleneck is provided by the manufacturer, and the container should not be dispensed if these are missing or there is evidence of prior removal and reapplication.

For ointments, it is the sealing of the tube or the carton holding the tube such that the contents cannot be used without providing visible evidence of destruction of the seal.

9.10 QUALITY CONTROL

The finished ophthalmic product may be subjected to a series of tests to evaluate its quality, safety and efficacy. Depending on the type of product, the parameters evaluated may be pH, isotonicity, viscosity, eye compatibility, clarity, particulate matter, particle size, uniformity of volume, uniformity of content, uniformity of weight and sterility.

Particulate matter: Apart from visual inspection, the presence of foreign particulate matter in ophthalmic solutions may be detected by the light obscuration particle count test or the microscopic particle count test as described in the USP. The product must comply with the standards prescribed for each test.

Particle size: Ophthalmic suspensions and semisolids may be subjected to particle size evaluation. A suitable volume of eye drops or semisolid is placed into a counting cell or onto a microscope slide and scanned under a microscope, an area corresponding to 10 μg of the solid phase. At least 50 representative fields are scanned.

Leakage test: This test is recommended for ophthalmic semisolids packaged in tubes. Select 10 tubes of ointments, with seals when specified. Thoroughly clean and dry the exterior surfaces of each tube with an absorbent cloth. Place the tubes in a horizontal position on a sheet of absorbent blotting paper in an oven maintained at a temperature of 60 ± 30° C for 8 hours. To comply with the pharmacopoeia standards, no significant leakage must occur during or at completion of the test.

Uniformity of volume: As per the IP, this test is appropriate for eye drops. For this test the contents of each container are poured completely into calibrated volume measures of the appropriate size. The volume of the contents of 10 containers are measured.

Uniformity of content: As stated by the BP this test is appropriate for powders for eye drops and eye lotions. Unless otherwise prescribed or justified and authorized, single-dose powders for eye drops and eye lotions with a content of active substance less than 2 mg or less than 2 per cent of the total mass must comply with the test. If the preparation has more than one active substance, the requirement applies only to those substances that correspond to the above condition. Using a suitable analytical method, the individual contents of active substance(s) of 10-dosage units taken at random are determined. The results obtained must be within the limits prescribed in the BP.

Uniformity of weight: According to the IP, a sample of 10 filled containers free of labeling are selected at random. The outer surfaces of the containers are cleaned and dried, and then each container was weighed. The contents from each were removed and weighed quantitatively. If necessary, the container was cut open and washed with a suitable solvent, taking care to ensure that the closure and other parts of the container are retained. The empty container was dried and weighed again together with its parts which may have been removed. The difference between the two weights is the net weight of the contents of the container and must comply with the limits in the IP.

Sterility test: This test may be carried out using the technique of membrane filtration or by direct inoculation of the culture media with the product to be examined as described in the IP.

Appropriate negative controls are to be included. The test must be carried out under aseptic conditions designed to avoid accidental contamination of the product during testing. For achieving these conditions, a grade A laminar air flow cabinet or an isolator is recommended. The test environment has to be adapted to the way in which the tests are performed. The reader may refer to the brief description of this test given under the chapter, "Parenteral Dosage Forms".

REVIEW QUESTIONS

Long Essays

1. Classify and describe ophthalmic dosage forms.
2. List out and describe the desirable characteristics of ophthalmic preparations.
3. Explain the formulation and preparation of eye drops.
4. What are the packaging materials used for ophthalmic dosage forms? Explain the various types of packaging.
5. How are ophthalmic dosage forms evaluated?

Short Essays

1. Explain the effect of pH and the use of buffers in eye drops.
2. What are the characteristics that define the stability of ophthalmic preparations? Explain.
3. Define ophthalmic ointments. Explain the formulation and manufacture of eye ointments. How are they packaged?
4. Explain the significance of sterility and the use of antimicrobial agents in ophthalmic preparations.
5. Write a short note on the methods of sterilization of eye drops.
6. How are eye drops packaged? Explain.
7. Write a short note on the formulation, preparation and labelling of eye lotions.

10

PHARMACEUTICAL AEROSOLS

Learning Objectives

After going through this chapter, you would be able to:

1. Enumerate and explain the different components of aerosol.
2. Describe the different components of valve.
3. Explain the formulation of aerosols.
4. Describe different filling process of pharmaceutical aerosols.
5. Discuss the stability test and other quality control tests of aerosols.

10.1 INTRODUCTION

Pharmaceutical aerosols are pressurized dosage forms. Aerosols are colloidal dispersions containing one or more active ingredients in gaseous medium that upon actuation emit a fine dispersion of liquid or solid. Aerosol is a system that depends on the power of compressed or liquefied gas to expel the contents from the container.

Pharmaceutical aerosols may be defined as aerosol products containing therapeutically active ingredients dissolved, suspended or emulsified in a propellant or a mixture of solvent and propellant, and intended for topical administration, for administration into one of the body cavities, such as the ear, rectum and vagina, or intended for administration orally or nasally as fine solid particles or liquid mists via the respiratory system, nasal passages or sublingually.

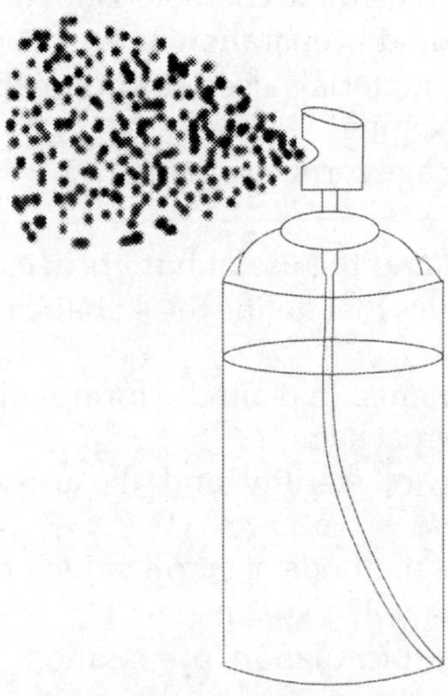

Fig. 10.1: Aerosol

10.1.1 Advantages of Aerosols over Other Dosage Forms

1. Rapid onset of action._
2. The dose can be withdrawn without contaminating the rest of the product.
3. Stability is improved for compounds that are adversely affected by oxygen or moisture.
4. While a dosage is being dispensed, sterility can be maintained.
5. Medication can be administered directly to the affected area in a desired form, such as spray, stream, quick breaking foam, and stable foam.
6. Irritation caused by the mechanical application of topical medication is minimised or eliminated.
7. Bypass or avoid first pass effect.
8. Degradation of drug in GI tract is avoided.
9. Alternate route when therapeutic agents may interact chemically or physically with other medications that are required at the same time.
10. When the drug exhibits variable pharmacokinetics upon oral or parenteral administration, this is an alternative.
11. Adjusting the dose of a medication to individual needs can be achieved.
12. Through use of metered valves, doses of drugs can be delivered accurately.

10.2 COMPONENTS OF AEROSOL PACKAGE

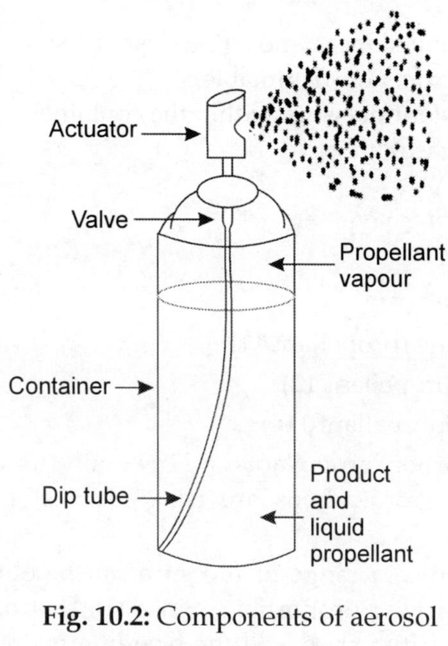

Fig. 10.2: Components of aerosol

An aerosol product consists of the following:

1. Propellants
2. Container
3. Valve and actuator
4. Product concentrate

10.2.1 Propellants

Propellant is responsible for

- Creating the right amount of pressure within the container.
- It expels the product when the valve is opened.
- Aids in the atomization or foam production of the product.
- The propellant must also act as a solvent and diluents.

Various types of propellants are utilized which can be classified as:

1. Liquefied gases
2. Hydrocarbons
3. Hydrocarbon ether
4. Compressed gases

***Liquefied gases*:** Liquefied gases at room temperature and atmospheric pressure exist in the gaseous or vapour state and can be liquefied easily by lowering the temperature or by increasing the pressure.

Most gases can be liquefied, only those that can be liquefied at a relatively low pressure or at a temperature close to room temperature are useful as aerosol propellants. When liquefied gases are placed into a sealed container, they immediately separate into a liquid and a vapour phase.

Advantages:

1. They disperse active substances into a fine mist or foam extremely well.
2. They are inert, non-toxic, non-flammable.
3. They maintain a constant pressure within the container.

Commonly used liquefied gases are:

Chlorofluorocarbons (CFCs)

Hydrochlorofluorocarbons (HCFC)

Hydrofluorocarbons (HFC)

Chlorofluorocarbons (CFCs)

Trichloromonofluoromethane (propellant 11)

Dichlorodifluoromethane (propellant 12)

Dichlorotetrafluoroethane (propellant 114)

Blends of various fluorocarbon propellants are generally used for pharmaceutical aerosols. The fluorinated hydrocarbons are used in most aerosols for oral and inhalational use.

As with the fluorocarbons, a range of pressure can be obtained by mixing the various hydrocarbons in varying proportions. Since the hydrocarbons are naturally occurring products, their purity varies, and the blending is done on the basis of the desired final pressure and not on the percentage of each component present. The pressure of each individual component varies, depending on the degree of purity.

The vapour pressure of a mixture of propellants can be calculated according to Dalton's law, which states that "the total pressure in any system is equal to the sum of the individual or partial pressure of the various components".

Raoult's law states that "the depression of the vapour pressure of a solvent upon the addition of solute is proportional to the mole fraction of solute molecules in the solution".

The vapour pressure of a mixture consisting of two individual propellants is equal to the sum of the mole fraction of each component present multiplied by the vapour pressure of each pure propellant at the desired temperature. This relationship can be shown mathematically.

$$P_a = \frac{n_a}{n_{a+n_b}} P_A O = N_A P_A O$$

where,

P_a = Partial vapour pressure of propellant A

$P_A O$ = Vapour pressure of pure propellant A

n_a = Moles of propellant A

n_b = Moles of propellant B

N_A = Mole fraction of component A

To calculate the partial vapour pressure of propellant B

$$P_b = \frac{n_a}{n_b + n_a} P_B O = N_B P_B O$$

The total vapour pressure of the system is then obtained from

$$P = P_a + P_b$$

P = is the total vapour pressure of the system.

***Hydrocarbons* (HCs):** Hydrocarbon propellants have replaced fluorocarbons for topical pharmaceutical aerosols.

Propane (A-108)

Butane (A-17)

Isobutane (A-31)

Hydrocarbon's ethers (HEs)

Properties

- Less toxic, less dense, flammable
- Lower cost than flourinated hydrocarbons
- Greater range of solubility
- Chemically more stable
- Flammability hazard can be reduced by using various combinations of fluorocarbons, hydrocarbons, and a vapour-tap valve.
- Density is less than 1, being lighter than water, the hydrocarbon remains on top of the aqueous layer and serves to push the content out of the container.
- They have extreme chemical stability (are not subjected to hydrolysis), so they are useful in making water based aerosols.

***Compressed gases*:** Compressed gases such as nitrogen, nitrous oxide, carbon dioxide have been used as aerosol propellants.

- Compressed gases have little expansion power and produce a fairly wet spray and less stable foam as compared to liquefied gases.
- Compressed gases are used in products such as dental creams, hair preparations, ointments, aqueous antiseptic and germicidal aerosols.
- Compressed gases have found widespread use in the pharmaceutical industry, due to aesthetics and excellent compatibility with drugs, glass, stainless steel, and aluminium containers.

10.2.2 Containers

Various materials have been used for the manufacture of aerosol containers, which must withstand pressure as high as 140 to 180 psig at 130°F.

A. Metal

1. Tin plated steel
   (a) Side-seam (three piece)
   (b) Two-piece of drawn
   (c) Tin-free steel
2. Aluminium
   (a) Two-piece
   (b) One-piece (extruded or drawn)
3. Stainless steel

B. Glass

1. Uncoated glass
2. Plastic coated glass

Tinplate containers: To produce an aerosol container that is light and relatively inexpensive, tin plated.

The three-piece tin plated steel container finds use in topical pharmaceutical aerosols. An internal organic coating has been used to decrease the compatibility problems. This coating generally consists of a film made of vinyl or epoxy resins. These materials are resistant to many of the pharmaceutical ingredients and can be successfully formulated with topical pharmaceuticals. Tinplated steel container consists of a sheet of steel plate that has been electroplated on both sides with tin. The thickness of the tin coating is described in terms of its weight (# 25, # 50)

Aluminium containers: Many topical pharmaceutical aerosols use an aluminium container. Aluminium also is preferred for use with most metered dose inhalers (MDIs).

Aluminium is used to manufacture extruded (seamless) aerosol containers. Many existing pharmaceuticals are packaged in aluminium containers because of:

1. Lower risk of incompatibility, due to its seamless nature.
2. Greater resistance to corrosion.
3. Extremely light weight.

Stainless steel containers: These containers are limited to the smaller sizes due to

1. Production problems
2. Cost
3. Extremely strong
4. Resistant to most materials

Stainless steel containers have been used for inhalation aerosols.

Glass containers: Glass aerosol containers have been used for a large number of aerosol pharmaceuticals. Glass containers with or without plastic coatings are available. The plastic coating may be totally adhered or non-adhered and vented. Glass containers can only be used for products with a low pressure and a low propellant proportion.

Glass aerosol containers are preferable for:

- Absence of incompatibilities
- Aesthetic value
- Corrosion problems are eliminated
- Glass provides a larger degree of container design flexibility

10.2.3 Valves

The valve mechanism, via which the contents of the package are expelled, is the most basic part of every aerosol or pressurised container. Performance of a pressurised package is determined by the valve, together with the formulation.

Aerosol valve is multifunctional in that:

- It can be easily opened and closed.
- Is capable of delivering the content in the desired form.

Example: For inhalation therapy, a liquid preparation must be delivered as a fine spray.

For topical application, an emulsion must be dispensed as a foam.

- In the case of pharmaceuticals, the valve is expected to deliver a required amount of medication.
- Valves regulate the flow of product from the container.
  1. Continuous spray valve
  2. Metering valves

Continuous Spray Valves: Spray valves have been used for a large number of aerosol pharmaceutical products. The particle size of the emitted spray can be varied depending on the formulation and design of the valve and actuator. Fine to coarse wet spray can be obtained, including foams.

An aerosol valve consists of many different parts and is assembled using high speed production techniques. Various materials are used to manufacture the many components of the valve. Valve assemblies consist of the following parts.

1. Ferrule or mounting cup

The ferrule or mounting cup is used to attach the valve properly to the container.

- Use containers having a one-inch opening, the cup is made from tin plate steel, aluminium also can be used.
- The valve cup is exposed to the contents of the container and to the effects of oxygen trapped in the head space, a single or double epoxy or vinyl coating can be added to increase resistance to corrosion.
- Ferrules are used with glass bottles or small aluminium tubes and are usually made from a softer metal such as aluminium or brass.
- The ferrule is attached to the container either by rolling the end under the lip of the bottle or by clinching the metal under the lip.

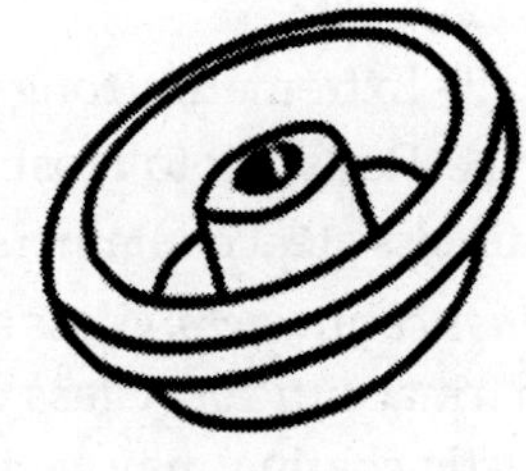

Mounting cup

2. Valve body or housing

- Housing is generally manufactured from Nylon or Delrin.
- Contains an opening at the point of the attached otothe dip tube, ranges from 0.013 inch to 0.080 inch.
- The housing may or may not contain another opening referred to as the "vapour tap".
- With the introduction of the "vapour tap" valve a greater degree of freedom is possible in formulating aerosols.
- The vapour tap allows for the escape of vaporized propellant along with the liquid product in order to produce a spray with a greater degree of dispersion.

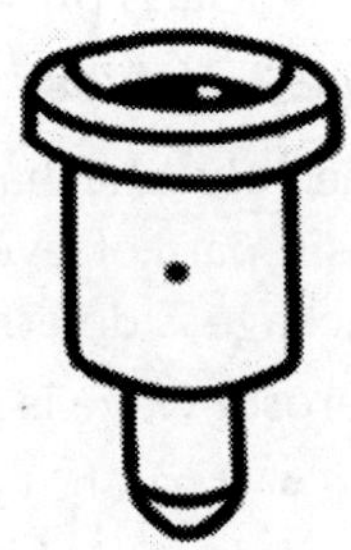

Housing

- Vapour tap further produces:
  1. Fine particle size.
  2. Prevents valve clogging with product containing insoluble materials.
  3. Allows for the product to be satisfactorily dispensed with the container in the inverted position.
  4. Reduces the chilling effect of the propellant on the skin.
- Vapour tap openings are available in size, ranging from 0.013 inch to 0.080 inch.
- Vapour tap valves are used with powder aerosols, water based aerosols, aerosols containing suspended materials, that would tend to clog the valve.

3. Stem

- Stem is made from Nylon or Delrin.
- Metals such as brass and stainless steel can also be utilized.
- One or more orifices are set into the stem, they range from one orifice of about 0.013 inch to 0.030 inch, to three orifices of 0.040 inch each.

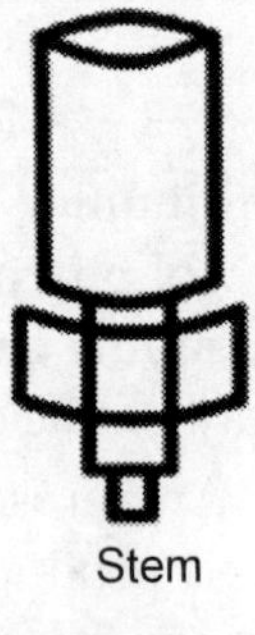

Stem

4. Gasket

- The gasket is made from Buna-N and Neoprene. These are compatible with most pharmaceutical formulations.

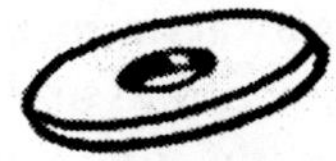

Gasket

5. Spring

Spring serves to hold the gasket in place

- When the actuator is depressed and released, it returns the valve to its closed position.
- Spring is made from stainless steel.

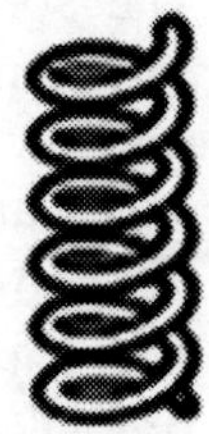

Spring

6. Dip tube

- Dip tubes are made from polyethylene or polypropylene. The polypropylene tube is more rigid.
- Inside diameter of the commonly used dip tube is about 0.120 inch to 0.125 inch.
- Capillary dip tubes are about 0.050 inch, and dip tubes for highly viscous products may be as large as 0.195 inch.
- Viscosity and the desired delivery rate play an important role in the selection of the inner diameter of the dip tube.

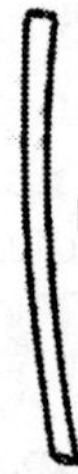

Dip tube

Metering valves

- Metering valves are used to dispense potent medications.
- Amount of medication dispensed is determined on the size of a chamber. The chamber is sealed via the metering gasket and the stem gasket. In the actuated position, the stem gasket will allow the contents of the metering chamber to be dispensed, while the metering gasket will seal off any additional product from entering the chamber.
- Accuracy of dosage can be achieved by use of metering valve.
- 50 to 150 mg + 10% of liquid material can be dispensed at one time with the use of metering valves.

10.2.4 Actuators

To deliver the aerosol product in proper and desired form, a specially designed button, i.e., actuator must be fitted to the valve system. Actuator is an integral part of almost every aerosol package.

- The actuator provides a rapid and convenient means of releasing the contents from a pressurized container.
- The valve can be opened and closed quickly with the help of an actuator.
- Aid in the production of the desired product discharge.

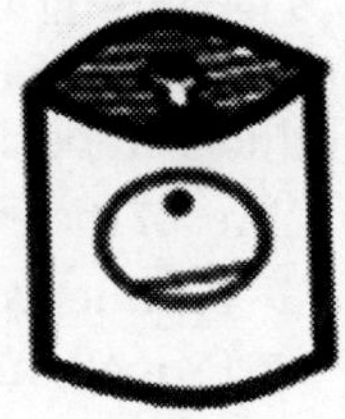

Actuator

There are many different types of actuators

1. Spray actuators
2. Foam actuators
3. Solid stream actuators
4. Special actuators

Spray actuator: It is an actuator that is capable of dispersing the stream of the product concentrate and propellant into relatively small particles by allowing the stream to pass through various opening of 0.016 inch to 0.040 inch in diameter.

The spray can be delivered in the appropriate particle size range using a combination of propellant vaporisation, actuator orifice, and internal channel. Spray type actuator can be used with pharmaceuticals intended for topical (such as spray on bandages, antiseptics, local anaesthetics).

When these spray actuators are used with aerosol product containing low amount of propellants, the product is dispensed as a stream rather than as a spray, since the propellant present in the product is not sufficient to dispense the product fully. For these products, a mechanical breakup actuator is required, which is capable of "mechanically" breaking a stream into fine particles by causing the stream to "swirl" through various channels built in the actuators.

Foam actuators: These actuators dispense the product in the form of foam. These actuators consist of relatively large orifices ranging from approximately 0.070 inch to 0.125 inch. The orifices allow for passage of the product into a relatively large chamber, where it can expand and dispense through the large orifice.

Solid stream actuators: These actuators are used for dispensing semisolid products such as ointments. Large openings allow for the passage of product through the valve stem and into the actuator. These are similar to foam actuators.

Special actuators: Many pharmaceutical and medicinal aerosols require a specially designed actuator. Special actuator is designed to deliver the medication to the appropriate site of action (throat, nose, eye, vaginal tract).

10.3 FORMULATION OF PHARMACEUTICAL AEROSOLS

An aerosol system consists of a product concentrate, propellant, container, and suitable valve. The concentrate can be of the solution, dispersion, emulsion, or semisolid type, while the propellant can be either a liquefied or a compressed gas.

Depending on the nature of the propellant and product concentrate, the combination of these two components with the appropriate valve and actuators, the product can be dispensed as spray, foam or semisolid.

An aerosol formulation consists of two essential components:

1. Product concentrate
2. Propellant

The product concentrate consists of active ingredients or mixture of active ingredient and other agents such as solvents, antioxidants, surfactants, and propellants.

The propellant may be a single or a blend of various propellants. The propellant is selected to give the desired vapour pressure, solubility, particle size. Blend of solvents is used to achieve desired solubility characteristics, or various surfactants are mixed to give the proper HLB valve for an emulsion system. Formulator must be familiar with physico-chemical properties of surfactants, solvent, suspending agents and with propellants and the effect of propellant upon the finished product. Propellants can be combined with active ingredients in many different ways, producing products with varying characteristics.

The pharmaceutical aerosol can be dispensed as a fine mist, wet spray, quick-breaking foam, stable foam, semi-solid, depending on the type of aerosol system used. The type of system selected depends on many factors such as:

- Physical, chemical, pharmacological properties of active ingredients.
- Site of application

10.4 TYPES OF SYSTEMS

10.4.1 Solution System/Two-phase System

- This system, also known as a two-phase system, has a vapour phase and a liquid phase.
- These aerosols consist of a solution of therapeutically active ingredients in pure propellant or a mixture of propellant and solvents. The solvent is used to dissolve the active ingredients and to retard the evaporation of the propellant. When active ingredients are soluble in the propellant, no other solvent is required.
- When the valve is depressed, liquid propellant containing dissolved active ingredients and other solvents are released. Because of the large expansion of the propellant at room temperature and atmospheric pressure, a fine mist or wet spray is produced depending on the nature of the propellants used, the quantity of propellant present, and the valve mechanism.
- This system is used to formulate aerosols for inhalation or nasal application. Propellants 11, 12, and 114 are used for inhalation aerosols.
- The propellant may consist of propellant 12 or a mixture of propellant 12 and other propellants, depending on the type of spray required. Other propellants with vapour pressures lower than that of propellant 12 are added to propellant 12, the pressure of the system decreases, resulting in the production of large particles.
- Lowering of the vapour pressure also produced through the addition of less volatile solvents such as ethyl alcohol, propylene glycol, ethyl acetate, glycerine and acetone.
- Amount of propellant vary from 5% for foam to 95% for inhalation product.
- When a spray is produced with large particles, a decrease is noted in the number of fine particles, decreasing the danger of inhaling.
- These sprays are also useful for topical preparations, since they tend to coat the affected area with a film of active ingredients.
- This type of formulation is usually packaged in a 15 to 30 mL stainless steel, aluminium, or glass container.

10.4.2 Water Based System/Three-phase System

- This system allows a greater use of liquid components not miscible with the propellants.

- Water can be utilised to replace all or part of the non-aqueous solvents included in aerosols.
- Since propellant and water are not miscible, the system is called three-phase system (propellant phase, water phase, vapour phase).
- Depending on the type of formulation, the product is emitted as a spray or foam.
- The formulation must consist of a dispersion of active ingredients and other solvents in an "emulsion" system in which the propellant is in an external phase, to produce a spray.
- When the product is dispensed, the propellant vaporizes and disperses the active ingredients into minute particles.
- To achieve the desired fine particle size with products containing large amounts of water and a low proportion of propellant, a mechanical break-up actuator must be used along with a "vapour tap valve".
- Ethanol has been used as a solvent to solubilize some of the propellant in the water.
- Surfactants have been extensively utilised to achieve a homogeneous dispersion, 0.5 to 2.0% of surfactant is used.
- Propellant content varies from about 25 to 60% but can be as low as 5% depending on the nature of the product.

10.4.3 Two-layer System/Aquasol System

- This system is designed to dispense pressurized products efficiently and economically using small amount of hydrocarbon, HFA, HCFC propellants.
- In this system the liquid propellant, vaporized propellant, and the aqueous solution of active ingredients make up the three phases. Since the liquid propellant and water are not miscible, hydroalcohol mixture is used, the propellant and hydroalcohol solution will mix and form a single layer. Since hydrocarbons are lighter than water, it will float on top of the aqueous layer.
- In this system the vapour phase of the propellant and the product enter the mixing chamber of the actuator through separate ducts or channels moving at tremendous velocity, the vaporized propellant enters the actuator while the product is forced into the actuator by the pressure of the propellant. At this point, product and vapour are mixed with violent force, resulting in a uniform, finely dispersed spray.
- Water based aerosols developed for use in this system have the advantage, since only active ingredient and water are dispensed, propellant is in vapour state and present only in extremely small quantity, the chilling effect associated with liquefied gas systems is eliminated. Since only vaporised propellant is dispensed, less propellant is required in the container with greater use of water as a solvent for active ingredients a greater range of products can be developed.

10.4.4 Suspension or Dispersion System

- To overcome the difficulties encountered for those substance that are insoluble in the propellant or mixture of propellant and solvent, in those cases where a co-solvent is not desirable, the active ingredients are dispersed in propellant or mixture of propellants.

- Surfactants or suspending agents have been added to the systems to reduce the rate of settling of the dispersed particles.
- These systems have been developed primarily for use with oral inhalation aerosols and has been used successfully to dispense anti-asthmatic aerosols, steroids, and antibiotics.

The physical stability of an aerosol dispersion can be increased by

1. Use of active ingredients having low solubility in propellant system.
2. Control of moisture content.
3. Use of dispersing agents.
4. Initial particle size reduces to less than 5 microns.
5. Adjustment of propellant density.

The formulation of this type of aerosol is not without difficulty. Problems arise as to caking, agglomeration, particle size growth and clogging of the valve.

The rate of agglomeration of the suspensoid determines the physical stability of a dispersed system. This rate is affected by the initial particle size of the drug, which must be in the range of 1 to 5 microns.

Various surfactants and lubricants have been used to control the rate of agglomeration. Isopropyl myristate and mineral oil have been added to reduce agglomeration and to act as a lubricant for the particles passing through the valve orifices. To decrease the danger of valve clogging vapour tap valves have been used.

10.4.5 Foam System

- Emulsion and foam aerosols consist of active ingredients, aqueous or non-aqueous vehicle, propellant and surfactants, and are dispensed as a stable or quick breaking foam. When the valve is depressed, the emulsion is forced through the nozzle, and in the presence of warm air and at atmospheric pressure, the entrapped propellant reverts to the vapour and converts the emulsion into a foam.
- The liquefied propellant is emulsified and is generally found in the internal phase.
- Aerosol emulsions are dispensed as foams, and this can be advantageous for applications of irritating ingredients, or when material is applied to a limited area.
- Several topical pharmaceuticals, shave creams and shampoos, have been formulated as foam aerosols.

  Aqueous stable foams

  Non-aqueous stable foams

  Quick breaking foams

  Thermal foams.

Aqueous Stable Foams: In this system total propellant content is usually about 8 to 10% v/v or 3 or 5% w/w

- As the amount of hydrocarbon propellant, A-70, A-46 increases, a stiffer and dryer foam is produced. Lower propellant concentration yields wetter foams.
- Several different steroids, antibiotics may be dispersed in this manner. Both hydrocarbons and compressed gas propellant may be used.

Non-aqueous stable foams: Non-aqueous stable foams may be formulated through the use of various glycols such as polyethylene glycol. Glycol = 91-92.5% w/w, Emulsifying agent = 4% w/w, Hydrocarbon propellant = 3.5-5.0% w/w,

Quick Breaking Foams: In this system, the propellant is in the external phase.

- When the product is dispensed, it is released as a foam, which eventually collapses into a liquid.
- This method is particularly useful for topical medications that may be administered to smaller or large areas without the use of mechanical force to disperse the active components.

  Ethyl alcohol = 46-66% w/w

  Surfactant = 0.5-5% w/w

  Water = 28-42% w/w

  Hydrocarbon propellant = 3-15% w/w

Thermal foams: Are used to produce a warm foam for shaving. They were soon discontinued, owing to inconvenience of uses, expense, and lack of effectiveness.

This system would be advantageous in dispensing medicated foams in which the application of heat would be desirable.

Intranasal aerosols: Drug delivery systems are designed for the deposition of medication into the nasal passageways and have been used to administer medications that have either a local or systemic effect.

The modes of administering intranasal preparations have been limited to nasal drops, non-pressurized nasal sprays, inhalants, intranasal gels, creams and ointments. A new preparation is gaining popularity, called the pressurized metered nasal aerosol. The intranasal aerosol offers numerous advantages such as:

1. The delivery of a precisely calculated dosage of medication.
2. Excellent depth of penetration into the nasal passageway.
3. Reduced droplet or particle size.
4. Lower dosage than comparable systemic preparations.
5. Sterility is maintained from dose to dose.
6. Increased patient compliance.
7. Mucosal irritability is reduced.
8. Greater flexibility in product formulation.

10.5 MANUFACTURE OF PHARMACEUTICAL AEROSOLS

To prepare and package pharmaceutical aerosols special knowledge, skills and equipment are required. Operations must be carried out under strict supervision and adherence to rigid quality control. The equipment used for the compounding of liquids, suspensions, emulsions, creams and ointments, specialized equipment capable of handling and packaging materials at relatively low temperature (about –40°F) or under high pressure must be available. This equipment is usually limited to aerosol or pressurized packaging, cannot be used for other pharmaceutical operation.

10.5.1 Pressure Filling Apparatus

- By the pressure method, the product concentrate is quantitatively placed in the aerosol container. The pressure filling method is carried out at room temperature utilizing pressure equipment.
- Pressure filling apparatus consists of a pressure burette capable of metering small volumes of liquefied gas under pressure into an aerosol container.
- The propellant is added into the burette through the inlet valve, which is situated at the bottom or top.
- Trapped air is allowed to escape through the upper valve.
- Under its own vapour pressure, the required amount of propellant is permitted to flow through the aerosol valve into the container.
- When the pressure is equalized blow the burette and container, the propellant stops flowing.

Procedure: When first developed, was generally slower than the cold filling method with the development of newer technology, the speed of this method has been greatly increased.

The concentrate is added to the container at room temperature and the valve is crimped in place, the propellant is added through the valve. Since the valve contains extremely small opening (0.018 inch to 0.030 inch), this step is slow and limits production.

With the development of rotary filling machines and newer filling heads, which allows propellants to be added around and through the valve stem, the speed has been increased.

For those products adversely affected by the air that may be trapped within the container, the air in the head space is evacuated prior to adding the propellant.

10.5.2 Cold Filling Apparatus

It consists of an insulated box fitted with copper tubing that has been coiled to increase the area exposed to cooling, which must be filled with dry ice/acetone prior to use. This system can be used with metered valve as well as with non-metered valve.

Procedure: The cold method requires the chilling of product concentrate and propellant to temperature of -30 or -40 °F.

Cold filling method is restricted to non-aqueous products and to those products not adversely affected by low temperature in the range of -40° F

- Product concentrate is chilled to -40°F and added to the chilled container.
- The chilled propellant is then added in one or two stages, depending on the amount.
- An alternating method of cold filling is to chill both concentrate and propellant in a pressure vessel to -40°F and then add their mixture to the aerosol container.

- A valve is then crimped in place. The container passes through a heated water bath in which the contents of the container are heated to 130°F to test for leaks and strength of container.
- This filling method is no longer used to any great extent and has been replaced by the pressure filling process.

10.6 COMPRESSED GAS FILLING APPARATUS

Since the compressed gases are under high pressure a pressure reducing valve is required. The apparatus consists of delivery gauge, attached to the delivery gauge is a flexible hose capable of withstand about 150 pounds per square inch gauge pressure and fitted with filling head. A flow indicator is attached b/w the gauge and flexible hose.

Procedure:

- The product concentrate is placed in the container, the valve is crimped in place, and the air is evacuated by means of a vacuum pump.
- The filling head is inserted in the valve opening, the valve is depressed, and the gas is allowed to flow into the container.
- When the pressure within the container is equal to the delivery pressure, the gas stops flowing.
- Carbon dioxide and nitrous oxide can be used for those products requiring an increased amount of gas or solubility of the gas in the product is necessary.
- The container is shaken manually during and after the filling operation or by using mechanical shaker, to obtain maximum solubility of the gas in the product.

10.7 STABILITY TESTING OF PHARMACEUTICAL AEROSOLS

Stability is the most important consideration in the formulation of pharmaceutical aerosols. Stability is directly concerned with the components used to prepare the pharmaceutical aerosol.

- Effect of the container and valve upon the product.
- Effect of product upon the container and valve must be considered.

Since a variety of different materials such as natural or synthetic rubber, plastic and stainless steel are used in the makeup of the container, valve and dip tube. The valve component of the aerosol package is made of different materials, such as natural or synthetic rubber, plastic and stainless steel. All these materials may produce an adverse effect on the product, it is difficult to determine whether a reaction takes place between the materials and the drug. All the materials must be studied separately and collectively. Container coatings and valves with different sub-components may be studied so that any reaction between the component and the product may be detected. Test must cover three areas:

1. Concentrate and propellant
2. Container
3. Valve

Concentrate and propellant

Immediately after preparation physico-chemical constants of the product are determined. Colour and odour, vapour pressure, viscosity, spray rate of valve, pH' density, refractive index, total weight, assay of active ingredients, infrared or gas chromatography curves. These are used for comparison during each evaluation of the product.

Container

The contents of the container are removed by chilling the contents to a temperature of 0°F or less and opening the container. The container is then examined for signs of corrosion. Attack upon tinplate, tin free steel or aluminium is generally visible to the naked eye and under a microscope, small pin holes can easily be detected. Containers have internal lacquering, the examination must ensure that the lacquer is not softened, dissolved, peeled or blistered by the concentrate. Special attention should be paid to the side seam and head space, as there is a greater danger of attack upon these areas.

When glass is used for the container, examination of the container can be omitted. Plastic container may require special testing to determine whether leaching or sorption has taken place.

Valve:

Valve should be examined to ensure that the product is dispensed correctly and that it closes easily.

- The valve cup should be examined for any signs of corrosion.
- The various valve subcomponents should also be examined for evidence of softening, cracking, elongation, or distortion.

Several of these effects can result in defective valve that will not operate properly.

10.8 QUALITY CONTROL FOR PHARMACEUTICAL AEROSOLS

Propellants

- Propellants used in pharmaceutical aerosols require special handling and special test procedures.
- Propellant vapour pressure, density, gas chromatography are determined and compared to specification.
- The purity and acceptability of the propellants is tested by moisture, halogen, and non- volatile residue determination.

Valve, actuators and dip tubes

- These parts are subjected to both physical and chemical inspection.
- The examination must determine whether the valves are fit to be used.

Three test solutions were prepared to rule out variations in valve delivery brought about by different formulation. These solutions consist of range of propellants and propellant concentration which are used in pharmaceutical aerosols.

The test solutions may be prepared in bulk and stored in hermetically sealed containers with suitable fitments for transferring the test solution in to the test units.

Transfer of the test solution should be made in such a manner that no change occurs in the proportion of the ingredients of the test solutions.

Test solution A	**% w/w**	**Test solution B**	**% w/w**
Isopropyl myristate	0.10	Isopropysmyristate	0.10
Dichlorodiflurormethane	49.95	alcohol USP	49.9
Dichlorotetrafluoroethane	49.95	dichlorodifluoromethane	25.0
Dichlorotetrafluoroethane	25.0		

Test solution C	**% w/w**
Isopropyl myristate	0.10
Trichloromonofluoromethane	24.9
Dichlorodifluoromethane	50.25
Dichlorotetrafluoroethane	24.75

Procedure

1. Twenty-five valves are selected.
2. Placed on suitable containers. These containers consist of specified test solution may be filled by pressure process.
3. A button type actuator with a 0.020 inch or larger orifice is attached.
4. This button remains in place throughout the test procedure.
5. The containers are placed in a suitable atmosphere at a temperature of 25+1°C.
6. When the product attains this temperature, the valve should be actuated to the full extent for at least 2 seconds for complete dispensing of a single delivery.
7. The test unit is weighed after single delivery.
8. The process is repeated by actuating the valve for second time.
9. The test unit is reweighed, and the difference between the new weight and the previous weight reflects the milligramme delivery.
10. Test procedure is repeated for a total of two individual deliveries from each of the twenty-five test units.
11. The individual delivery weights in milligrams are divided by the specific gravity of the test solution to obtain the valve delivery per actuation in microlitres.

Valve acceptance:

54 mL or less, the limits are +15%

55 mL to 200 mL, the limits are + 10%

- Out of 50 individual deliveries, if 4 or more are beyond the limits for the specified valve delivery valves are rejected.
- Three individual deliveries are beyond the limit another 25 valves are sampled, and the test is repeated. If more than one delivery is beyond the specifications the valves are rejected.

- If two deliveries from one valve are beyond the limits, another 25 valves should be taken. The valves are accepted if NMT one delivery is beyond the specifications.

Containers

- Both uncoated and coated metal containers must be examined for defects in the lining.
- For metal containers the degree of conductivity of an electric current is determined.
- Glass containers must be examined for flaws.
- The dimensions of the neck and other parts must be checked to determine conformity to specifications.
- The weight of the bottle also should be determined.

Weight checking

- Periodically Weight checking is done periodically while filling.
- Tared empty aerosol containers, which after being filled with concentrate, are removed and then accurately weighed.
- The same procedure is used to check the weight of the propellant that is being added.
- The finished container is weighed to check the accuracy of the filling operation.

Leak Test: Leak testing of each container after the filling operation is employed by the manufacturer.

- Inspecting the crimping of the valve to prevent defective containers due to leakage.
- For metal containers this is accomplished by measuring the "crimp" dimensions and ensuring that they meet specifications.
- The efficiency of the valve closure is accomplished by passing the filled containers through the water bath periodic checks are made of the temperature of the water bath, and these results are recorded.

Spray Testing: Many pharmaceutical aerosols are 100% spray tested.

- This serves to clear the dip tube containing pure propellant, and pure concentrate.
- To check for defects in the valve and the spray pattern.

10.9 TESTING OF PHARMACEUTICAL AEROSOLS

Since aerosols are "pressurized packages" many tests are necessary to ensure proper performance of the package and safety during use and storage.

Pharmaceutical aerosols can be evaluated by a series of physical, chemical and biologic tests.

A. Flamability and Combustibility

1. Flash point
2. Flame extension

B. Physico-chemical Characteristics

1. Vapour pressure
2. Density
3. Moisture content
4. Identification of propellant
5. Concentration of propellant ratio

C. Performance

1. Aerosol valve discharge rate
2. Spray pattern
3. Drug concentration
4. Dosage with metered valve
5. Net contents
6. Foam stability
7. Particle size determination

D. Biological Characteristics

Flame Projection: The product is sprayed for about 4 seconds into a flame, the flame is extended, depending on the nature of the formulation, the exact length being measured with a ruler. Test indicates the effect of an aerosol formulation on the extension of an open flame.

Flash Point: This is determined by use of the standard tag open cup apparatus. The aerosol product is chilled to a temperature of about –25° F and transferred to the test apparatus. The test liquid temperature is allowed to increase slowly, and the temperature at which the vapour ignites is taken as flash point.

Vapour pressure

Pressure can be measured with a pressure gauge and special equipment. Determination of pressure variation from container to container is important, since excessive variation indicates the presence of air in the head space.

Density

Determined through the use of a hydrometer or pycnometer. Methods, which have been used for the density of non-aerosols, have been modified to accommodate liquefied gas preparation.

A pressure tube is fitted with metal flanges and a choke valve, which allows for the introduction of liquid under pressure. The hydrometer is placed in the glass pressure tube. Sufficient sample is introduced through the valve to cause the hydrometer to rise halfway up the length of the tube. The density can be read directly.

Moisture

Karl Fischer method and gas chromatography has been used.

Aerosol valve discharge rate

Taking an aerosol product of known weight and discharging the contents for a given period of time using standard apparatus. By reweighing the container after the time limit, the change in weight per time dispensed is the discharge rate, which is expressed as gm/sec.

Identification of propellants

Gas chromatography and IR spectrometry have been used to know the proportion of each propellant in a blend and to identify the propellants.

Spray pattern

This method is based on the impingement of the spray on a piece of paper that has been treated with a dye-talc mixture. Depending on the nature of aerosol, an oil-soluble or water-soluble dye is used. The particles that strike the paper courses the dye to go into solution and to be absorbed on to the paper. This gives a record of the spray, which can then be used for comparison purposes. To control the amount of material coming into contact with the paper, the paper is attached to a rotating disk that has an adjustable slit.

Drug concentration

The drug concentration inside a pressurised container may be ascertained by releasing a portion of the contents under the surface of a suitable solvents, assaying for the amount of the drug (W1) and noting the weight loss (W2) from the container.

Dose with metered valves

1. Reproducibility of dosage each time the valve is depressed.
2. Amount of medication actually received by the patient.

1. Reproducibility of dosage may be determined by assay technique

Method A: One or two doses are dispensed into a solvent or onto a material that absorbs the active ingredients. This solution can be assayed, and the amount of active ingredients determined.

Method B: Accurate weighing of filled container followed by dispensing of several doses. The container can then be reweighed and the difference in weight divided by the number of doses dispensed gives the average dose.

2. Determination of the dose received by a patient is a rather difficult procedure, since all of the material dispensed is not carried to the respiratory tract.

Net content

Method A: The tared cans that have been placed on to the filling lines are reweighed, and the difference in weight is equal to the net contents.

Method B: It is a destructive method and consists of weighing a full container and then dispensing the contents the contents are then weighed.

Foam stability

The life of a foam can range from a few seconds to one hour or more depending on the formulation.

Several methods have been used, which include:

1. Use of rotational viscometer.
2. Time for the given rod that is inserted into the foam to fall.

3. Time for a given mass to penetrate the foam.
4. Visual evaluation.

Particle size determination

1. ***Light scattering method*:** Droplets and particle size can be monitored directly in the aerosol cloud by light scattering and diffraction method. The main disadvantage of this technique is that they do not distinguish between various chemical species in multicomponent aerosols.
2. ***Cascade impactor*:** The aerosols pass through a series of stages which have nozzles of decreasing size. Perpendicular to each nozzle and some distance downstream from it is located a collection plate. In order to prevent bouncing and blowing off of solid particles, the plate should be coated with a viscous fluid. The larger particles deposit on the first stage because their large momenta will force them to impinge upon the collection plate. The smaller particles follow the air streamlines around the first collection plate and then reach the second, smaller nozzle in which they gain higher velocity and hence higher momenta. Again, some particles will be collected on the second plate whereas the finer fraction continues to the lower stages. The final stage is an 'absolute filter' which should capture the remainder of any droplets or particles contained in the aerosol. The drug mass distribution as a function of the aerodynamic diameter may be calculated from the calibration curves for the individual stages. These curves are obtained by determining the collection efficiency of each stage with monodisperse aerosol.

Biological Testing

Biological testing of aerosol product should include a consideration of therapeutic efficacy and toxicity.

Therapeutic activity

The dosage of the product has to be determined for inhalation aerosols, and this must be related to particle size distribution.

Topical preparation is applied to test areas in the usual manner, and the absorption of therapeutic ingredients can be determined.

Toxicity:

Toxicity test should include both topical and inhalation effects. Aerosols applied topically may be irritating to the affected area and may cause a chilling effect. The degree of chilling effect depends on the type and amount of propellant present.

Thermistor probes attached to recording thermometers have been used to indicate the change in skin temperature when skin is sprayed with aerosol for a given period of time.

Inhalation toxicity must also be considered even though the product may be intended for topical administration. Accomplished by exposing test animals to vapours sprayed from an aerosol container.

REVIEW QUESTIONS

Long Essays

1. Explain the different types of aerosol system.
2. Explain in detail quality control tests for pharmaceutical aerosols.
3. Define pharmaceutical aerosols with their merits and demerits. Add a note on foam type aerosols.
4. Give a detailed account of testing of pharmaceutical aerosols.
5. Describe the various methods of aerosol filling process with merits and demerits.
6. Define aerosols. Explain in detail the formulation and filling of aerosols.
   (a) Write an elaborate note on three-phase systems of aerosols with examples.
   (b) Describe stability testing methods for pharmaceutical aerosols.

Short Essays

1. Define aerosols and write their advantages and disadvantages.
2. Explain two filling methods in manufacturing of pharmaceutical aerosols.
3. Explain the various methods of manufacture of pharmaceutical aerosols.
4. List out the ideal properties of a propellant. Add a note on fluorinated hydrocarbon propellants used in aerosols.
5. Briefly describe formulation of aerosols.
6. Write a note on propellants used for aerosols.
7. Cold filling process of aerosols.
8. Write a note on aerosol propellants and valve system.
9. Discuss and differentiate the pressure filling and cold filling of aerosols.
10. Quality control test for aerosols.

Short Answer

1. Significance of glass container in aerosols.
2. Pressure filling apparatus in aerosols.
3. Propellants of aerosols.
4. What are metered dose inhalers?
5. Define flash point and flame extension test.
6. List out the components of aerosol valve assembly. Give their functions.
7. Advantages of metered dose inhalers.
8. Write the merits and demerits of aerosols.
9. List evaluation test of aerosols.
10. Classify the propellants with suitable examples.

11

COSMETICS

Learning Objectives

After going through this chapter, you would be able to:

1. Define cosmetics and classify them.
2. Describe the formulation of lipsticks and their preparation.
3. Explain the role of surfactants and additives used in shampoo.
4. Describe the preparation of shampoos.
5. Explain the formulation of cold cream and vanishing cream.
6. Elaborate on the formulation of toothpaste.
7. Classify hair dyes and explain their formulation.
8. Explain the effects of UV radiation on the skin and the role of sunscreens.
9. Describe the components used in the formulation of sunscreen preparation.
10. Describe the components used in the formulation of sunscreen preparation.

11.1 INTRODUCTION

From historical times, both men and women have been known to make themselves look more attractive using various types of simple products such as *kohl* for the eyes and creams for the skin from beeswax and olive oil. Today, we have a wide range of cosmetics known for not only their quality but also for their performance.

According to the Drugs and Cosmetics Act, 1940, a cosmetic can be defined as, "Any article intended to be rubbed, poured, sprinkled or sprayed on, or introduced into, or otherwise applied to, the human body or any part thereof for cleansing, beautifying, promoting attractiveness, or altering the appearance, and includes any article intended for use as a component of cosmetic." Thus, a cosmetic is meant to alter appearance, cleanse or beautify but are not meant to produce biological changes anywhere on the body as drugs do. Articles meant to apply cosmetics such as brushes, sponges, applicators, blades, razors, etc., also do not come under the definition of cosmetics.

Cosmetics can be classified on the basis of the area on the body for application. For instance, cosmetics for the hair (hair oil, shampoo, conditioner, etc.), cosmetics for the skin (skin creams, face powder, makeup, etc.), cosmetics for the nails (nail lacquer, manicure preparations, etc.) and cosmetics for the mouth (toothpaste, tooth powder, etc.)

11.2 LIPSTICK

Lipsticks are dispersions of colouring matter in a base consisting of a blend of oils, fats and waxes. Lipstick is used to impart an attractive colour and appearance to lips accentuating their good points and disguising any bad ones. For example, narrow lips can be made to look wider and broad lips can be made to look narrow.

Lips look more attractive if they possess a slightly moist appearance. This can be achieved by the use of a greasy base which also has an emollient (skin softening) action. Apart from making lips attractive, lipsticks help in decreasing cracked and chapped lips, the crevices of which can lead to bacterial action.

11.2.1 Characteristics of a Good Lipstick

The following are the properties expected of a good lipstick:

1. *Should have an attractive appearance, i.e., should have a smooth surface of uniform colour free from defects such as pinholes, grittiness due to colour or crystal aggregates.
2. *Should retain the above characteristics during shelf life and usage, i.e., should not exude oil, develop bloom, flake, cake, harden, soften, crumble or become brittle over a wide range of temperatures during storage and use.
3. *Should be non-toxic, non-irritant both dermatologically and on oral ingestion.
4. *Should be easy to apply, giving a film that is not too greasy nor too dry.
5. *Should be reasonably permanent but easily removable.

11.2.2 Formulation

The materials used in the manufacture of a lipstick can be categorized as:

1. Colouring materials
   (a) Staining dyes
   (b) Pigments and lakes
2. Base
   (a) Dyestuff solvents
   (b) Fats and waxes
   (c) Perfumes
   (d) Preservatives
   (e) Antioxidants

Colouring materials

Colour of a lipstick is its major selling point. The shades may vary with the fashion of the times, but it is usual for the colour to contain some red which allows shades ranging between orange-yellow and purple-blue. Depth of colour and opacity also vary. Colour is imparted to the lips in two ways:

(i) By staining the skin: For this the dye in solution should be capable of penetrating the outer surface of the lips.

(ii) By covering the lips with a coloured layer which hides any surface imperfection and gives a smooth appearance. This is possible by using insoluble dyes and pigments which make the film more or less opaque.

Staining dyes or dyestuffs

Since insoluble pigments do not stain the lips, a lipstick coloured only with pigments will rub off the lips, leaving very little colour. Therefore skin penetrating dyes are required for lasting colour.

The most widely used staining dye is the water soluble eosin and other halogenated derivatives of fluorescein. They are popularly known as 'bromo acids'', since acid eosin is tetrabromofluorescein. Eosin is also known as D & C Red no. 21 which is an insoluble orange compound which changes to intense red salt when the pH is above 4, such as on application to the lip skin. On neutralization by the lip tissue, the dye produces a purple-red stain.

Apart from eosin, other bromo acids used are Dibromofluorescein or D & C Orange No. 5 (gives an orange-red stain), Diiodofluorescein or D & C Orange No. 10 and Tetrachloro-tetrabromofluorescein (D & C Red No. 27 (gives a bluish-red stain).

Disadvantage of bromo acids

1. May lead to allergic reactions or photo-sensitization leading to cheilitis (inflammation) in some people.
2. Shade variation because of difficulty in getting homogenous dispersion of the dye in the lipstick mass. This problem can be minimized by preparing amine salts of the bromo acids which are dissolved in mixtures of oils and waxes.

Pigments and lakes

Pigments and lakes are insoluble colouring materials. Unlike the dyes, they do not have a staining effect. Both inorganic and organic pigments and metallic lakes are used to give intensity and variation of colour. Pigments should be so finely divided so as to cause no gritty feeling when rubbed on the lips. Titanium dioxide is used as white pigment (up to 4%) for obtaining pink shades when used along with bromo acids. Also gives opacity to the film on the lips. The grade selected must be lipophilic. Lakes of many D&C dyes with metals such as aluminium, calcium, barium, and strontium are good pigments for lipsticks. For example, calcium lakes of D & C Reds No. 7, 31, aluminium lakes of D & C Reds. No. 2, 3 and 19. Pigments and lakes are used in levels of 8 -10%.

For iridescent lipsticks, mica coated with titanium dioxide or bismuth oxychloride (2%) may be used.

Base

Besides colour, quality of a lipstick is determined by the composition of the fatty base which determines the rheology of the mixture at various temperatures. The base is responsible for moulding and setting properties of the lipstick and acts as the vehicle for the colouring materials. During shelf life, the stick must remain rigid and stable and on using should soften sufficiently to spread easily on the lips. No single material has all the desired properties and therefore a combination of oils, fats and waxes is used.

Dyestuff solvents: Some part of the base should have solvent properties for the bromo acids and at the same time should be compatible with the rest of the base. Therefore, these materials should have some polar properties.

Vegetable oils such as olive and sesame oil have poor solvent properties and become rancid. Castor oil is an excellent solvent due to its high content of ricinoleic acid and also has high viscosity which delays pigment settling and the oiliness gives gloss and emollience. About 40-50% is used. However, it has poor wetting properties.

Fatty alcohols oleyl alcohol, hexadecyl alcohols are good solvents. Also stearyl, cetyl alcohols.

Esters: Butyl stearate is not a good solvent for bromo acids but acts as a good wetting agent for dyes and pigments. Isopropyl myristate, palmitate, diethyl sebacate are also used and have similar properties as butyl stearate.

Glycols are more polar than fatty alcohols and better dyestuff solvents. For example, propylene glycol is used in high stain lipsticks because of its ability to dissolve bromo acids and also has sweet taste and low toxicity. But since it is hygroscopic and immiscible with oils used in the base, it is coupled with propylene glycol monoesters for better compatibility. PEGs (polyethylene glycols) such as PEG 400, 4000, 1500 are also used.

Fats and waxes: They have high melting points and hardness which is necessary for giving good moulding properties, i.e., quick setting and good release with glossy surface and the strength to produce a rigid stick.

Waxes: e.g., Carnauba wax is the hardest vegetable wax, with a melting pt. of 85°C, gives rigidity, hardness and contraction properties for moulding. Also candelilla wax, beeswax, ozokerite wax, and microcrystalline wax.

Fats: Lanolin or hydrous wool fat has emollient properties, good solvent properties for bromo acid, also acts as binding agent and plasticizer, thereby preventing sweating and cracking of the stick. Other fats include petroleum jelly, acetoglycerides, and lecithin, glyceryl monostearate.

Perfumes: They are important for influencing consumer acceptance. Used to an extent of 2-4 % used. Should be free of irritation and should not have unpleasant taste. Perfume selected should mask the fatty odour of the base. Sometimes flavour is also included. Perfume should be stable and compatible with other ingredients. Usually, light florals are used, e.g., rose alcohols and esters. Also flavours such as aniseed, cinnamon, lemon, orange, strawberry, etc.

Preservatives: They are necessary to prevent microbial growth which may spoil the lipstick and affect its appearance and also produce unpleasant odour. Parabens such as methyl and propyl paraben may be used.

Antioxidants: The fats and oils used in lipsticks are prone to oxidation and may develop unpleasant rancid odours. This oxidation can be prevented by the use of a suitable antioxidant such as butylated hydroxyl anisole (BHA), butylated hydroxytoluene (BHT) and propyl gallate.

Formula

Ingredients	% w/w
Castor oil	60
Lanolin	0.7
Propylene glycol mono-ricinoleate	10
PEG 400	5
Beeswax	7
Candelilla wax	7
Ozokerite wax	3
Bromo acids	3
Lakes and pigments	10
Preservatives	0.2

11.2.3 Manufacture

Manufacturing process has three stages: (1) Preparation of component blends, i.e., oil blend, colour dispersion and wax blend, (2) blending of these intermediates to form lipstick mass, and (3) moulding of lipstick mass into sticks.

1. Preparation of component blends

Oils and dyestuff solvents are first blended together. Dyes and pigments should be milled or ground using ball mills, roller mills, etc. The soluble dyes are first blended with dyestuff solvents using heat if necessary and kept aside. For pigment dispersion, the pigments are ground with components of the base that have good wetting properties such as lanolin, glycols, etc. The pigment dispersion is then ground with dye solution. Remainder of fats and waxes are melted together in a steam jacketed kettle with slow speed stirrer.

2. Blending of intermediates to form lipstick mass.

The dye and pigment dispersion is blended with melted fats and wax blend in a steam jacketed mixing kettle to give the lipstick mass. The molten mass is slowly agitated to prevent incorporation of air. The mass is tested for shade and then the perfume and flavour are mixed. The mass is pumped into storage trays and allowed to cool until used further.

3. Moulding of the lipstick mass

When required, the lipstick mass is gently melted in a steam jacketed pan and agitated slowly for 30 minutes to allow any entrapped air to rise to the surface and thus prevent formation of pinholes in the final lipsticks. The molten mass is poured into cavities of lipstick moulds for casting. Moulds are filled in excess to prevent formation of depression in the centre of the sticks. After congealing, excess is scraped off and moulds are allowed to cool further to set completely without overcooling. After setting, sticks are removed from the moulds and stored for a week before filling into lipstick holders after which they are rapidly passed through a gas flame to melt the surface layer to give a bright, smooth glossy surface. This is known as 'flaming'.

11.3 SHAMPOOS

Shampoos are preparations containing surfactants in a suitable form such as liquid, semisolid or powder used for the purpose of removing grease, dirt, debris and residues from hair grooming preparations from the hair and scalp without adversely affecting hair, scalp and other parts of the body. They are usually aqueous solutions or suspensions prepared by dissolving cleansing agents or detergents in a suitable liquid in which other agents are added to improve the functions of the shampoo.

A shampoo must leave the hair fragrant, lustrous, soft and manageable with a healthy look. Therefore the shampoo should have both cleansing and conditioning properties. Though cleansing is the primary objective, it should be selective and preserve a quantity of natural oil that coats the hair and scalp. There should be a balance between cleansing and conditioning.

11.3.1 Characteristics of a Good Shampoo

1. Should be effective in small quantities.
2. Should remove grease, dirt and skin debris from hair and scalp.
3. Should be non-toxic, non-irritant and should not damage the skin and the eyes.
4. Should produce adequate foam in soft and hard water.
5. Should give pleasant fragrance after use.
6. Should be easily washed off with water.
7. Should leave the hair soft, lustrous and manageable.

11.3.2 Formulation

The ingredients used in a shampoo can be categorized as follows:

1. Principal surfactants (cleansing and foaming agents)
2. Auxiliary surfactants (foam boosters and stabilizers)
3. Additives (to complete formulation and give special effects)
   (a) Conditioning agents
   (b) Sequestering agents
   (c) Opacifiers
   (d) Clarifying agents
   (e) Viscosity modifiers
   (f) Preservatives
   (g) Fragrance
   (h) Colour
   (i) Stabilizers
   (j) Special additives

Principal Surfactants

These are primarily used as cleansing agents and provide detergency and foam. Detergency is important for cleansing action by the following processes.

(i) Lowers the surface tension and wets both hair and the dirt/oil on its surface.

(ii) Reduces interfacial tension between dirt/oil and hair and therefore displaces it.

(iii) Disperses the dirt particles so that they are readily washed away.

Surfactants used in shampoos may be non-ionic, anionic and cationic in nature.

Anionic surfactants

Anionics are the most commonly used because of their superior foaming properties and low cost. Although there are several chemical classes coming under this group, not all are suitable. For instance, metallic or alkanolamine salts of fatty acids commonly referred to as 'soaps' were the first surfactants used in shampoos but are no longer used because of their alkaline nature which makes the hair appear rough, dull and unmanageable. The preferred anionics are as follows:

Alkyl sulphates

These surfactants have the advantages of being easily perfumed, freedom from rancidity, easily rinsed out and reasonably cheap. The best being those derived from lauryl and myristyl alcohols. Lauryl sulphates produce greater volume of lather and myristyl sulphates give greater richness of lather. A mixture of these may be used in shampoos.

Sodium lauryl sulphate is superior to all alkyl sulphates because of its flash foam and foam volume. It is poorly water soluble, but its solubility increases with temperature resulting in concentrated solutions. Therefore it gives shampoos of high viscosity such as in cream and powder shampoos. But it has a defatting effect and is a mild irritant.

Alkanolamine salts are preferred to sodium lauryl sulphate because they are milder, less defatting and more water soluble. They are used as 30-40% solutions and are yellow viscous fluids. Hence, they are used in liquid and lotion shampoos, for example: Monothanol amine, triethanolamine lauryl sulphate.

Alkyl ether sulphates

These anionic surfactants have better solubility, and lower cost. They also have good foaming properties, foam produced is lighter and collapses readily in presence of grease. Therefore, they require foam boosters and stabilizers in addition. However, they are good cleansers, good solvents for fatty additives and fragrances. They are also stable at broader pH range, better mildness and lesser irritancy. They may not leave the hair in good condition, for example: Sodium lauryl ether sulphate.

Sulphosuccinates

These are average foamers and detergents and have some conditioning effects. Monoesters are very mild to the skin, produce lower eye irritancy, with good foaming and detergent properties. The diesters are superior for their wetting properties. Generally used along with alkyl ether sulphates to produce mild shampoos, e.g., baby shampoos.

Isothionates, taurides and sarcosinates

Isothionates are exceptionally mild to the skin and eyes, and are tolerant to hard water. Methyl taurides are less mild, but leave the hair in good condition after washing. Sarcosinates foam well, produce good feel to skin and hair and are used as auxiliaries to lauryl sulphates or amphoterics. They are also stable at low pH and compatible with a wide range of cationics.

Cationic surfactants

The surfactants in this group are good detergents but are normally incompatible with anionics, and are unlikely to be used in shampoo systems containing the former. However, in the absence of anionics they may be used as conditioning agents or as preservatives.

Auxiliary Surfactants

These are surfactants which may not be effective detergents on their own but significantly improve the detergency and foaming power of the principal surfactants. Hence they are also known as 'foam boosters' and stabilizers.

Non-ionics are often used because they are good foam boosters and stabilizers and also have excellent resistance to hard water and are mild.

They are not usually the major ingredient of a shampoo. They are important, however, as co-surfactants, rheology modifiers and solubilizers for insoluble components such as fragrance oils.

Fatty acid alkanolamides

They are not used alone, but used as additives to anionic detergents especially with the monoalkanolamides.

Monoalkanolamides are waxy solids, insoluble in water but easily soluble in detergent solutions with warming. About 15% may be used in a formula. They are commonly used with lauryl sulphates and increase their solubility as well as the viscosity of the solutions, e.g., Stearic ethanolamide is used as a pearlescent thickener.

They are also known to improve the after-effects on hair due to softening properties, e.g., Oleic ethanolamide is used as a conditioning agent.

Monoalkanolamides improve the volume and richness of the lather produced by the alkyl sulphates.

Diethanolamides have better solubility, e.g., Oleic diethanolamide is used as an emulsifier but their synergistic properties are not as good as that of monoalkanolamides.

Polyglyceryl ethers

These non-ionics offer good foaming properties and can be used as main surfactants. They are also free of irritancy to the skin and the eyes.

Other non-ionics such as sorbitol esters (tweens) are mostly used as solubilizes and emulsifiers in shampoos.

Amphoteric surfactants

These are surface active agents that have both anionic and cationic charges in the hydrophilic head groups of the molecule. The negative group is usually carboxylic and the positive group is amino. They are compatible with all classes of surfactants.

They are used in combination with anionics, and have beneficial effects on foam and viscosity and there is also a synergistic effect on mildness. They also contribute to the conditioning effects on hair. They include the N-alkyl amino acids, betaines and the alkyl imidazolines.

N-alkyl amino acids

They show good foaming, cleansing and conditioning properties, e.g., Asparagine derivatives.

Betaines

They are used as co-surfactants, and have the ability to modify rheology and foam character, conferring mildness to the shampoos through their synergistic effects.

Alkyl imidazolines

They have very low irritation potential and are utilized in baby or other mild shampoo systems. They possess good foaming properties and can be used with all surfactants.

Additives

Several additives may be included in shampoos to provide additional properties, improve performance, appearance and stability.

Conditioning agents

These are substances that coat the hair with a very small amount of material that either improves the handling characteristics of hair fibre or lubricates the hair for better slip and smoothness. They include surfactants (cationics), fatty materials (lanolin, mineral oil), natural products (polypeptides, herbal additives, egg derivatives) and synthetic resins (phosphate salts of polyacrylic acid aminoethyl ester) which improve manageability, feel and lustre of the hair.

Cationics: the quaternary ammonium salts condition hair by reducing the electrostatic charge on hair fibre.

Water-soluble proteins such as hydrolysed collagen.

Smoothness and gloss by super fatting agents such as ethoxylated lanolin derivatives, silicones, mineral oil, sesame oil, jojoba oil. They deposit onto the keratin fibre during shampooing and lubricate it.

Sequestering agents

These are compounds that prevent the formation and deposition of calcium and magnesium soaps onto hair when using the shampoo with hard water, e.g., EDTA salts, citric acid, tripolyphosphate – 1%

Viscosity modifiers

These are agents that thicken or thin down shampoos. Thickening can be achieved by:

Electrolytes: 1-4% ammonium or sodium chloride in alkyl ether sulphate shampoos.

Natural gums: Tragacanth, acacia, alginate.

Cellulose derivatives: CMC, HPMC, Na CMC.

Carboxy vinyl polyners or carbopols (93, 941).

Others: PVP, PVA, phosphate esters.

Viscosity of shampoos can be reduced by addition of small amounts of solvents (alcohols), or sodium xylene sulphonate.

Opacifying agents

Opacity or pearlescence to the shampoo can be provided by alkanolamides of higher fatty acids (stearic), cetyl or stearyl alcohols, insoluble salts of stearic acid, finely dispersed zinc oxide or titanium dioxide. A clear liquid shampoo can be converted to liquid cream or lotion shampoo by the addition of an opacifier.

Clarifying agents

These are solubilizing agents which are used when the transparency of the shampoo needs to be improved and stabilized. They are often used in clear liquid shampoos. They should be non-toxic, and non-irritant to the eyes. For example, solubilizing alcohols such as ethanol, isopropanol, propylene glycol and phosphates, nonionic solubilizers such as polyethoxyated alcohols and esters.

Preservatives

Early shampoos which were soap based did not require the use of preservatives. Modern shampoos are milder and the use of non-ionic surfactants, gums and natural additives increases the risk of microbial contamination. Microbial growth can lead to breakdown of detergents resulting in discolouration and development of odours, e.g., Formaldehyde - 0.1 - 0.15 % , Bronidox, p-hydroxy benzoic acid esters.

Sulphated detergents and perfume oils also possess antibacterial activity.

When selecting a preservative, it must be kept in mind the possibility of surfactants in the shampoo interfering with its bactericidal action.

For example, quatenary ammonium salts. Their bactericidal action is reduced in the presence of non-ionic surfactants.

Perfumes

Perfumes are important for sales appeal. The fragrances used in shampoos may vary from herbal, fruity, or floral by using essential oils. The perfume selected must be evaluated for solubility, compatibility, non-irritancy, effect of oxidation, pH, temperature, sunlight, and effect on viscosity or stability.

Colours

Only certified colours approved by Drugs & Cosmetics Act are used in shampoos. The dye selected usually matches with the function of the shampoo, e.g., yellow dye in egg shampoos, green for herbal shampoos.

pH Stabilizers and antioxidants

Shampoos may require their pH to be balanced usually between pH 5.6 and 6.2. Small amounts of acids may be added to achieve this, e.g., citric acid.

Antioxidants prevent unpleasant odours which arise from unwashed hair and scalp due to sebum maturation.

Special additives

These are special ingredients included in shampoos to improve the appearance of the hair or for enhancing growth, e.g., Panthenol (provitamin of pantothenic acid or vitamin B5) is essential for normal hair growth. Panthenol has also been shown to improve body and texture of hair together with a moisturizing capability.

Other additives may include anti-dandruff agents, e.g., zinc pyrithione (ZPT), piroctone olamine (PO), selenium sulphide and salicylic acid.

Types of shampoos

1. Clear liquid shampoos
2. Liquid cream or lotion shampoos
3. Solid cream and gel shampoos
4. Conditioning shampoos
5. Baby shampoos
6. Anti-dandruff and medicated shampoos
7. pH balanced shampoos
8. Herbal shampoos

Formula for conditioning (egg) shampoo

Ingredients	% w/w
Sodium lauryl sulphate (30% solution)	20
Coconut diethanolamide	5
Glycol stearate	1
Methyl paraben	0.1
Sodium chloride	0.25
Yellow dye - q.s.	q.s
Perfume – q.s	q.s
Egg powdered or whole	2
Water	100 mL

11.3.3 Manufacture of Liquid Shampoo

The basic detergents used in the manufacture are available from the detergent manufacturer as solutions. Clear liquid shampoos can be made from preformulated concentrated solutions available from the detergent manufacturer. These are diluted, coloured and perfumed. The dilutions can be done in a stainless steel tank with a slow speed stirrer.

If an alkanolamide is used, it should be dissolved in about half the total amount of the detergent by gentle heating. The remaining detergent solution is added slowly. Perfume is dissolved in cold concentrated detergent. Colour and preservative are dissolved separately in water and added to the mix. The remaining water is added with slow stirring to make up the volume. The viscosity of the shampoo can be controlled by adding electrolytes as solutions in small proportions, stirring after each addition until maximum viscosity is reached.

11.4 COLD CREAM

Cold cream is one of the oldest cosmetic emulsions known to man. The Greek physician, Galen was considered to be the inventor of cold cream which at that time was mainly made from natural waxes such as beeswax and vegetable oils such as olive oil. Since the product was unstable and subject to rancidity, mineral oil was substituted in the place of vegetable oil and borax was included to give better stability since it reacted with free fatty acids in beeswax to form sodium soaps, therefore producing an emulsifier *in situ*. Hence, cold cream or 'ceratum refigerans' is a beeswax-borax type of emulsion.

11.4.1 Characteristics

The term 'cold' is used because when applied on the skin, they produce a cooling effect due to evaporation of water. Cold cream is a white cream, of high luster, free from graininess, has a firm consistency and on application, they liquefy and spreads easily. It is a w/o emulsion.

11.4.2 Formulation

The basic ingredients are beeswax, mineral oil, borax and water. Other ingredients are normally added to modify or improve the properties of the basic formula, such as secondary emulsifiers, perfume, preservative, etc. The quantity of borax used is 5-6% of the weight of beeswax and the amount of beeswax used can vary from 5-16%. Lower levels produce softer creams. Mineral oil has an occlusive effect and helps to hydrate the skin, keeping it soft. It also forms the oil phase. In beeswax-borax systems, both w/o and o/w creams can be produced without the use of secondary emulsifiers, depending upon the ratio of oil to water, proportion of beeswax saponified, constituents of the cream and the temperature. A water level of 45% was considered the critical level. Below this level, the creams were w/o and above it they were o/w. For most cold creams it was below 45%.

Typical formula

Ingredients	% w/w
Beeswax	16
Mineral oil	50
Borax	0.8
Water	33.2
Perfume	q.s

11.4.3 Method of Preparation

Melt the beeswax and mineral oil together and bring to a temperature of 70°C. Dissolve borax in water and heat to the same temperature. Add the aqueous phase to the oil phase with rapid stirring. After the addition of water, agitate slowly while cooling. Add the perfume at a temperature of 50°C. Fill into jars when the cream has cooled to 42°C.

The formation of an emulsion can be explained as follows: When a borax solution is mixed with molten beeswax, the sodium salts of the wax acids will be formed at the oil-water interface, emulsifying the water into the oil phase.

Use: To hydrate and soften dry skin, keeping it soft and smooth.

11.5 VANISHING CREAM

These are emollient creams which spread easily and seem to disappear rapidly when rubbed on the skin. This disappearing or 'rub-in' effect is due to the fact that vanishing creams contain in their oil phase, emollient esters which leave little apparent film on the skin, and for this reason also a low percentage of oil phase is usually chosen. The traditional formula for a vanishing cream is based on high quality stearic acid in the oil phase. This provides an oil phase which melts above body temperature and crystallizes in a suitable form so as to be invisible in use and gives a non-greasy film and also imparts a very attractive appearance to the product. The emulsifier is a soap which is formed *in situ* by adding sufficient alkali to neutralize a portion usually 20-30% of stearic acid.

11.5.1 Characteristics

Vanishing creams are o/w emulsions and can be easily washed off with water. They are prepared by emulsification of stearic acid and water by means of alkali such as potassium hydroxide, borax or triethanolamine. These creams are actually suspensions of stearic acid in a gel of stearate soap (hydrogel suspension). With stearic acid, white creams are produced and because of this whiteness, they are also referred to as 'snows'. The pearly white shiny appearance is due to the presence of free stearic acid.

11.5.2 Formulation

'Triple pressed' stearic acid is used in vanishing cream. It is a mixture of 55% palmitic acid and 45% stearic acid. Earlier it was obtained by pressing a mixture of fatty acids to exclude unsaturated fatty acids. The name, 'single', 'double' or 'triple' pressed is given on the basis of the number of pressings made to obtain stearic acid. Today, good quality stearic acid is obtained by solvent crystallization or hydrogenation or vacuum distillation. The total proportion of stearic acid used in the cream should not exceed 25%. The texture of the cream depends on the amount of stearic acid saponified and the alkali used. Creams made with sodium hydroxide are harder than those with potassium hydroxide. Triethanolamine produces excellent creams and can be mixed with emollients such as isopropyl myristate. Glycerine used as humectant, should not exceed 10%. It helps to minimize water loss by evaporation from the cream, since these creams are o/w emulsions (water is in the dispersed phase) and therefore prevents the cream from drying out in the container. Improved formulas of vanishing cream include extra moisturizing agents, UV absorbers and additional emollients. The soapiness of the cream may be overcome by the use of agents such as dimethicone polyols. To prevent dryness, secondary emulsifiers such as PEG esters and fatty alcohol ethers may be used.

Formula

Ingredients	% w/w
Stearic acid	15
Potassium hydroxide	0.7
Glycerin	8
Water	76.3
Perfume	q.s

11.5.3 Method of Preparation

Melt stearic acid and add glycerin and bring to 70°C. Dissolve potassium hydroxide in water and heat to 70°C. Add this aqueous phase to the oil phase with constant stirring until saponification is complete. Triturate the preparation well to improve the appearance of the cream. Add perfume and preservative.

Creams produced with such formulae contain partly saponified stearic acid, free stearic acid and water. Improved formulas of vanishing cream contain in addition, extra moisturizing agents, UV absorbers, additional emollients, etc.

Use: To improve complexion of the facial skin; as a base for face powder and makeup and useful to absorb excess oil in people with oily facial skin.

11.6 TOOTHPASTE

Toothpastes are dentifrices in paste form, used with a tooth brush for cleaning the accessible surfaces of the teeth. They are packed in collapsible tubes. Though the primary function of toothpaste is cleansing, the secondary results of the cleaning are reduction of tooth decay, maintenance of healthy gums and reduction of mouth odours.

11.6.1 Basic Requirements of a Toothpaste

1. When used with a toothbrush, should clean teeth adequately and remove food debris, plaque (mucous coating on teeth produced by bacteria and saliva) and stains.
2. It should leave the mouth with a fresh clean sensation.
3. The cost should be reasonable.
4. It should be harmless, pleasant and convenient to use.
5. Should be stable during storage.
6. Should conform to accepted standards in terms of abrasivity to enamel and dentine.

11.6.2 Formulation

Additives used are: abrasives, detergents, humectants, gelling agents, flavours, sweeteners, preservatives, colours, bleaches, cariostatic agents.

Abrasives: They are insoluble materials which along with the brush provide the necessary friction to remove adherent matter from teeth. Their functions are (a) removal of debris and residual stains from teeth, and (b) polishing of the tooth surface. They should not scratch the enamel or damage the tooth surface. Some abrasives are calcium carbonate, calcium pyrophosphate, insoluble sodium meta phosphate, silicates. Commonly used are calcium carbonate or precipitated chalk and dicalcium phosphate dihydrate (DCP). Insoluble sodium metaphosphate is useful in fluoride containing toothpaste since it contains no calcium ions which may react with fluoride to give insoluble calcium fluoride. Transparent toothpaste or gel toothpaste use abrasives that appear transparent such as silica in the form of hydrated xerogel and sodium aluminium silicate

Detergents: Surfactants are required to bring about wetting of the tooth surface and necessary to help in penetration and removal of adherent film on teeth by reducing interfacial tension and suspend the removed matter in the foam produced. The foam makes teeth cleaning more pleasant. Soap is not used but synthetic detergents are used, e.g., sodium lauryl sulphate, sodium N-lauroyl sarcosinate, sodium lauryl ether sulphate.

Humectants: They prevent drying of toothpaste especially if the cap is not replaced properly. They also help in mixing of solids and giving suitable consistency. Best humectant is glycerin since it is stable, non-toxic, slightly sweet and has some solubilizing properties. Helps to give a glossy paste. Other examples are 70% sorbitol syrup, and propylene glycol.

Gelling agents: Since the paste is a high solid suspension, it is necessary to maintain stability, i.e., they prevent separation of components by increasing viscosity with the addition of a binding or gelling agent. They are hydrophilic colloids, e.g., natural gums such as Irish moss, gum tragacanth, sodium alginate. Synthetic cellulose derivatives are preferred since they are non-coloured, non-toxic and tasteless, e.g., sodium CMC, methyl cellulose, HEC. Also carbopol, polyox, etc.

Flavours: Flavour of a toothpaste is an important characteristic that influences consumer acceptance. Flavours selected should be those that leave a fresh sensation in the mouth and lasting awareness that the mouth has been cleaned e.g., oils of wintergreen, peppermint, spearmint which are supplemented with a trace of menthol to give a cooling effect. Also clove oil, aniseed oil, etc.

Sweeteners: All flavours require sweeteners. Artificial sweeteners used such as sodium saccharin, a form of saccharin. Unlike sugar, saccharin doesn't promote tooth decay. Some toothpastes contain xylitol, a natural type of sweetener known as a sugar alcohol. Important flavour additive (improves flavour of flavouring agent) is chloroform which also acts as preservative and also has sweet taste.

Preservatives: Toothpastes must be preserved especially due to the presence of gelling agents which support microbial growth in the presence of moisture. They are included to prevent the growth of microorganisms in the toothpaste. Commonly used preservatives are sodium benzoate, methyl paraben, and ethyl paraben.

Colours: Only permitted colours and dyes are used (approved by the Drugs and Cosmetics Act, 1940) red, blue, green used in gel toothpaste and striped toothpaste.

Bleaches/whitening agents: These agents enhance the whitening action of toothpaste on teeth and help in removing stains. They are typically oxidizing agents such as sodium perborate, magnesium peroxide, hydrogen peroxide-urea compounds.

Cariostatic and therapeutic ingredients

They are included to control tooth decay or caries and improve oral hygiene. They have bacteriostatic, bactericidal action (e.g., chlorophyll, fluorides) or as enzyme inhibitors (e.g., sodium n-lauroyl sarcosinate) and acid neutralizing agents (e.g., Urea). Fluorides increase the resistance of teeth against caries by the fluoride uptake of the tooth enamel which gives hardness and lasting tooth structure, e.g., sodium fluoride, stannous fluoride, and sodium monofluorophosphate.

The proportions of these additives used in toothpastes are as follows:

Additives	% w/w
Abrasives	15 - 50
Detergents	1 - 2
Humectants	10 - 30
Gelling agents	1
Sweeteners	0.1 - 0.2
Flavours	1 - 1.5
Preservative	0.1 - 0.5
Miscellaneous (prophylactic)	1.1 - 1
Purified Water to	100

Formula

Calcium carbonate	20
Sodium carboxymethyl cellulose	1
Glycerin	25
Sodium saccharin	0.2
Peppermint oil	1.5
Sodium lauryl sulphate	2
p-hydroxy benzoate	0.3
Colour	q.s
Purified water up to	100

11.6.3 Manufacture of Toothpaste

There are two steps in the manufacture of a toothpaste.

1. Hydration of the gelling agent.
2. Dispersion of the abrasive in the gel.

Hydration of the gelling agent

The gelling agent is dispersed in a mixture of glycerin and part of the water in which sweetener and preservative are already dissolved, under vigorous agitation. This mixture is allowed to swell to form a homogeneous gel.

Dispersion of the abrasive in the gel

The abrasive powder is added to the gel in a vessel that can withstand heavy duty mixing. The final mixing is done under vacuum to de-aerate the product. The active agent if present is added later. Surfactant (detergent) and flavour are added and mixed last with slow mixing. This is to avoid excessive foaming and reduce loss of flavour during evacuation. The paste is allowed to stand for 24 hours and then tubed.

11.7 HAIR DYES

Hair dyes or hair colourants are preparations used to change the natural colour of hair. They are also used to colour white hair which appear with age.

11.7.1 Requirements of a Good Hair Dye

1. Must not be injurious to general health.
2. Must be non-injurious to the hair shaft.
3. Should colour the hair without impairing the natural texture and gloss.
4. Should be non-irritant and non-toxic to the skin and free of sensitizing properties.
5. Should produce shades that are natural in colour and reasonably lasting.
6. Must be compatible with other treatments such as hair straightening, hair setting and hair waving.
7. Should have adequate physical and chemical stability on hair, i.e., air, sunlight, sweat.
8. Should be stable over time in the formulation product in which they are sold or used.

11.7.2 Hair Colouring Formulations

Hair colouring systems are classified into three categories:

A. Temporary colouring

They are colouring preparations which can be removed at the first shampooing. Also known as 'colour rinses'. They use colours of high molecular weight which get deposited on the surface of the hair without penetrating into the cortex.

B. Semi-permanent colouring.

They are colours which resist several shampooings (3-6) but whose fastness is poorer than permanent colours. They are direct dyes of low molecular weight having a good affinity for hair keratin. Therefore, they are capable of penetrating the cortex.

C. Permanent colouring

These products provide effective permanent colouration resistant to shampooing and other external factors such as brushing, friction, light, etc. They are most widely used. Here, uncoloured intermediates are used which by a series of chemical reactions (usually oxidation), produce the desired colour *in situ* in the hair.

Temporary hair dyes

These products include coloured rinses, shampoos, powders, crayons, etc., all should be easily removable and have no appreciable effect on the texture or other characteristics of normal hair. Dye stuffs used are generally basic dyes, disperse dyes, pigments or metallized dyes belonging to the chemical classes of azo, anthraquinone, triphenyl methane phenazine.

Colour rinses

In these products, dyestuffs are used in the form of simple aqueous solutions or aqueous-alcoholic solutions. They are sold as ready to use or in concentrated form meant to be diluted in water and used by pouring repeatedly over hair until practically all the tint has disappeared from the water.

Colour shampoos

Azo dyes can be combined with shampoos of different types. They are based on synthetic surfactants with wetting and detergent properties such as sulphonated oils. Newer colour shampoos use nitro dyes and anionic detergents such as sodium lauryl sulphate with the addition of a fatty acid alkanolamide to increase solubility.

Crayons

These are sticks or blocks of colouring similar to mascara used mainly for retouching new growth of hair between applications of permanent dyes. Either rubbed directly onto wet hair or transferred to the hair with a brush. They are made of mixtures of natural or synthetic waxes with a soap such as triethanolamine stearate into which dyes or pigments were incorporated.

Formula

Ingredients	% w/w
Gum Arabic	27.5
Sodium stearate	15
Glycerol	15
Water	26.5
Colour	16

Method: Mix water and glycerol. Add Gum Arabic to half of this solution and allow to stand. Add sodium stearate to the remainder and warm mixture until it is dissolved. Mix all the ingredients, add colour and mill thoroughly. Pour into moulds and dry in heat.

Semi-permanent dyes

They are actually direct dyes without bleaching action and are usually applied as shampoos. They can colour a good percentage of white hairs, but their prime effect is to impart highlights to naturally coloured hair. Their presence is often indispensable in the formulation of the permanent colours, the oxidation dyes. Some of them are capable of providing hair shades ranging from yellow to orange shades which are impossible to obtain with oxidation dyes and whose contribution is necessary to provide complete range of shades. The dyestuffs used are:

Nitro dyes such as the nitrophenylene diamines and the nitroamino phenols, e.g., nitro-p-phenylene diamine produces an orange red dye, 4-nitro o-phenylene diamine produces an orange yellow shade.

Amino anthraquinone dyes which have good affinity to hair keratin and stable to light, e.g., 1-amino 4 methylamino anthraquinone.

Reactive dyes are colours which work by chemically reacting with the hair fibre and thus the dye part of the molecule is firmly held by the fibre, e.g., azo dyes, azo metal complexes with nickel or cobalt ions, polysulphites, etc.

Semi-permanent dyes are formulated as foaming lotions or as anionic or cationic shampoos as creams or liquids. For solution types, solvents such as benzyl alcohol, butanol and phenoxyethanol are used.

Formula using nitro dye

Ingredients	% w/v
Monoethanolamine lauryl sulphate	20
Ethylene glycol monostearate	5
2-nitro p-phenylene diamine	1.5
Diethanolamine coconut fatty acid	3
Perfume/preservative	q.s
Water q.s	100

Permanent hair dyes

They are based almost entirely on the use of oxidation dyes, i.e., para dyes. Para dyes are substances that are colourless at the time of application to the head (precursors) and are transformed into a coloured material *in situ* on the hair as a consequence of a chemical reaction. They are easily applied, produce natural looking shades and have no adverse effect on normal hair and have gradually replaced 'hennas' in beauty parlours and at home.

They are applied cold and depend on hydrogen peroxide for development of the shade or any other compound that readily liberates oxygen. The chemical reactions involved are oxidation reactions and coupling or condensation effected at alkaline pH (due to ammonia) by the action of an oxidizing agent, usually hydrogen peroxide or one of its solid derivatives such as melamine peroxide or urea peroxide. The hydrogen peroxide brings about a bleaching action on the hair which occurs simultaneously and independent of the dyeing of the hair. The bleaching action makes the hair lighter and allows it to be dyed to the new shade.

11.7.3 Formulation

Dyes (intermediates)

These compounds are used as bases called intermediates because their actual dyeing properties are developed only on oxidation, e.g., o- and p-diamine, aminohydroxy compounds of benzene such as p-aminodiphenyl amine.

Modifiers

These are other related compounds which modify or stabilize certain shades, e.g., metadiamines and several polyphenols such as 7,4-diaminoanisole, pyrogallol, resorcinol.

Alkalizers

Amino dyes work more efficiently in an alkaline medium. Ammonium hydroxide is the best alkali for dyes because it helps to soften the hair and leave no foreign residue. The amount to be added should be carefully controlled so that it does not exceed 1-2% in the final mixture to be applied.

Developer

Although all amino or oxidation dyes darken on exposure to light and air, a developer is always used with permanent dyes to bring the time required for the oxidizing process within reasonable limits, e.g., hydrogen peroxide as 5-6% solution. Developer is made as clear, cloudy or creamy fluid in a large bottle in which dye is mixed.

Antioxidants

Since amino dyes oxidize rapidly especially in the presence of air, all manufacturing processes should be protected from access of air. An antioxidant is added such as sodium sulphite. Amount added depends on the total amount of oxidizable intermediates. Ascorbic acid 0.2-0.3% also used.

Other adjuvants

To improve a good dye solution, substances with special properties are added, i.e., small amounts of soap, ammonia and certain wetting agents which help the penetration of the dye into the hair. They should be compatible and not interfere in the dyeing process.

Different forms of permanent dyes are clear liquids, shampoo tints, cream dyes and colour shampoos. Whatever be the form, the materials for any single application are packaged in two units; one containing the dye and the other containing the developer.

Formula

Ingredients	% w/v
Intermediate	
p-amino diphenyl amine	0.05
4-amino 2 dinitrophenol	0.10
p-aminophenol	0.2
2-nitro – p - phenylene diamine	0.1

p-phenylene diamine	2.1
Modifiers	
Pyrogallol	0.2
Resorcinol	1.4
Antioxidants	
Sodium sulphite	0.5
Solvent for intermediates	
Ammonium hydroxide	10
Isopropanaol	2.5
Perfume	0.5
Base	
Oleic acid	35
Polyoxyethylene sorbitan monooleate	10
Non-ionic surfactant	3.5
Lanolin	1.75
Lecithin	1.25
Chelating agent	0.25
Water to make	100

11.7.4 Method of Preparation

The intermediates are dissolved in the solvent mixture which acts as an emulsifier for the base. The ingredients of the base are combined and added to the dissolved intermediates cold. Agitation should be steady but slow. The pH of the final mixture should be adjusted at 9.0 to 9.2. The base consists of detergents, wetting, foaming and conditioning agents.

11.8 SUNSCREENS

Sunlight may show beneficial or harmful effects on the exposed skin depending on length and frequency of exposure to sunlight. These effects are largely due to the UV radiation component of sunlight.

Sunscreen, also known as sunblock, sun cream or suntan lotion, is a lotion, spray, gel, foam, stick or other topical product that absorbs or reflects some of the sun's ultraviolet (UV) radiation and thus helps protect against sunburn.

Regular use of sunscreen can also slow or temporarily prevent the development of wrinkles, moles and sagging skin.

11.8.1 Effects of UV Radiation

Ultraviolet radiation (UVR) reaching the earth's surface can be divided into UVB (290–320 nm, UVA (320–400 nm) and UVC <290 nm. UVA radiation is responsible for development of slow natural tan and may augment the effects of UVB. UVB is the principal cause of acute sunburn and tanning as well as being immunosuppressive, mutagenic, and carcinogenic. Although UVC has the potential for the greatest skin damage, it does not reach the earth's surface since it is completely absorbed by ozone in the highest part of the earth's atmosphere.

Moderate exposure may stimulate blood circulation, increase haemoglobin production and activate 7-dehydrocholesterol (pro vitamin D3) in skin to form vitamin D. Prolonged exposure to UV rays of sunlight can be harmful and cause skin damage, premature skin aging and even lead to cancer. Skin damage from radiation is cumulative whether sunburn occurs or not.

Sunburn is the term used to refer to red (erythematous), sometimes swollen, and painful skin caused by overexposure to ultraviolet (UV) rays from the sun.

Sun tanning or simply tanning is the process whereby skin colour is darkened or tanned due to excess production of the skin pigment melanin when exposed to UV radiation from the sun. Melanin protects the skin by absorbing UV radiation.

Protection against the effects of UVR in the skin is achieved by specially designed molecules (i.e., UV filters) incorporated in suitable formulations (sunscreens) such as creams or lotions, oils, gels, sticks, etc.

11.8.2 Sun Protection Factor (SPF)

The level of protection from sunburn provided by a topical product is described by the sun protection factor (SPF). Since SPF measures sunburn, it is therefore a measure of UVB protection.

The sun protection factor (SPF) is defined as the dose of UVR required to produce one minimal erythema dose (MED) on protected skin after application of 2 mg/cm^2 of product divided by the dose of UVR to produce one MED on unprotected skin. For example, a product of SPF 10 means that an individual using it would receive only one-tenth of the exposure than he or she would have received in the same time if unprotected.

11.8.3 Formulation of Sunscreen Products

A sunscreen product is formulated to contain the following ingredients:

1. Sunscreen agents
   (a) Organic
   (b) Inorganic
2. Waterproofing agents
3. Emollients and diluents
4. Miscellaneous ingredients

Sunscreen agents

An effective sunscreen must have the following attributes:

(i) Must absorb UV light over a broad or specified part of the spectrum without any chemical breakdown which can lead to reduction in efficacy or the production of toxic or irritant by-products.

(ii) Must possess suitable characteristics to allow it to be readily formulated into cosmetic vehicles and should be absorbed easily into the skin.

(iii) It must be resistant to removal by water or sweat.

(iv) It must not require too frequent re-application to be effective.

(v) It must be highly effective at low concentrations.

(vi) It must be non-toxic, non-irritant and non-sensitizing.

Organic sunscreens

They function primarily by absorbing UV energy and converting it into heat. Commonly used organic compounds as sunscreens are: PABA (para-aminobenzoic acid) and its esters, cinnamates and salicylates, camphor derivatives and dibenzoylmethanes.

PABA (para-aminobenzoic acid) is very effective in the UVB range (200-320 nm) and is most effective in concentrations of 5% in 70% ethanol. Maximum benefit is obtained when applied 60 minutes prior to exposure (to ensure penetration and binding to stratum corneum). However, they may stain clothing.

PABA esters such as Padimate A, Padimate O and Glyceryl PABA are also very effective in UVB range of 280-320 nm and most effective in concentrations of 2.5-8% in 65% alcohol.

Cinnamates and Salicylates are minimally effective, and generally used in combination with one of the above, e.g., 2-ethylhexyl-p-methoxycinnamate (Octylmethoxycinnamate) at levels up to 10%.

Camphor derivatives such as 3-(4-Methylbenzylidene) is widely used as a UVB sunscreen, in spite of its low peak absorbance wavelength of 300 nm. It has superior photostability and improves the photostability of other filters when used in combination with them. It is allowed up to a maximum concentration of 6%.

Dibenzoylmethanes are the most commonly used UVA absorbing materials, particularly in the EU.

The most widely used derivative is 4-t-butyl-4'-methoxydibenzoylmethane, which has its peak absorbance at 358 nm.

Inorganic/ Physical sunscreens

A physical sunscreen is an inorganic compound which has radiation scattering and reflective properties due to its physical form, e.g., natural minerals and pigments -- talc, mica, kaolin and metal oxides.

Iron oxides are frequently used in facial colour cosmetics at low levels and mica, or titanium dioxide coated micas, are used as pearlescent pigments in colour cosmetics and these either reflect or transmit light. Products containing zinc oxide offer a very broad UV protection, but also tend to give some visible light protection which may result in a white appearance of the product on the skin.

Waterproofing agents

An important requisite of any sunscreen product is that it should withstand water, either in the form of sweat, or from activities such as swimming. During swimming, the skin continues to be exposed to high levels of irradiation as UV light readily penetrates the water's surface. It is highly desirable therefore that the product is not easily washed off.

Oil based formulations or stick formulations have water repellency due to their non-aqueous nature. The majority of sun protection products are w/o emulsions which can contain very high levels of oil and therefore very greasy. Oil-in-water (o/w) emulsions are preferred since they are cosmetically more elegant and have a better skin feel.

Silicone oils are used such as dimethicone 350, cyclomethicone and dimethicone/trimethylsiloxysilicate.

Emollients and diluents

Most sunscreen users prefer to avoid heavy, greasy materials and those which impart a tacky feel. On the other hand, the formulation must not be too thin and insubstantive. On application, they must produce a uniform and continuous film on the skin which is desirable to ensure complete protection.

Branched chain esters, because of their spreadability, are more likely to produce a more even protective film and also improve the skin feel and acceptability of a product.

Miscellaneous ingredients

Rheology modifiers are important since they affect not only the ease with which the product is applied, but also the efficiency of both inorganic and physical sunscreens.

Moisturization is achieved by humectant materials rather than by occlusion, in order to be more acceptable to the consumer. Humectants such as sorbitol, glycerol or propylene glycol are essential to skin-care products unless some of the more sophisticated materials are to be used.

Antioxidant vitamins E, C act as free radical scavengers, inhibiting the peroxidation of unsaturated lipids due to UVA radiation.

11.8.4 Types of Sunscreen Products

Gels

These are extremely attractive and elegant formulation type. However, their main drawbacks lie in their potential irritancy when alcohol is part of the formula, and their relatively low SPF and water-resistant properties.

Sticks

These are meant for direct application of sunscreens to a specific small area such as the nose, lips, forehead good water repellents due to the presence of oils and waxes, but are often expensive to prepare. They may contain opaque sunscreens.

Oils

They are convenient to use and have good water resistance due to their oily nature. However, their disadvantage is that they give low SPFs, due to the limitation of sunscreen solubility and the production of a very thin transparent film on the skin. They are relatively expensive and are sticky and greasy.

Emulsions

Emulsions are the most popular formulation type for sunscreen products. They are highly convenient and cosmetically acceptable. They are usually formulated as thick creams to light milks. May be oil-in-water, water-in-oil or more complex emulsions and are able to achieve the highest SPF of all formulation types because they deposit a uniform non-transparent film on the skin. These products also have the ability to penetrate the skin's horny layer to some degree, thus increasing their efficacy and durability.

Formula

Oil-in-water lotion used with high SPF

Ingredients	% w/w
Phase A	
Lanolin	4.5
Cocoa butter	2.0
Glyceryl monostearate	3.0
Stearic acid	2.0
Octyl dimethyl PABA	7.0
Oxybenzone	3.0
Phase B	
Deionized water	71.6
Sorbitol liquid	5.0
Triethanolamine	1.0
Methyl paraben	0.3
Propyl paraben	0.1
Phase C	
Benzyl alcohol	0.5

Heat phases (A) and (B) and homogenize together. Cool to below 50ºC and add benzyl alcohol, which is heat-sensitive.

REVIEW QUESTIONS

Long Essays

1. How are lipsticks formulated and manufactured? Give a formula for a lipstick.
2. Explain the formulation and preparation of toothpaste.
3. Define and classify shampoos. Describe the ingredients used in the formulation of shampoos.

Short Essays

1. Explain the formulation of vanishing cream.
2. Describe the formulation of sunscreens. What is SPF?
3. Write a note on permanent hair dyes.
4. What are the ideal characteristics of lipsticks?
5. What are cold creams? Explain their formulation.
6. Explain the formulation and preparation of toothpaste.

12

PACKAGING MATERIALS SCIENCE

Learning Objectives

After going through this chapter, you would be able to:

1. Appreciate the importance of packaging in the pharmaceutical industry.
2. Enlist and explain the properties of packing materials.
3. Select the suitable packaging material based on drug product properties.
4. Describe quality requirements for packing materials.
5. Describe quality requirements for packing materials.

12.1 INTRODUCTION

In the pharmaceutical sector, it is critical that the packaging chosen sufficiently preserves the product's integrity. Pharmaceutical packaging is the combination of components necessary to contain, preserve, protect, and deliver a safe, efficacious drug product, such that at any point of time before expiration date of the drug product, a safe and efficacious dosage form is available. The selection of a package thus begins with an assessment of the product's physical and chemical properties, protective needs, and marketing requirements. The materials chosen must have the following properties:

1. protect the preparation from environmental conditions,
2. not be reactive with the product,
3. not impart flavours or odours to the product,
4. be nontoxic,
5. be FDA approved,
6. meet applicable tamper-resistance requirements, and
7. be adaptable to commonly used high-speed packaging equipment.

12.1.1 Levels of Packaging

Packaging in the pharmaceutical industry varies from drug to drug and normally there are three levels of packaging commonly referred to as the primary, secondary, and tertiary packaging.

1. **Primary packaging:** Primary packing system is the material that first envelops the product and holds it, i.e., those package components and subcomponents that actually come in contact with the product, or those that may have a direct effect on the product shelf-life, e.g., ampoules and vials, prefilled syringes, IV containers, blister packs, etc.
2. **Secondary packaging:** Secondary packing system is placed outside the primary packaging and used to group primary packages together, e.g., cartons, boxes, shipping containers, injection trays, etc.

3. **Tertiary packaging:** Tertiary packaging system is employed for bulk handling and shipping of the pharmaceutical products, e.g., barrel, container, edge protectors, etc.

12.1.2 Materials used for Packaging of Pharmaceutical Products

It is important to have a basic knowledge of all packaging materials, their properties, characteristics, etc., and the processes by which they are fabricated/decorated as a packaging container or component, as well as how these and any subsequent processes may affect their properties, e.g., sterilization by ethylene oxide can lead to ethylene oxide and ethylene glycol residues. Gamma irradiation of low-density polyethylene not only marginally reduces material flexibility owing to molecular cross-linkage but can give rise to formic acid and formaldehyde residues.

Packaging types, styles and systems can be broadly defined by the material of construction, e.g., glass, plastic, metal, rubber, paper, etc., and the process used for fabrication, e.g., blow moulding, injection moulding, etc.

12.1.3 Glass Containers

Glass is commonly used in pharmaceutical packaging because it possesses superior protective qualities, it is economical, and containers are readily available in a variety of sizes and shapes. It is essentially chemically inert, impermeable, strong, and rigid, and has FDA clearance. Glass does not deteriorate with age, and with a proper closure system, it provides an excellent barrier against practically every element except light. Coloured glass, especially amber, can give protection against light when it is required. The major disadvantages of glass as a packaging material are its fragility and its weight.

Composition of Glass: Glass is composed principally of sand, soda ash, limestone, and cullet. The sand is almost pure silica, the soda ash is sodium carbonate, and the limestone, calcium carbonate. The composition of glass varies and is usually adjusted for specific purposes. The most common cations found in pharmaceutical glassware are silicon, aluminium, boron, sodium, potassium, calcium, magnesium, zinc, and barium. The only anion of consequence is oxygen. Many useful properties of glass are affected by the kind of elements it contains.

Glass is basically of three types: neutral, (type I), surface-treated soda lime glass (type II) and soda lime glass or alkali glass (types III and NP). These materials may be converted into components by pressing, blowing into a mould, or the shaping of glass cane (tubular containers). Typical compositions of type I (neutral) and type III (soda or alkali) glass are as follows (Table 12.1).

Table 12.1

Compound	Type I glass	Type III glass
Silica	66-74%	66-75%
Lime	1-5%	6-12%
Soda	7-10%	12.5-19%
Alumina	4-10%	1-7%
Boric oxide	9-11%	-

Type I: Borosilicate Glass (Neutral glass)

Although glass is a virtually inert material and is used to contain strong acids and alkalis as well as all types of solvents, it has a definite and measurable chemical reaction with some substances, notably water. The sodium is loosely combined with the silicon and is leached from the surface of the glass by water. In type I glass the alkaline element is largely eliminated using boric oxide to neutralize the oxides of potassium and sodium. Neutral glass has a higher melt temperature (around 1750°C) and a narrower working temperature range, which, together with the higher cost of boric oxide and the greater likelihood of imperfections, usually means a cost of two to three times that of soda glass for containers made by the blow moulding process.

Type II: Surface Treated Soda-Lime Glass

Surface-treated glass (type II) is made by treating the hot surface of type III (soda) glass with sulphur dioxide, ammonium sulphate or, in some countries, ammonium chloride. This neutralizes some of the surface alkali radicals, producing a more neutral surface. The process, which may also be referred to as sulphuring or sulphating, invariably leaves a hazy surface bloom (normally sodium sulphate) and so washing is essential prior to use.

Type III: Soda-Lime Glass or alkali glass

Soda glass (type III) is the most widely used material where extraction of alkali metal ions is not critical to the product.

Type NP: General-Purpose Soda-Lime Glass

Type IV or NP (non-parenteral) glass has similar composition to type III, but it cannot be guaranteed to have the same quality.

Coloured Glass – Light Protection: Glass containers for drugs are generally available in clear flint or amber colour. For decorative purposes, special colours such as blue, emerald green, and opal may be obtained from the glass manufacturer. Only amber glass and red glass are effective in protecting the contents of a bottle from the effects of sunlight by screening out harmful ultraviolet rays. The USP specifications for light-resistant containers require the glass to provide protection against 2900 to 4500 angstroms of light. Amber glass meets these specifications, but the iron oxide added to produce this colour could leach into the product. Therefore, if the product contains ingredients subject to iron-catalysed chemical reactions, amber glass should not be used.

12.1.4 Plastic Containers

Plastics in packaging have proved useful for several reasons, including the ease with which they can be formed, their high quality, and the freedom of design to which they lend themselves. Plastic containers are extremely resistant to breakage and thus offer safety to consumers along with reduction of breakage losses at all levels of distribution and use. Plastic containers for pharmaceutical products are primarily made from the following polymers: polyethylene, polypropylene, polyvinyl chloride, polystyrene, and to a lesser extent, polymethyl methacrylate, polyethylene terephthalate, polytrifluoroethylene, the amino formaldehydes, and polyamides. Plastic containers consist of one or more polymers together with certain additives. Those manufactured for pharmaceutical purposes must be free of substances that can be extracted in significant quantities by the product contained therein.

Polyethylene: High-density polyethylene (HDPE) is the material most widely used for containers by the pharmaceutical industry and will probably continue to be for the next several years. It is a good barrier against moisture, but a relatively poor one against oxygen and other gases. Most solvents do not attack polyethylene, and it is unaffected by strong acids and alkalis. Lack of clarity and a relatively high rate of permeation of essential odours, flavours, and oxygen militate against the use of polyethylene as a container material for certain pharmaceutical preparations. Despite these problems, polyethylene in all its variations offers the best all-around protection to the greatest number of products at the lowest cost. The density of polyethylene, which ranges from 0.91 to 0.96, directly determines the four basic physical characteristics of the blow moulded container: (1) stiffness, (2) moisture vapour transmission, (3) stress cracking, and (4) clarity or translucency. As the density increases, the material becomes stiffer, has a higher distortion and melting temperature, becomes less permeable to gases and vapours, and becomes less resistant to stress cracking. Since these polymers are generally susceptible to oxidative degradation during processing and subsequent exposure, the addition of some antioxidant is necessary. Usually, levels of hundreds of parts per million are used. Antioxidants generally used are butylated hydroxy toluene or dilauryl thiodipropionate. Antistatic additives are often used in bottle grade polyethylenes. Their purpose is to minimize airborne dust accumulation at the surface bottle during handling, filling, and storage. These antistatic additives are usually polyethylene glycols or long chain fatty amides and are often used at 0.1 to 0.2% concentration in high-density polyethylene.

Polypropylene: Polypropylene has recently become popular because it has many of the good features of polyethylene, with one major disadvantage either eliminated or minimized. Polypropylene does not stress-crack under any conditions. Except for hot aromatic or halogenated solvents, which soften it, this polymer has good resistance to almost all types of chemicals, including strong acids, alkalis, and most organic materials. Its high melting point makes it suitable for boilable packages and for sterilizable products. Lack of clarity is still a drawback, but improvement is possible with the construction of thinner walls. Polypropylene is an excellent gas and vapour barrier. Its resistance to permeation is equivalent to or slightly better than that of high-density or linear polyethylene.

Polyvinyl Chloride (PVC): Clear rigid polyvinyl chloride bottles overcome some of the deficiencies of polyethylene. They can be produced with crystal clarity, provide a good oxygen barrier, and have greater stiffness. In its natural state, polyvinyl chloride is crystal clear and stiff, but has poor impact resistance. It can be softened with plasticizers. Various stabilizers, antioxidants, lubricants, or colourants may be incorporated. Polyvinyl chloride is seldom used in its purest form. It is an inexpensive, tough, clear material that is relatively easily processed. It must not be overheated because it starts to degrade at 280°F, and the degradation products are extremely corrosive. Polyvinyl chloride yellows when exposed to heat or ultraviolet light unless a stabilizer is included by the resin supplier. Polyvinyl chloride is an excellent barrier for oil, both volatile and fixed alcohols, and petroleum solvents. It retains odour and flavours quite well and is a good barrier for oxygen. Rigid polyvinyl chloride is a good barrier for moisture and gases in general, but plasticizers reduce these properties. Polyvinyl chloride is not affected by acids or alkalis except for some oxidizing acids. Its impact resistance is poor, especially at low temperatures.

Other selected materials find specialized usages for containers, devices, components, plies or coatings. These include nylon (PA), arcylonitrile butadiene styrene (ABS), styrene acrylonitrile (SAN), polycarbonate (PC), polysulphone, polyvinylidene chloride (PVdC), poly-monochloro-trifluoroethylene (PCTFE), polyester (PET) and polytetrafluoroethylene (PTFE).

12.1.5 Disadvantages

In theory plastics appear to have certain disadvantages, e.g., possible extraction, interaction, adsorption, absorption, lightness and hence poor physical stability; all are permeable to some degree to moisture, oxygen, carbon dioxide, etc, and most exhibit electrostatic attraction, allow penetration of light rays unless pigmented black, etc. It is necessary to be aware of other possible negative features. These include:

1. ***Stress-cracking:*** A phenomenon related to low-density polythene and certain stress cracking agents such as wetting agents, detergents, and some volatile oils.
2. ***Panelling or cavitation:*** Whereby a container shows inward distortion or partial collapse owing to absorption of gases from the headspace, absorption causing swelling of the plastic, or dimpling following a steam autoclaving operation.
3. ***Crazing:*** A surface reticulation which can occur particularly with polystyrene and certain chemical substances (isopropyl myristate first causes crazing, which ultimately reaches a state of total embrittlement and disintegration).
4. ***Poor key of print:*** Certain plastics, such as the polyolefins, need pre-treating before ink will key. Additives that migrate to the surface of the plastic may also cause printing problems.
5. ***Poor impact resistance:*** Both polystyrene and PVC have poor impact resistance. This can be improved by the inclusion of impact modifiers, such as rubber in the case of polystyrene and methyl methacrylate butadiene styrene for PVC.

12.1.6 Metal and Metal Containers

Metal, mainly as tin plate, or aluminium was at one time widely used for rigid containers for tablets, capsules, pastilles, powders, and even liquid products. A significant part its usage has been lost to other materials over the last few years. Light flexible gauges of metal (aluminium, tin, and tin-coated lead) were widely used for collapsible tubes. Thin gauges of aluminium are widely used as foil in combination with other support or heat-sealing polymer films. Although all the above uses for metals still exist, there has been a gradual reduction in their use other than for foil and for aerosols. In addition to containers, tin plate, aluminium, and aluminium alloys have been widely employed for ancillary components, including closures. Although the use of tin plate and certain types of aluminium screw closures has reduced, the special aluminium alloy developed for rolled-on and rolled-on pilfer-proof closures has remained in use owing mainly to recent events related to security and tamper evidence. The production of collapsible tubes made by a process known as impact extrusion has been static recently, first because of the growth in plastic tubes, and more recently because of the introduction of a multi-ply lamination, once known as 'Glaminates'. Metal collapsible tubes in the UK are largely made of aluminium (plain or lacquered) with a few in pure tin. As aluminium work hardens during impact extrusion (i.e., it becomes less flexible and springier) aluminium tubes have to undergo an annealing process to ensure that the metal becomes flexible and capable of being shaped and folded. If any interaction between the product and metal is likely an internal protective lacquer, usually based on vinyl or epoxide resins, can be added. As metal tubes have a shoulder bearing an orifice (which takes a closure) and an open end (through which the contents are filled and after which the metal is folded and crimped), they have in effect two closures and two areas of seal. Whereas the dispensing end can be sealed, with a blind nozzle and/or a screw cap to make a good seal, the folded metal is less reliable in terms of thin or mobile products. The fold can therefore be improved by the addition of a latex or heat-seal band. Although the number of folds in the filling end can also be varied (e.g., saddleback (triple) fold, double fold, etc.) the longer tube length required for the former (say + 9 mm) will add to the cost. Tubes with elongated nozzles and a controlled orifice size are used for eye ointments. Nearly all caps on metal tubes are waddles, being plastic and moulded in polyethylene and polypropylene.

12.1.7 Rubber Based Components

The main types of rubber used for pharmaceutical products include natural rubber, neoprene, nitrile, butyl, chlorobutyl, bromo butyl and silicone. Among them, silicone is the most expensive and, although the most inert, is readily permeable to moisture, gases and absorbent to certain preservatives. Rubber components are likely to contain more additives than plastics. most rubber formulations are relatively complex and may contain one or more of the following: vulcanizing agents (many of which are sulphur based), accelerators, fillers, activators, pigments, antioxidants, lubricants, softeners, or waxes. They are therefore tested by basically similar extractives and product contact procedures before they are used for injectable products. Rubber gaskets are also found in aerosols and metered-dose pump systems.

Paper, Paperboard, and Cardboard

The most common applications of paper, paperboard, and cardboard are in blister lidding stock and in over the counter (OTC) outer packaging. Because paper, paperboard, and cardboard offer virtually no moisture or gas barrier, they are typically part of the secondary pharmaceutical container. To provide additional protection, paper can be laminated or coated with a variety of materials. More commonly, when paper is involved in critical packaging functions, it is the only one component of a multicomponent system that offers optimal environmental protection to the drug environment. Although paper does not offer high shear strength, its relatively high tensile strength makes it an easy barrier to overcome if one intends to do so but is an exceedingly confounding one for a child. Paper also simplifies printing on the blister itself. Other uses of paper, paperboard, and cardboard are as secondary packaging or for shipping packaging (e.g., corrugated cardboard).

12.2 FACTORS INFLUENCING CHOICE OF CONTAINERS

Before a pack can be selected and the relevance of the various hazards considered, it is necessary to establish a thorough background brief which covers consideration of the product, the market, the distribution system, manufacturing facilities and other considerations. These are discussed below.

12.2.1 The Product

Product detail must include chemical and physical characteristics of the drug entity, the excipients, and the formulation. It must also cover any recognized routes of deterioration or degradation, the dosage and frequency of dosage, the mode of administration and type of patient (baby, child, teenager, adult, elderly, infirm. etc.), any of which could influence the product and pack style and any controlling legislative detail. Whether the product is seasonal or has a year-round use may be a further influence on pack selection.

12.2.2 The Market

The eventual channels of sale should be considered, i.e., where, when, how and by whom it is to be used or administered (e.g., doctor, dentist, nurse, patient, etc.). Where the product may be used (i.e., clinic, home, hospital), whether for home trade and/or export, the quantity per pack and the predicted sales for initial launch and follow-up sales, must all be carefully considered during pack design and selection.

12.2.3 The Distribution System

The distribution system should be carefully thought out, for example, conventional wholesale/retail outlets, or direct to selected outlets. How a product is to be distributed may be more relevant to export markets where less sophisticated transport systems (mules, donkeys, camels, etc.) may be used, and where climatic conditions may be more severe, particularly if intermediate storage facilities are non-existent (e.g., no dockside warehouses) so that the consignment will be directly exposed to the atmosphere.

12.2.4 Manufacturing Facilities

The suitability of the manufacturing facilities may have to be considered for several reasons, i.e., new pack, increased sales, improvements in GMP, revised product, new product, etc. For example, can the envisaged product be manufactured and packed with existing facilities, or are new plant, equipment and buildings required? If the latter applies, then the likely profit must be balanced against the likely cost of the venture. For example, an entirely new facility for the introduction of a packed product by an aseptic or a terminal autoclaving process would be more expensive than that required for a solid or liquid dosage form.

12.2.5 Drug-Plastic Considerations

A packaging system must protect the drug without in any way altering the composition of the product until the last dose is removed. The selection of a suitable package for a drug is not an easy task, in as much as an error can lead to serious consequences. Drug-plastic considerations have been divided into five separate categories: (1) permeation, (2) leaching, (3) sorption, (4) chemical reaction, and (5) alteration in the physical properties of plastics or products.

12.2.6 Permeation

The transmission of gases, vapours, or liquids through plastic packaging materials can have an adverse effect on the shelf-life of a drug. Permeation of water vapour and oxygen through the plastic wall into the drug can present a problem if the dosage form is sensitive to hydrolysis and oxidation. Temperature and humidity are important factors influencing the permeability of oxygen and water through plastic. An increase in temperature reflects an increase in the permeability of the gas. Molecules do not permeate through crystalline zones; thus, an increase in crystallinity of the material should decrease permeability. Two polyethylene materials may therefore give different permeability values at various temperatures. Materials such as nylon, which are hydrophilic in nature, are poor barriers to water vapour, while such hydrophobic materials as polyethylene provide much better barriers.

12.2.7 Leaching

Since most plastic containers have one or more ingredients added in small quantities to stabilize or impart a specific property to the plastic, the prospect of leaching, or migration from the container to the drug product, is present. Problems may arise with plastics when colouring agents in relatively small quantities are added to the formula. Dyes may migrate into a parenteral solution and cause contamination, and a toxic effect.

12.2.8 Sorption

This process involves the removal of constituents from the drug product by the packaging material leading to serious consequences. Since drug substances of high potency are administered in small doses, losses due to sorption may significantly affect the therapeutic efficacy of the preparation. A problem commonly encountered in practice is the loss of preservatives that exert their activity at low concentration, and their loss through sorption may be great enough to leave a product unprotected against microbial growth.

12.2.9 Chemical Reactivity

Certain ingredients that are used in plastic formulations may react chemically with one or more components of a drug product. At times, ingredients in the formulation may react with the plastic. Even micro-quantities of chemically incompatible substances can alter the appearance of the plastic or the drug product.

12.2.10 Polymer Modification

The physical and chemical alteration of the packaging material by the drug product is called modification. Such phenomena as permeation, sorption, and leaching play a role in altering the properties of the plastic and may also lead to its degradation. Some solvent systems have been found to be responsible for considerable changes in the mechanical properties of plastics. Oils, for example, have a softening effect on polyethylene, fluorinated hydrocarbons attack polyethylene and polyvinyl chloride.

12.3 LEGAL AND OFFICIAL REQUIREMENTS FOR CONTAINERS

12.3.1 FDA Regulations

Under the provisions of the Federal Food, Drug and Cosmetic Act, however, no specifications or standards for containers or container closures are provided. Under the Act, it is the responsibility of the manufacturer to prove the safety of a packaging material and to get approval before using it for any food or drug product. The FDA does not approve containers as such, but only the materials used in the container. A list of substances considered "generally recognized as safe" (GRAS) has been published by the FDA. In the opinion of qualified experts, they are safe under specified conditions, assuming they are of good commercial quality. A material that is not included under GRAS or prior sanction, and is intended to be used with food, must be tested by the manufacturer, and the data must be submitted to the FDA. The FDA has published regulations (part 133) that implement the Current Good Manufacturing Practice requirements of section 501 (a) of the Act. Part 133.9 of these regulations sets forth criteria with respect to product containers, which manufacturers, processors, packers, or holders of drugs use as guidelines. The specific FDA regulation relative to drugs states that "containers, closures and other component parts of drug packages, to be suitable for their intended use, must not be reactive, additive or absorptive to an extent that the identity, strength, quality or purity of the drug will be affected." Any drug container must be approved for such use, along with the drug, before going on the market. The drug manufacturer must include data on the container and package components in contact with the pharmaceutical product in its New Drug Application (NDA). If the FDA can determine that the drug is safe and effective, and that the package is suitable, it approves the drug and package.

12.3.2 Stability Aspects of Packaging Materials

Information on stability is given in the guidelines for stability testing of pharmaceutical products containing well-established drug substances in conventional dosage forms. For primary packaging, it is necessary to know the possible interactions between the container and the contents. Normally, product/component stability and compatibility are confirmed during the primary research and development stage. While excluding the effect of external factors on the product, the packaging itself should not interact with it to introduce unacceptable changes.

There are numerous possibilities of interactions between (primary) packaging materials and pharmaceutical products, such as:

- release of chemicals from components of the packaging materials,
- release of visible and/or subvisible particles,
- absorption or adsorption of pharmaceutical components by the packaging materials,
- chemical reactions between the pharmaceutical product and the packaging materials,
- degradation of packaging components in contact with the pharmaceutical products, and
- influence of the manufacturing process (e.g., sterilization) on the container.

The active pharmaceutical ingredients should remain within their specification limits over the shelf-life of the pharmaceutical product. The question of whether a packaging will provide the required protection for the pharmaceutical product and the required stability over a certain period can only be answered by means of real-time stability studies. Such studies must evaluate the changes in the quality of the product, in contact with its packaging, during a period equivalent to its intended shelf-life.

In addition, packaging must meet the following requirements. It must

- preserve the physical properties of all dosage forms and protect them against damage or breakage,
- not alter the identity of the product,
- preserve the characteristic properties of the product, so that the latter complies with its specifications, and
- protect the product against undesirable or adulterating chemical, biological or physical entities.

12.4 QUALITY CONTROL OF PACKAGING MATERIALS

The USP defines the container closure system as that device that holds the drug and is or may be in direct contact with the drug. The immediate container is that which is always in direct contact with the drug. The closure is a part of the container. Packaging materials should not interact physically or chemically with the finished product to alter the strength, quality, or purity beyond specified requirements.

The compendium provide specifications and test procedures for light resistance: well closed, tightly closed, and four different types of glass containers. Specifications and test methods are designed for containers based on tests performed on the product in the container. The following features are to be considered in developing container specifications.

- Properties of container tightness.
- Moisture and vapour tightness regardless of container construction.
- Toxicity and chemical/physical characteristics of materials needed in container construction.
- Physical or chemical changes of container upon prolonged contact with product.
- Compatibility between container and product.

Good manufacturing practices require that stability data be submitted for the finished dosage form of the drug in the container closure system in which it is to be marketed. Quality control parameters for various containers are enlisted in the Table 12.2.

Table 12.2: Quality control profile of various packaging materials as per USP

Sl No.	Item	Function	Test Required
1.	High-density polyethylene containers	Containers for capsules and tablets	Multiple internal reflectance, thermal analysis, light transmission, water vapour permeation, extractable substances, non-volatile residue, heavy metals.
2.	Highly resistant, borosilicate glass (Type II)	Parenteral use	Light transmission, chemical resistance, powdered glass test.
3.	Treated soda-lime glass (Type II)	Acidic and neutral parenteral preparation	Light transmission, chemical resistance,water attack at 121° test.
4.	Soda-lime glass (Type III)	Parenteral and non-parenteral preparation	Light transmission, chemical resistance, powdered glass test.
5.	General purpose soda-lime glass	Non-parenteral articles, i.e., oral, or topical use	Light transmission, chemical resistance, powdered glass test.
6.	Elastomeric closure	Parenteral use	Biologic test—acute systemic toxicity, intracutaneous reactivity.

12.5 QUALITY CONTROL OF GLASS CONTAINERS

12.5.1 Evaluation Parameters

(a) ***Crushed-glass test:*** This test is official in USP. The container is crushed and sieved to produce uniform particles of which a definite weight is taken. The control of the particle size and weight of powder ensures that a constant surface area is exposed to the solution. Because all the glass (not just the surface layer) is examined and extraction is enhanced by the rough surfaces of the particles, this is a severe test, and, if a glass passes through this test, it is unlikely that containers made from it will give trouble while in use. Nevertheless, the technique is tedious and is not applicable to surface treated containers (sulphured or siliconized) because crushing would expose the alkaline glass below the surface. This test can be used for determining the nature of a glass or for distinguish between two types of glasses, such as neutral or surface treated.

(b) ***Whole-container test:*** This test is official in European, British and International Pharmacopoeias. It is used in the USP for treated soda-lime containers only. The containers are simply filled with the test solution and exposed to the test conditions. Glassware may pass the whole container test more easily because the surface layer of a container is smooth and less reactive.

In this test, surface area does not increase as much as volume with the increase in container size, consequently, the small sized containers are more attacked by the leaching of the alkali from the surface. The limits are given in Table 12.3.

Table 12.3: Surface area limits for glass containers which supplies alkali to each millilitre of the solution

Container	Surface area which supplies alkali to each millilitre of the solution.
Ampoule (1 mL)	5.9 cm^2
Ampoule (10 mL)	2.9 cm^2
Bottle (1000 mL)	0.5 cm^2

(c) ***Chemical resistance of test:*** USP and IP provide two tests to determine the chemical resistance of glass containers. Limits for alkalinity of glass containers are given in Table 12.4.

Table 12.4: Table shows limits of alkalinity for glass containers

Tests	Containers	Limits ml of 0.02 N Sulfuric acid
1. Powdered Glass Test	Type I	1.0
	Type III	8.5
	Type NP	15.0
2. Water Attack Test	type II (100 mL of less)	0.7
	type II (over 100 mL)	0.2

(d) ***Powdered Glass Test:*** From the glass containers, alkaline constituents (oxides of sodium, potassium, calcium, aluminium, etc.) are leached into purified water under conditions of elevated temperatures. When the glass is powdered the leaching of alkali can be enhanced in the powdered is critical.
The principle involved in the powdered glass test in estimate the amount of alkali leached from the glass powder. The amount of acid that is necessary to neutralize the released alkali (a specified limit) is specified in the pharmacopoeia. The basic analysis is acid-base titration using methyl red indicator.

(e) ***Water Attack Test:*** This test is used only with containers that have been exposed to sulphur dioxide fumes under controlled humidity conditions. Such a treatment neutralizes the surface alkali. Now the glass becomes chemically more resistant. The principle involved in the water attack test is to determine whether the alkali leached from the surface of a container is within the specified limits or not. Since the inner surface is under test, the entire container (ampoule) must be used. The amount of acid that is necessary to neutralize the released alkali from the surface is estimated, the leaching of alkali is accelerated using elevated temperature for a specified time. Methyl red indicator is used to determine the end point. The basic is acid-base titration.

12.6 QUALITY CONTROL OF PLASTIC CONTAINERS

Parenteral and non-parenteral preparations

1. **Leakage test**: Fill ten containers with water. Fit with intended closures and keep them inverted at room temperature for 24 hours. There are no signs of leakage from any container.
2. **Collapsibility test:** This test is applicable to containers. Which are to be squeezed in order to remove the contents. A container by collapsing inwards during use yields at least 90% of its nominal contents at the required rate of flow at ambient temperature.
3. **Clarity of aqueous extract:** Select unlabelled, unmarked and non-laminated portions from randomly selected containers. Cut pieces of sufficient surface area on both sides and cut them into strips none of which has a total area of more than 20 sq.cm. Wash the strips free from extraneous matter by shaking them with at least two separate portions of distilled water for about 30 seconds in each case, then draining off the water thoroughly.
4. **Transparency test:** Fill five empty containers to their nominal capacity with diluted suspension as described in IP 1966. The cloudiness of the diluted suspension in each container is detectable when viewed through the containers as compared with a container of the same type filled with water.
5. **Water vapour permeability test:** Fill five containers with nominal volume of water and heat seal the bottles with an aluminium foil-polyethylene laminate or other suitable seal. Weigh accurately each container and allow to stand (without any overwrap) for 14 days at a relative humidity of 60+5% and a temperature between 20 and 25 ^{0}C Reweigh the containers. The loss in weight in each container is not more than 0.2%.

Biological Tests

The USP has provided its procedures for evaluating the toxicity of plastic materials. This tests has three phases:

1. Implantation test: Implanting small pieces of plastic material intramuscularly in rabbits and observed for erythema.
2. Systemic injection test: Injecting eluates using sodium chloride injection, with and without alcohol intravenously in mice and injecting eluates using polyethylene glycol 400 and sesame oil intraperitoneally in mice.
3. Intracutaneous test: Injecting all four eluates subcutaneously in rabbits. The reaction from test samples must not be significantly greater than nonreactive control samples.

12.7 QUALITY CONTROL OF RUBBER CLOSURES

1. **Penetrability:** This is measured to check the force required to make a hypodermic needle penetrate easily through the closure. It is measured by using the piercing machine. The piercing force must not exceed a stated value. If it exceeds that stated value, the hypodermic needle can be damaged because of undesirable hardness of the closures.

2. **Fragmentation test**: This test is performed on 20 closures. Each closure is penetrated with hypodermic needle in a piercing machine five times within a limited area and needle is washed to transfer any fragment present. The contents are filtered through coloured paper that contrasts with the rubber and the fragments counted. On an average there should not be more than three fragments per unit.
3. **Self sealability test:** Applicable to multidose containers, fill 10 vials with water close them with prepared closures and secure with a cap. For each closure use a new hypodermic needle and pierce 10 times each time at different sites, immerse the vials upright in methylene blue (0.1%) solution and reduce external pressure for 10 minutes. Restore the atmospheric pressure and leave the vials immersed for 30 minutes. Rinse the outside of the vials. None of the vials contains any trace of coloured solution.
4. **Extractive test:** In this test, the closure is boiled with water for four hours under reflux and the water evaporated to dryness. The residue must not exceed the specified amount.
5. **Compatibility test:** This test is performed to check the compatibility of the rubber closures with various types of the substances, since it is necessary to ensure that there is no interaction between the contents of the bottle and the closure.
6. **Light absorption:** Filter extractive test solution through membrane filter. Measure the light absorbance of filtrate in the range 220 to 360 nm using a blank solution (prepared in the same manner as test solution). The absorbance is not more than 2.

REVIEW QUESTIONS

Long Answers

1. Explain pharmaceutical packaging materials and their standards.
2. Write in detail about plastics used in pharmaceutical packaging.
3. Explain the factors determining the choice of a packaging system.

Short Answers

1. Define packaging and what are the levels of packaging?
2. Explain the quality control test for glass containers.
3. Discuss the quality control test for plastic containers.
4. Write about HDPE as a packing material.
5. Write a note on rubber closures.
6. What are the problems associated with plastic containers?

13

PILOT PLANT SCALE-UP TECHNIQUES

Learning Objectives

After going through this chapter, you would be able to:

1. Understand the general considerations of pilot plant scale-up.
2. Understand the features of processing equipment for production and process control.
3. Discuss the pilot plant scale-up requirements for solid, liquids and semi-solid dosage forms.
4. Explain the pilot plant scale-up considerations for raw materials, personnel and space requirements.
5. Understand the SUPAC guidelines.
6. Know the pharmaceutical platform technology.
7. Know the pharmaceutical platform technology.

13.1 INTRODUCTION

"Defined as a part of the pharmaceutical industry where a lab scale formula is transformed into a viable product by the development of liable practical procedure for manufacture."

Why conduct pilot plant studies?

- A pilot plant allows investigation of a product and process on an intermediate scale before large amounts of money are committed to full-scale production.
- It is usually not possible to predict the effects of a manifold increase in scale.
- It is not possible to design a large complex food processing plant from laboratory data alone with any degree of success.

A pilot plant can be used for

- Evaluating the results of laboratory studies and making product and process corrections and improvements.
- Producing small quantities of product for sensory, chemical, microbiological evaluations, limited market testing or furnishing samples to potential customers, shelf-live and storage stability studies.
- Determining possible saleable by-products or waste stream requiring treatment before discharge.
- Providing data that can be used in making a decision on whether or not to proceed to a full-scale production process; and in the case of a positive decision, designing and constructing a full-size plant or modifying an existing plant.

Considerations in pilot plant development

- Kind and size: depend on goals; evaluating product and process; producing samples of product for evaluation; market testing or furnishing to potential customers.
- Location: Near R&D facility? At an existing plant? Close liaison between R&D and pilot plant staff is essential.
- Labor requirements and costs: engineering staff, skilled operations and maintenance staff-pilot plant costs may exceed those of usual plant production costs. The pilot plant may be used for training personnel for a full-scale plant.

Objectives of scale-up

"Find mistakes on small scale and make profit on large scale."

- To produce physically and chemically stable therapeutic dosage forms.
- Review of the processing equipment.
- Guidelines for production and process control.
- Evaluation and validation.
- To identify the critical features of the process.
- To provide master manufacturing formula.

Pilot p studies include the close examination of the formulations to determine:

- Its ability to withstand batch scale.
- Process modification.
- Compatibility of the equipment with the formulation.
- Cost factor.
- Availability of raw materials meeting the specifications required to produce the product.
- Market requirement.
- Physical space required and the layout of the related functions.

Thus, during the scale-up efforts in the pilot plant:

- Production and process controls are evaluated, validated and finalized. Product reprocessing procedures are developed and validated.
- Appropriate records and reports are issued to support cGMP.

In short, all critical features of a process must be identified so that as the process is scaled up, it can be adequately monitored to provide assurance that the process is under control and that the product produced at each level of the scale-up maintains the specified attributes originally intended.

13.2 PILOT PLANT DESIGN

A pilot plant design should support three key strategic objectives:

- Formulation and process development.
- Clinical supply to manufacture.
- Technology evaluation, scale-up and transfer.

Attributes playing a key role in achieving the above objectives are:

- cGMP compliance.
- A flexible highly trained staff.
- Equipment to support multiple dosage form development.
- Equipment at multiple scales based on similar operating principles to those in production.

The pilot plant design should be according to cGMP norms. The layout should be according to the need for flexibility (portable equipment installed, use of multipurpose rooms), restricted access, personnel flow and material flow. The facility and equipment should be able to capture critical process information. Intermediate sized and full-scale production equipment should be available in order to evaluate the effects of scale-up of research formulations. Adequate space required to carry out each function smoothly (e.g., cleaning of pilot plant equipment). The final design should result in a facility that supports the key strategic objectives and should have low maintenance and operating costs.

Although the pilot plant design must simulate the manufacturing environment in which the new product will ultimately be produced, there are many differences in operation because of the specific objectives of the two types of facilities, i.e., the pilot plant facilitates product development activities, whereas the manufacturing plant routinely fabricates products for the market.

13.3 PILOT PLANT OPERATION

Operational aspects of pilot plant includes:

Validation
Training
Engineering Support
Maintenance
Calibration
Material Control
Inventory
Orders
Labelling

Validation: A validation master plan should be developed that addresses:

- Design qualification
- Installation qualification
- Operational qualification
- Performance qualification

A fully validated pilot plant should ensure compliance with cGMP and should meet current FDA standards.

Training: Training in four major areas required:

- Compliance with quality standards such as cGMP
- Safety and environmental responsibilities
- Compliance with SOPs
- Technical skills and knowledge

Engineering Support: It is required for:

- Design, construction, commissioning and validation of the pilot plant facility.
- Coordination, scheduling and direction of ongoing operations.

Maintenance: It is required to:

- Meet cGMP norms.
- To ensure data integrity and equipment reliability during the development process.
- The maintenance programme should be documented and written procedure established.

Calibration: Calibration of critical instruments/equipment is required for:

- Compliance with cGMP.
- Maintaining the integrity of data generated during the development process.
- Calibration should be performed by well trained and expert staff.

Material Control: More flexible and efficient computer based system is required for material control in a pilot plant.

Inventory: Inventory should be maintained in a computer based inventory ordering dispensing system.

Orders: All orders must be placed through the computer system. For placement of the order, First in First out (FIFO) criteria is followed.

Labelling: Labels should comply with GMP-GLP requirements. Computer system must be used for labelling.

Process and manufacturing activities:

- Formulation and process development studies.
- Clinical supply manufacture.
- Technology evaluation, scale-up and transfer.
- Precise documentation of each trial has to be made.

Quality assurance and A-Quality control:

AQ Activities

- Auditing pilot plant.
- Auditing and approval of component suppliers.
- Reviewing, approving and maintaining batch records for clinical supplies.
- Sampling and release of raw materials and components required for clinical supplies.
- Release of clinical supplies.

- Maintaining and distributing facility and operating procedures (SOPs).
- Review and approval of validation and engineering documentation.

QC Activities

- Release testing of finished products.
- Physical, chemical, and microbiological testing of finished clinical products.
- Components and raw materials.
- Testing for validation and revalidation programmes.
- QC in-process testing during development, scale-up, and technology transfer activities.

13.4 GENERAL CONSIDERATIONS

Personnel Requirements

- Scientists with experience in pilot plant operations as well as in actual production area are the most preferable.
- As they have to understand the intent of the formulator as well as understand the perspective of the production personnel.
- The group should have some personnel with engineering knowledge as well as scale-up also involves engineering principles.

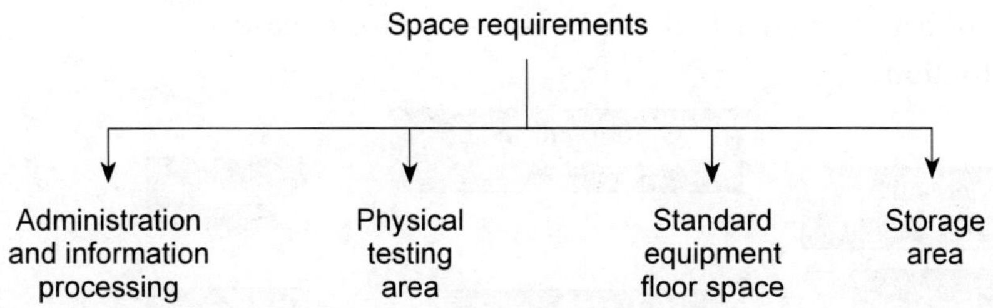

- Separate provisions for API and excipients further segregated into approved and unapproved areas according to GMP.
- Storage area for in-process materials, finished bulk products, retained samples, experimental production batches, packaging materials (segregated into approved and unapproved areas).
- Controlled environment space allocated for storage of stability samples.

Review of the formula

- A thorough review of the each aspect of formulation is important.
- The purpose of each ingredient and its contribution to the final product manufactured on the small-scale laboratory equipment should be understood.
- Then the effect of scale-up using equipment that may subject the product to stresses of different types and degrees can more readily be predicted, or recognized.

Raw materials

One purpose/responsibility of the pilot plant is the approval and validation of the active ingredient and excipients raw materials. Raw materials used in the small-scale production cannot necessarily be the representative for the large-scale production.

Relevant processing equipment

- The most economical and the simplest and efficient equipment which are capable of producing product within the proposed specifications.
- The size of the equipment should be such that the experimental trial runs should be relevant to the production size batches.
- If the equipment is too small the process developed will not scale-up, whereas if the equipment is too big then there may be wastage of the expensive active ingredients.

Production rates

It can be determined by the immediate future market requirements.

Equipment and the process should be chosen on the basis of production of a batch at frequency that takes into consideration:

1. Product loss in the equipment during manufacture.
2. The time required to clean the equipment between batches.
3. The number of batches that need to be tested for release.

Process evaluation:

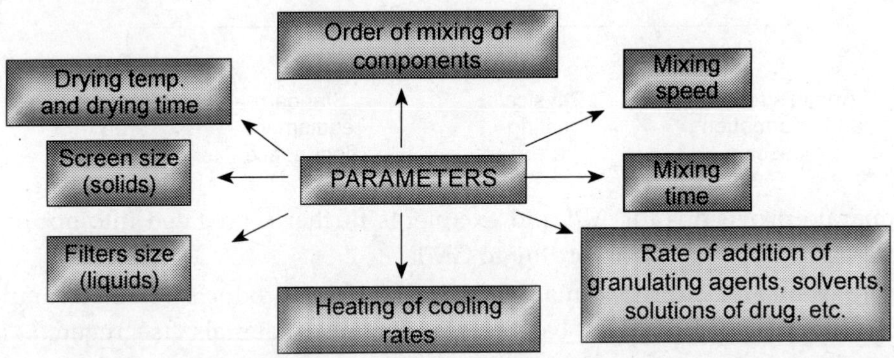

- It is the basis of process validation documentation of the process to be done. Process is validated only if there are no changes in the formula, quality of the ingredients, or the equipment configuration.
- Revalidation needs to be done to ensure that changes have not taken place.

Preparation of master manufacturing procedures: It includes:

- The chemical weigh sheets. It should clearly identify the chemicals required in a batch and present the quantities and the order in which they will be used.
- The sampling directions.
- In-process and finished product specifications.

- Manufacturing directions should be in a language understandable by the operator.
- Batch record directions should include specifications for addition rates, mixing times, mixing speeds, heating and cooling rates, and temperature.
- Proper documentation should be carried out.

Product stability and uniformity:

- The primary objective of the pilot plant is the physical as well as chemical stability of the products.
- Hence, each pilot batch representing the final formulation and manufacturing procedure should be studied for stability.
- Stability studies should be carried out in finished packages as well.

13.5 GMP CONSIDERATIONS

GMP items that should be a part of scale up are:

- Equipment qualification
- Process validation
- Regularly scheduled preventative maintenance
- Regularly process review and revalidation
- Relevant written standard operating procedures
- The use of competent technically qualified personnel
- Adequate provision for training of personnel
- A well-defined technology transfer system
- Validated cleaning procedures
- An orderly arrangement of equipment so as to ease material flow and prevent cross- contamination

Transfer of analytical methods to quality assurance

Analytical methods developed in research must be transferred to QA department. Transfer process includes:

1. Review the process to make sure that proper analytical instrument is available.
2. Personnel should be trained to perform the test.
3. Reliability of the test should be checked.
4. At last assay procedure should be reviewed before transfer.

Scale-up techniques

Scale-up: The are for designing of prototype using the data obtained from the pilot plant model.

13.6 STEPS IN SCALE UP

Define product economics based on projected market size and competitive selling and provide guidance for allowable manufacturing costs

↓

Conduct laboratory studies and scale-up planning at the same time

↓

Define key rate-controlling steps in the proposed process

↓

Conduct preliminary larger-than-laboratory studies with equipment to be used in rate-controlling step to aid in plant design

↓

Design and construct a pilot plant including provisions for process and environmental controls, cleaning and sanitizing systems, packaging and waste handling systems, and meeting regulatory agency requirements

13.6.1 Pilot Plant Design for Tablets

- The primary responsibility of the pilot plant staff is to ensure that the newly formulated tablets developed by product development personnel will prove to be efficiently, economically, and consistently reproducible on a production scale.
- The design and construction of the pharmaceutical pilot plant for tablet development should incorporate features necessary to facilitate maintenance and cleanliness.
- If possible, it should be located on the ground floor to expedite the delivery and shipment of supplies.
- Extraneous and microbiological contamination must be guarded against by incorporating the following features in the pilot plant design:
- Fluorescent lighting fixtures should be the ceiling flush type.
- The various operating areas should have floor drains to simplify cleaning.
- The area should be air-conditioned and humidity controlled.
- High-density concrete floors should be installed.
- The walls in the processing and packaging areas should be enamel-cement finish on concrete.
- Equipment in the pharmaceutical pilot plant should be similar to that used by production division-manufacture of tablets.

1. Material handling system

- In the laboratory, materials are simply scooped or poured by hand, but in intermediate- or large-scale operations, handling of materials often becomes necessary.

- If a system is used to transfer materials for more than one product steps must be taken to prevent cross contamination.
- Any material handling system must deliver the accurate amount of the ingredient to the destination.
- The type of system selected also depends on the characteristics of the materials.
- More sophisticated methods of handling materials such as vacuum loading systems, metering pumps, screw feed system, etc.

2. Dry Blending

- Powders to be used for encapsulation or to be granulated must be well blended to ensure good drug distribution. Inadequate blending at this stage could result in discrete portion of the batch being either high or low in potency.
- Steps should also be taken to ensure that all the ingredients are free of lumps and agglomerates.
- For these reasons, screening and/or milling of the ingredients usually makes the process more reliable and reproducible.

The equipment used for blending are:

- V-blender
- Double cone blender, ribbon blender, slant cone blender.
- Bin blender
- Orbiting screw blenders vertical and horizontal high intensity mixers.

3. Granulation

The most common reasons given to justify granulating are:

- To impart good flow properties to the material.
- To increase the apparent density of the powders.
- To change the particle size distribution.
- Uniform dispersion of active ingredient.

Traditionally, wet granulation has been carried out using:

- Sigma blade mixer.
- Heavy-duty planetary mixer.

Wet granulation can also be prepared using tumble blenders equipped with high-speed chopper blades. More recently, the use of multifunctional "processors" that are capable of performing all functions required to prepare a finished granulation, such as dry blending, wet granulation, drying, sizing and lubrication in a continuous process in a single equipment.

Fluidized bed granulations:

1. Process inlet air temperature
2. Atomization air pressure
3. Air volume
4. Liquid spray rate
5. Nozzle position and number of spray heads
6. Product and exhaust air temperature

7. Filter porosity
8. Cleaning erequency
9. Bowl capacity

4. Binders

- Used in tablet formulations to make powders more compressible and to produce tablets that are more resistant to breakage during handling.
- In some instances, the binding agent imparts viscosity to the granulating solution so that transfer of fluid becomes difficult.
- This problem can be overcome by adding some or all binding agents in the dry powder prior to granulation.
- Some granulation, when prepared in production sized equipment, take on a dough-like consistency and may have to be subdivided to a more granular and porous mass to facilitate drying.
- This can be accomplished by passing the wet mass through an oscillating type granulator with a suitably large screen or a hammer mill with either a suitably large screen or no screen at all.

5. Drying

- The most common conventional method of drying a granulation continues to be the circulating hot air oven, which is heated by either steam or electricity.
- The important factor to consider as part of scale-up of an oven drying operation are airflow, air temperature, and the depth of the granulation on the trays.
- If the granulation bed is too deep or too dense, the drying process will be inefficient, and if soluble dyes are involved, there may be migration of the dye to the surface of the granules.
- Drying times at specified temperatures and air flow rates must be established for each product, and for each particular oven load.
- Fluidized bed dryers are an attractive alternative to the circulating hot air ovens.
- The important factors considered as part of scale-up fluidized bed dryer are optimum loads, rate of air flow, inlet air temperature and humidity.

Tray dryer parameters to be considered for scale-up are:

1. Air flow
2. Air temperature
3. Depth of the granulation on the trays
4. Monitoring of the drying process by the use of moisture and temperature probes
5. Drying times at specified temperatures and air flow rates for each product

Fluidized bed dryer: Parameters to be considered for scale-up are:

1. Optimum load
2. Air flow rate
3. Inlet rir temperature
4. Humidity of the incoming air

6. Reduction of Particle Size

- Compression factors that may be affected by the particle size distribution are flowability, compressibility, uniformity of tablet weight, content uniformity, tablet hardness, and tablet colour uniformity.
- First step in this process is to determine the particle size distribution of granulation using a series of "stacked" sieves of decreasing mesh openings.
- Particle size reduction of the dried granulation of production size batches can be carried out by passing all the material through an oscillating granulator, a hammer mill, a mechanical sieving device, or in some cases, a screening device.
- As part of the scale-up of a milling or sieving operation, the lubricants and glidants, which in the laboratory are usually added directly to the final blend, are usually added to the dried granulation during the sizing operation. This is done because some of these additives, especially magnesium stearate, tend to agglomerate when added in large quantities to the granulation in a blender.

7. Blending

Type of blending equipment often differs from that used in laboratory.

In any blending operation, both segregation and mixing occur simultaneously. These are functions of particle size, shape, hardness, and density, and of the dynamics of the mixing action.

Particle abrasion is more likely to occur when high-shear mixers with spiral screws or blades are used.

When a low dose active ingredient is to be blended it may be sandwiched between two portions of directly compressible excipients to avoid loss to the surface of the blender.

In scale-up of blending, following parameters should be considered:

1. Blender loads
2. Blender size
3. Mixing speeds
4. Mixing times
5. Bulk density of the raw material (must be considered in selecting blender and in determining optimum blender load).
6. Characteristics of the material

8. Specialized Granulation procedures

Slugging (Dry Granulation)

- A dry powder blend that cannot be directly compressed because of poor flow or compression properties. This is done on a tablet press designed for slugging, which operates at pressures of about 15 tonnes, compared with a normal tablet press, which operates at pressure of 4 tonnes or less.

- Slugs range in diameter from 1 inch, for the more easily slugged material, to ¾ inch in diameter for materials that are more difficult to compress and require more pressure per unit area to yield satisfactory compacts.
- If an excessive amount of fine powder is generated during the milling operation the material must be screened and fines recycled through the slugging operation.

Dry Compaction

- Granulation by dry compaction can also be achieved by passing powders between two rollers that compact the material at pressure of up to 10 tonnes per linear inch.
- Materials of very low density require roller compaction to achieve a bulk density sufficient to allow encapsulation or compression.
- One of the best examples of this process is the densification of aluminium hydroxide.
- Pilot plant personnel should determine whether the final drug blend or the active ingredient could be more efficiently processed in this manner than by conventional processing in order to produce a granulation with the required tableting or encapsulation properties.

Compression

The ultimate test of a tablet formulation and granulation process is whether the granulation can be compressed on a high-speed tablet press. During compression, the tablet press performs the following functions:

1. Filling of empty die cavity with granulation.
2. Pre-compression of granulation (optional).
3. Compression of granules.

Ejection of the tablet from the die cavity and take-off of compressed tablet.

- When evaluating the compression characteristics of a particular formulation, prolonged trial runs at press speeds equal to that to be used in normal production should be tried.
- Only then are potential problems such as sticking to the punch surface, tablet hardness, capping, and weight variation detected.
- High-speed tablet compression depends on the ability of the press to interact with granulation.

Following are the parameters to be considered while choosing speed of press.

1. Granulation feed rate.
2. Delivery system should not change the particle size distribution.
3. System should not cause segregation of coarse and fine particles, nor it should induce static charges.

The die feed system must be able to fill the die cavities adequately in the short period of time that the die is passing under the feed frame. The smaller the tablet, the more difficult it is to get a uniform fill at high press speed. For high-speed machines, induced die feed systems is necessary.

These are available with a variety of feed paddles and with variable speed capabilities, so that optimum feed for every granulation can be obtained.

After the die cavities are filled, the excess is removed by the feed frame to the centre of the die table. Compression of the granulation usually occurs as a single event as the heads of the punches pass over the lower and under the upper pressure rollers.

This causes the punches to penetrate the die to a preset depth, compacting the granulation to the thickness of the gap set between the punches.

The rapidity and dwell time in between this press event occurs is determined by the speed at which the press is rotating and by the size of compression rollers.

Larger the compressions roller, the more gradually compression force is applied and released. Slowing down the press speed or using larger compression rollers can often reduce capping in a formulation. The final event is ejection of compressed tablets from die cavity. During compression, the granulation is compacted to form tablet, bonds within compressible material must be formed which results in sticking.

High level of lubricant or ove- blending can result in a soft tablet, decrease in wettability of the powder and an extension of the dissolution time. Binding to die walls can also be overcome by designing the die to be 0.001 to 0.005 inch wider at the upper portion than at the centre in order to relieve pressure during ejection.

Tablet Coating

Sugar coating, carried out in conventional coating pans, has undergone many changes because of new developments in coating technology and changes in safety and environmental regulations.

The conventional sugar coating pan has given way to perforated pans or fluidized bed coating columns.

The development of new polymeric materials has resulted in a change from aqueous sugar coating and more recently, to aqueous film coating.

The tablets must be sufficiently hard to withstand the tumbling to which they are subjected in either the coating pan or the coating column.

Some tablet core materials are naturally hydrophobic, and in these cases, film coating with an aqueous system may require special formulation of the tablet core and/or the coating solution. A film coating solution may have been found to work well with a particular tablet in small lab coating pan but may be totally unacceptable on a production scale.

This is because of increased pressure and abrasion to which tablets are subjected when batch size is large and different in temperature and humidity to which tablets are exposed while coating and drying process.

Scale-up for liquid orals

- The physical form of a drug product that is pourable displays Newtonian or pseudoplastic flow behaviour and conforms to its container at room temperature.

- Liquid dosage forms may be dispersed systems or solutions.
- In dispersed systems there are two or more phases, where one phase is distributed in another.
- A solution refers two or more substances mixed homogeneously.

Steps of liquid manufacturing process

1. Planning of material requirements:
2. Liquid preparation
3. Filling and packing
4. Quality assurance

13.6.2 Critical Aspects of Liquid Manufacturing

Physical Plant

Heating, ventilation and air controlling system

The effect of long processing times at suboptimal temperatures should be considered in terms of consequences on the physical or chemical stability of ingredients as well as product.

Solution

Parameters to be considered are:

1. Tank size (diameter)
2. Impeller type
3. Impeller diameter
4. Rotational speed of the impeller
5. Number of impellers
6. Number of baffles
7. Mixing capability of impeller
8. Clearance between impeller blades and wall of the mixing tank
9. Height of the filled volume in the tank
10. Filtration equipment (should not remove active or adjuvant ingredients)
11. Transfer system
12. Passivation of SS (pretreating the SS with acetic acid or nitric acid solution to remove the surface alkalinity of the SS).

Suspension:

Parameters to be considered are:

1. Addition and dispersion of suspending agents (lab scale sprinkling method and production scale – vibrating feed system)
2. Hydration/wetting of suspending agent
3. Time and temperature required for hydration of suspending agent
4. Mixing speeds (high speed leads to air entrapment)
5. Selection of the equipment according to batch size
6. Versator (to avoid air entrapment)

7. Mesh size (the one which is chosen must be capable of removing the unwanted foreign particulates but should not filter out any of the active ingredients. Such a sieve can only be selected based on production batch size trials.)

Emulsion

Parameters to be considered are:

1. Temperature
2. Mixing equipment
3. Homogenizing equipment
4. In-process or final product filters
5. Screens, pumps and filling equipment
6. Phase volumes
7. Phase viscosities
8. Phase densities

Formulation aspects of oral liquids

Solutions:

Protecting the API	Buffers, antioxidants, preservatives
Maintaining the appearance	Colourings, stabilizers, co-solvents, antimicrobial preservatives
Taste/smell masking	Sweeteners, flavourings.

Suspensions

Purpose	Agent
Facilitating the connection between API and vehicle	Wetting agents Salt formation ingredients
Protecting the API	Buffering systems, polymers, antioxidants
Maintaining the suspension appearance	Colourings, suspending agent, flocculating agent.
Masking the unpleasant taste/smell	Sweeteners, flavourings

Emulsions:

Purpose	Agent
Particle size	Solid particles, droplet particles
Protecting the API	Buffering systems, antioxidants, polymers
Maintaining the appearance	Colourings, emulsifying agents, penetration enhancers, gelling agents
Taste/smell masking	Sweeteners, flavourings

13.6.3 Pilot Plant Scale-up for Semi-solid Products

The following parameters are to be considered during the scale-up of semisolid products:

1. Mixing equipment (should effectively move semi-solid mass from outside walls to the centre and from bottom to top of the kettle).
2. Motors (used to drive mixing system must be sized to handle the product at its most viscous stage)
3. Mixing speed
4. Component homogenization
5. Heating and cooling process
6. Addition of active ingredients
7. Product transfer
8. Working temperature range (critical to the quality of the final product)
9. Shear during handling and transfer from manufacturing to holding tank to filling lines
10. Transfer pumps (must be able to move viscous material without applying excessive shear and without incorporating air)
11. While choosing the size and type of pump
    (a) Product viscosity
    (b) Pumping rate
    (c) Product compatibility with the pump surface
    (d) Pumping pressure required should be considered.

13.6.4 Scale-up of Liquid and Semi-solid Manufacturing Processes

In mixing and semi-solid manufacturing, mixing is an important operation.

Flow regimes in pharmaceutical system undergoing mixing process may range from laminar to turbulent to transitional flow. The flow regime in the vicinity of an impeller is often turbulent while the flow regime elsewhere in the system can be laminar or transitional.

For turbulent flow regime, power is ρN3D2 (ρ = density; N = rotational speed; D = Diameter of impeller).

For laminar flow regime, power is ηN2 (η = viscosity)

Scale-up of solutions: Three methods can be applied.

1. Power Law Approach

N2 = N1 (1 ÷ R)n

n is power law exponent

N1 & N2 are rotational speed of impeller

R is geometric scaling factor such as: D1T1 or D2T2 (D = impeller diameter and T is mixing tank diameter); Z1T1 or Z2T2 (Z = height of liquid in the mixing tank)

2. Dimensionless Numbers

Reynolds number (the ratio of inertial to viscous forces in a flow)

Re = (D2ρN ÷ η)

Froude number (the ratio of inertial stress to the gravitational force per unit area in a liquid)

Fr = (DN2 ÷ g)

It is a means of correlating process characteristics at various production scales.

D = Diameter of impeller; N = Rotational speed of impeller

η = Viscosity; ρ = Density; g = Acceleration gravity

3. Scale of agitation approach

Applicable only if system shows Newtonian flow and geometric similarity. The rheological behaviour of shear-thinning (pseudoplastic) systems may be described by the Ostwald-de Wale equation between the shear rate extremes corresponding to the zero-shear viscosity, η_0 and to the infinite shear viscosity, $\eta\infty$

T = Kγa

In which T is the shear stress, γ is the rate of shear and, K and a are constants.

The ratio of η:η_0 corresponding to the ratio of T:T0 would then be used to facilitate scaling.

13.6.5 Scale-up and Post-approval Changes (SUPAC)

Approval of ANDA is the start of generic drug product history. Changes are made frequently to chemistry and manufacturing controls after approval throughout the scale-up, post-approval changes (SUPAC) and post-marketing surveillance in the life term of product.

Manufacturing may bring changes in drug formulation, batch size, process, equipment; mfg. site may affect the identity, strength, quality, purity and potency of the finished product.

- Changes to approved ANDA may be done as per revised market forecast: change in batch size, qualification of new API, source optimization of manufacturing process.
- Upgrade of container/closure.
- Enhancement of analytical method.
- Change made may have adverse effects depending on the type or dosage form or product.

For example, change in container/closures (solid/parenterals), conc. of inactive (immediate release/sustained release) impacts bioavailability.

Frequent and numerous changes may render the product substantially different from the one approved in original ANDA. Supportive data is to be submitted and comparison with original exhibit batch/bio batch will be done.

SUPAC guidelines

- Prior to FDAMA, basis of revision of FD&C Guidance for Industry: Scale-up & post approval changes (SUPAC). Provided the clear, definitive language regarding regulatory notification process and requirements for post-approval changes, reduced regulatory burden on industry. Classified into levels, provided requirements for each level.

- SUPAC expanded 21 CFR 314.70 and defined in much detail the types of changes and reporting category required.

In the following areas the change is likely

- Components and composition of the drug product
- Manufacturing site change
- Scale-up of the drug product
- Manufacturing equipment
- Packaging

SUPAC describes 3 levels of changes

Recommends chemistry, manufacturing and control tests, *in vitro* dissolution tests, and bioequivalence tests for each level.

Level and Definition

1. Changes those are unlikely to have any detectable impact on formulation quality and performance.
2. Changes that could have a significant impact on formulation quality and performance.
3. Changes those are likely to have a significant impact on formulation quality and performance.

13.6.6 Current Requirements for Post-approval Changes

1. Components/composition
2. Site changes
3. Change in batch size
4. Manufacturing
5. Specifications
6. Packaging

1. Components/Composition

- Changes to the qualitative/quantitative composition of the formulation are considered major changes.
- These changes must be considered carefully before implementation. Such changes require a "Prior Approval Supplement" unless otherwise exempted by regulation or guidance documents.
- Current guidance for industry, changes to an approved ANDA or NDA, does not address components/composition in detail.
- SUPAC guidance remains in effect for defining components and composition changes and the reporting category.
- Addition or deletion of an ingredient can have an adverse effect on the dissolution profile of the finished product and on the *in vivo* bioequivalence to the RLD.
- Addition or deletion of an ingredient must be filed as a Prior Approval Supplement.

- Exceptions - colours (removed/reduced).
- Some cases - less stringent reporting.

2. Site Changes

- The sponsor of an ANDA include in its application the site of manufacture, where the drug product will be produced, tested, packaged, and/or labelled.
- A change in any of these sites can adversely affect the identity, strength, quality, purity, or potency of the finished product.
- Any site change under SUPAC-IR calls for the new site to be in compliance with good manufacturing practice (cGMP) regulations.
- A stand-alone packaging operation site change, utilizing container (s)/closure(s) in the approved application, may be submitted as a "Change Being Effected Supplement".
- Facility should also have a current and satisfactory cGMP compliance profile with FDA.
- If the facility has not received a satisfactory cGMP Inspection within the previous two years for the type of packaging operation involved, a "Prior Approval Supplement" with the same commitment for stability is recommended.
- Supplement should also contain a commitment to place the first production batch of the product on long-term stability studies using the approved protocol in the application and to submit the resulting data in annual reports.

3. Change in Batch Size

- Change in batch size from pivotal/pilot scale bio-batch to larger or smaller production batches tends to change the operating parameters. Therefore, all the parameters, such as mixing time, speed, etc., are adjusted according to the equipment (large or small) used in the process.
- This requires proper validation of the batches before submission of additional information in the application.
- Any change in the production batch for which the operating parameter falls within the range established for the ANDA batch and validation batches will be regarded as a level 1 change.
- If it falls outside the validation ranges, the change would be permitted under SUPAC-IR as level 2 changes.
- Regardless, SUPAC-IR does not address scale-down below 1,00,000 units.

4. Manufacturing

This includes any change made in equipment and the process used in manufacturing a drug product.

Equipment change

- Any change in manufacturing equipment other than that used in the approved application requires appropriate validation studies to demonstrate that the new equipment is similar to the original equipment.
- Equipment within the same class and subclass would be considered to have the same design and operating principle under SUPAC-IR.

  E.g: Change in diff Mfr of V-cone blender isacceptable.

- Change from one class of equipment to another would be considered a change in design and operating principle and would be considered different under SUPAC-IR.

  E.g: V-cone blender to ribbon blender.
- A guidance for industry, SUPAC-IR/MR: Immediate Release and Modified Solid Oral Dosage Forms Manufacturing Equipment Addendum, 1999 (3), explains in detail about various changes in equipment and the regulatory requirement.
- The two different levels of change and regulatory requirements on change.

Process change

- Change in manufacturing process or technology may have adverse effects on the identity, strength, quality, purity, or potency of a drug product.
- The safety or effectiveness of the product depends on the type of the manufacturing process and the changes being instituted for the drug substance or drug product.
- Any fundamental change in the manufacturing process, e.g., dry to wet granulation or change from one type of drying process to another (e.g., oven tray, fluid bed) is considered a major change, whereas change in mixing time, operating speed, etc., within an approved range is considered a minor change.

Specifications

- Specifications are the standards a drug product must meet to ensure conformance to predetermined criteria for consistency, reproducibility, and quality.
- Such changes generally require a "Prior Approval Supplement" unless the specification is tightening or otherwise exempted by regulation guidance documents.
- Prior approval is required on the following major changes in specification except as provided in the SUPAC-IR guidance.
  - Relaxing an acceptance criterion
  - Deleting any part of a specification
- Changing or establishing a new regulatory analytical procedure that does not provide the same or increased assurance of the identity, strength, quality, purity, or potency of the material being tested as the analytical procedure described in the approved application.
- At 30 days changes being effected supplement needs to be filed in case of moderate changes in specifications, e.g., change in regulatory analytical procedures other than editorial or identified as major change.
- A change in analytical procedure or deletion of a test for raw materials used in drug substance.
- The following changes in specifications that are considered to have minimal potential for an adverse effect on the identity, strength, quality, purity, or potency of a product as they may relate to the safety or effectiveness of the product, and therefore can be submitted in an annual report:

- Change in specification made to comply with an official compendium.
- Change in analytical procedure for testing raw material, drug substance or drug product that provides the same or increased assurance of identity, strength, purity, or potency of the material being tested as the analytical procedure described in the approved application.
- Tightening of acceptance criteria.

5. Packaging

A container/closure system for a solid oral dosage form tends to be low risk and will have little impact on the shelf life of the finished product. Therefore, under the new guidance for industry, and the stability guidance, the requirements for packaging changes have been relaxed significantly.

Comparability Protocols

A comparability protocol is a plan for anticipated future CMC changes. FDA recently published a draft guidance, Comparability Protocols Chemistry, Manufacturing, and Controls Information, to provide recommendations on preparing and using comparability protocols for post-approval changes in the CMC section of an NDA or ANDA.

According to the guidance, "A comparability protocol is a well defined, detailed, written plan for assessing the effect of specific CMC changes in the identity, strength, quality, purity, and potency of a specific drug product as these factors relate to the safety and effectiveness of the product. A comparability protocol describes the changes that are covered under the protocol and specifies the tests and studies that will be performed, including analytical procedures that will be used, and acceptance criteria that will be achieved to demonstrate that specified CMC changes do not adversely affect the product."

A comparability protocol may be submitted with an ANDA or NDA application or as a Prior Approval Supplement (post-approval).

The benefit of the comparability protocol is that an FDA request for additional information to support a change is less likely when the change is covered under an approved protocol.

Thus, the sponsor could implement a CMC post-approval change as described in the comparability protocol.

Post-Marketing Surveillance

- Once the FDA approves a generic drug product, manufacturers are responsible for conducting post-marketing surveillance.
- Post-marketing reporting requirements for an approved ANDA are set forth in the US Federal Code of Regulations, 21 CFR 314.80 (5) and 314.98.
- The main component of this requirement is the reporting of adverse drug experiences (ADEs).
- According to 21 CFR 314.80(a), an adverse drug experience is defined as "any adverse event associated with the use of a drug in humans, whether or not considered drug related".

- The definition continues by stating that adverse events include those that occur in the course of the use of a drug product in professional practice, occur from drug overdose (accidental or intentional), abuse, or withdrawal, or involve failure of expected pharmacological action.
- According to the definition, it is irrelevant whether or not an event is considered drug related.
- The fact that an adverse event occurred while a person was using a drug product is reason enough to consider it an ADE.

Platform technology

A platform is a group of technologies that are used as a base upon which other applications, processes or technologies are developed.

Platform technologies such as sustained release and combination products, and in key platforms to enhance drug delivery system capabilities. These technologies enhance the drug's safety and its efficacy by a targeted therapy approach. In some instances, the convenience of patients is an important factor. The strategic aim is to formulate differentiated products that overcome the key.

Nanotechnology

- Nanotechnology has been adapted to develop targeted therapies for diseases like cancer. It involves employing nano-size particles to deliver drugs to specific types of cells such as cancer cells.
- The particles are engineered so that they are attracted to diseased cells which allow direct treatment of those cells. We have been successful in developing and manufacturing a number of nanotech based products such as paclitaxel, fenofibrate and sirolimus, amongst others.
- The aim is to prevent unwanted toxicity due to wide distribution, improve patient compliance and thus provide favourable clinical outcomes.
- Nanotechnology addresses the challenges of undesirable physiochemical properties of certain drugs which lead to poor pharmacokinetics. Nanoparticulate drug delivery systems show a promising approach to obtain desirable drug-like properties by altering the biopharmaceutics and pharmacokinetics properties of the molecule.

Microsphere

Microsphere technology is used to develop differentiated formulations for targeted delivery. We aim to use this technology for a site specific action, to eliminate inconvenience of repeated injections and to decrease toxic side effects.

Liposomes

Liposomal technology is another method to improve the delivery of drugs. Liposomes offer excellent opportunity to selectively target drugs; which is expected to optimize the pharmacokinetic parameters, the pharmacological effect and to reduce the toxicity of the drugs. These are minute spherical sacs of phospholipids molecules enclosing a water droplet, especially as formed artificially to carry drugs or other substances into the tissues.

Sustained Release Formulations

- Osmoticcontrolled Release Oral Delivery System (OROS) technology is used to deliver once-daily tablets.
- This advanced technology uses osmotic pressure to deliver the drug in several therapeutic areas. It can lead to improved safety profile, stable drug concentrations, and uniform drug effects and reduced dosing frequency.
- OROS technology enables the use of an effective starting dose and eliminates the need for dose titration. This allows symptom control much earlier than immediate-release tablets.

Orally Disintegrating Formulations Technology

Orally disintegrating tablets which disintegrate rapidly when placed upon the tongue and ensure faster onset of action.

Sprinkles

Innovative oral granule formulation called 'sprinkles' especially for paediatric patients. They can be sprinkled over a child's food making the drug palatable. This formulation addresses the issue of compliance, a key challenge in pediatric therapy. This technology may be used to develop anti-HIV therapy for children.

Examples of the commercially available platform technology products:

Example 1:

Liquid Dispensing Technology (LDT)

Understand the potential of a highly capable process for difficult-to-manufacture tablets

Develop high quality tablets of high potency compounds safely and reproducibly

Deliver high potency products rapidly to the clinic and to the market from a novel manufacturing process

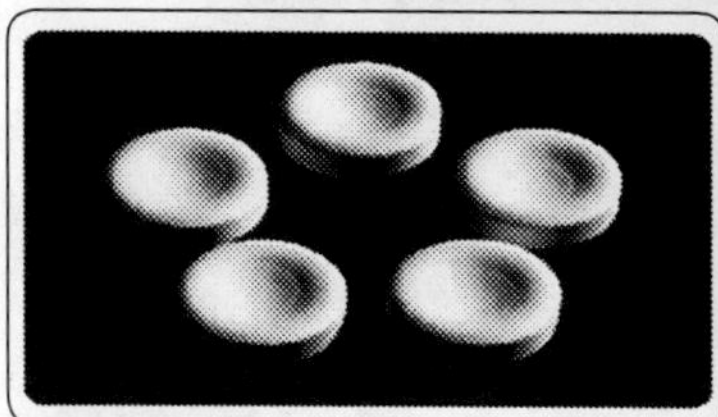

LDT is a novel manufacturing platform technology developed by GlaxoSmithKline to aid in the rapid development and manufacture of low-dose and/or highly potent products. Drug product is prepared in a liquid form and then applied to placebo tablets. The solution preparation significantly reduces the potential risk for operator exposure and eliminates or minimizes the need for extensive and costly containment facilities. LDT is for use with immediate release products and suitable for doses in the range of 1 microgram to 5 milligrams.

Example 2:

DiffCORE™ Accelerating the Development of Controlled Release Products

Understand drug substance and drug product properties that influence oral in-vivo performance

Develop tablets with a controlled release profile showing optimum efficacy and safety for the patient

Deliver rapidly, an innovative and differentiated dosage form for clinic and market

REVIEW QUESTIONS

1. Explain the pilot plant scale-up considerations for the manufacturing of solid dosage forms.
2. Define pilot plant in pharmaceutical industry. Discuss the personnel requirements and space requirements with relevant documentation.
3. Describe the general pilot plant scale-up considerations for liquid orals with relevant documentation.
4. Write the pilot plant scale-up considerations for semi-solids.
5. Explain the types of equipment qualifications.
6. Write the pilot plant considerations for raw materials.
7. Write about the significance of pilot plant scale-up technique in pharma industry.
8. Explain the significance of SUPAC guidelines.
9. Define SUPAC and explain the guidelines.
10. Discuss the SUPAC guidelines for drug components and site changes.
11. Write the SUPAC guidelines for manufacturing and batch size changes.
12. Write the SUPAC changes for manufacturing and packaging.
13. Explain the platform technology to pharmaceutical product development.

14

Technology Development and Transfer

Learning Objectives

After going through this chapter, you would be able to:

1. Understand the concept of technology transfer in pharma industry.
2. Understand the documentation of technology transfer for APIs, excipients.
3. Explain the validation process and qualification of equipment.
4. Understand the roles of different technology transfer agencies.

14.1 INTRODUCTION

Transfer of processes to an alternative site occurs at some stage in the life cycle

- Development
- Scale-up
- Manufacturing
- Production and launch
- Post-approval phase

Transfer of technology is defined as "a logical procedure that controls the transfer of any process together with its documentation and professional expertise between development and manufacture or between manufacture sites".

- Systematic procedure
- Passes documented knowledge and experience
- Experience gained during development or commercialization
- Technology transfer embodies
- Transfer of documentation

Demonstrated ability of the receiving unit (RU) to effectively perform the critical elements of the transferred technology. This should be to the satisfaction of all parties and any applicable regulatory bodies.

- Literature
- Little information available from national or regional regulatory bodies
- Guidance available from ISPE
- Business strategies of pharmaceutical companies involve intra- and intercompany transfers of technology for additional capacity, relocation of operations, consolidations, and mergers.

The guidance was issued in the year 2011 in TRS 961 Annex 7. 9 Prepared by Drug Regulations a Not for Profit Organization.

Transfer of technology requires:

- Documented, planned approach
- Trained and knowledgeable personnel
- Compliant quality system
- Documentation of data: Development, production and quality control.

Usually there is a:

- Sending unit (SU)
- A receiving unit
- Unit managing the process, which may or may not be a separate entity.

For the transfer to be successful, the following general principles and requirements should be met:

- The project plan should encompass the quality aspects of the project transfer.
- Should be based on the principles of quality risk management.
- The capabilities of the SU and at the RU should be similar, but not necessarily identical.
- For the transfer to be successful, the following general principles and requirements should be met:
- Facilities and equipment should operate according to similar operating principles.
- A comprehensive technical gap analysis between the SU and RU should be performed (technical, quality, regulatory).
- Adequately trained staff should be available or should be trained at the RU.
- For the transfer to be successful, the following general principles and requirements should be met:
- Regulatory requirements in the countries of the SU and the RU, should be considered.
- Regulatory requirements where product is intended to be supplied, should also be considered.
- There should be effective process and product knowledge transfer.

Technology transfer can be considered successful when there is a:

- Documented evidence.
- RU can routinely reproduce the transferred product, process or method against a predefined set of specifications.
- In the event that the RU identifies particular problems, the RU should communicate them back to the SU to ensure continuing knowledge management.

Technology transfer projects have legal and economic implications.

- Intellectual property rights
- Royalties

- Pricing
- Conflict of interest
- Confidentiality

These should be addressed before and during planning and execution of the transfer.

Any lack of transparency may lead to ineffective transfer of technology.

Some of the principles outlined here may also be applicable to manufacturing investigational pharmaceutical products.

Some of the responsibilities outlined here for the SU may also be considered to be part of the management unit responsibilities.

The definitions given below apply to the terms used in these guidelines.

Acceptance criteria

Measurable terms under which a test result will be considered acceptable.

Active pharmaceutical ingredient (API)

Any substance or mixture of substances intended to be used in the manufacture of a pharmaceutical dosage form and that, when so used, becomes an active ingredient of that pharmaceutical dosage form. Such substances are intended to furnish pharmacological activity or other direct effect in the diagnosis, cure, mitigation, treatment, or prevention of disease or to affect the structure and function of the body.

Bracketing

An experimental design to test only the extremes of, for example, dosage strength. The design assumes that the extremes will be representative of all the samples between the extremes.

Change control (C/C)

A formal system by which qualified representatives of appropriate disciplines review proposed or actual changes that might affect a validated status. The intent is to determine the need for action that would ensure that the system is maintained in a validated state.

Commissioning

The setting up, adjustment and testing of equipment or a system to ensure that it meets all the requirements, as specified in the user requirement specification, and capacities as specified by the designer or developer. Commissioning is carried out before qualification and validation.

Control strategy

A planned set of controls, derived from current product and process understanding, that assures process performance and product quality. The controls can include parameters and attributes related to materials and components related to drug substances and drug product materials and components, facility and equipment operating conditions, in-process controls, and finished product specifications.

Corrective action (C/A)

Any action to be taken when the results of monitoring at a critical control point indicate a loss of control.

Critical control point (CCP)

A step at which control can be applied and is essential to prevent or eliminate a pharmaceutical quality hazard or to reduce it to an acceptable level.

Design qualification (DQ)

Documented evidence that the premises, supporting systems, utilities, equipment and processes have been designed in accordance with the requirements of good manufacturing practices (GMP).

Design space

The multidimensional combination and interaction of input variables (e.g., material attributes) and process parameters that have been demonstrated to provide assurance of quality.

Drug master file (DMF)

Detailed information concerning a specific facility, process or product submitted to the medicines regulatory authority, intended for incorporation into the application for marketing authorization.

Finished pharmaceutical product (FPP)

A product that has undergone all stages of production, including packaging in its final container and labelling. An FPP may contain one or more APIs.

Gap analysis

Identification of critical elements of a process which are available at the SU but are missing from the RU.

Good manufacturing practices (GMP)

That part of quality assurance which ensures that pharmaceutical products are consistently produced and controlled to the quality standards appropriate to their intended use and as required by the marketing authorization.

In-process control (IPC)

Checks performed during production in order to monitor and, if necessary, to adjust the process to ensure that the product conforms to its specifications. The control of the environment or equipment may also be regarded as a part of in-process control.

Installation qualification (IQ)

The performance of tests to ensure that the installations (such as machines, measuring devices, utilities and manufacturing areas) used in a manufacturing process are appropriately selected and correctly installed and operate in accordance with established specifications.

Inter-company transfer

A transfer of technology between sites of different companies intra-company transfer. A transfer of technology between sites of the same group of companies.

Operational qualification (OQ)

Documented verification that the system or subsystem performs as intended over all anticipated operating ranges.

Performance qualification (PQ)

Documented verification that the equipment or system operates consistently and gives reproducibility within defined specifications and parameters for prolonged periods.

Process validation

Documented evidence which provides a high degree of assurance that a specific process will consistently result in a product that meets its predetermined specifications and quality characteristics.

Qualification

Action of proving and documenting that any premises, systems and equipment are properly installed, and/or work correctly and lead to the expected results. Qualification is often a part (the initial stage) of validation, but the individual qualification steps alone do not constitute process validation.

Qualification batches

Those batches produced by the RU to demonstrate its ability to reproduce the product.

Quality assurance (QA)

Quality assurance is a wide-ranging concept covering all matters that individually or collectively influence the quality of a product. It is the totality of the arrangements made with the objective of ensuring that pharmaceutical products are of the quality required for their intended use.

Quality control (QC)

Quality control covers all measures taken, including the setting of specifications, sampling, testing and analytical clearance, to ensure that starting materials, intermediates, packaging materials and finished pharmaceutical products conform with established specifications for identity, strength, purity and other characteristics.

Quality planning

Part of quality management focused on setting quality objectives and specifying necessary operational processes and related resources to fulfil the quality objectives.

Quality policy

Overall intentions and direction of an organization related to quality as formally expressed by senior management.

Quality risk management (QRM)

Quality risk management is a systematic process for the assessment, control, communication and review of risks to the quality of the pharmaceutical product throughout the product life-cycle.

Receiving unit (RU)

The involved disciplines at an organization where a designated product, process or method is expected to be transferred.

Sending unit (SU)

The involved disciplines at an organization from where a designated product, process or method is expected to be transferred.

Spiking

The addition of a known amount of a compound to a standard, sample or placebo, typically for the purpose of confirming the performance of an analytical procedure.

Standard operating procedure (SOP)

An authorized written procedure giving instructions for performing operations not necessarily specific to a given product or material (e.g., equipment operation, maintenance and cleaning, validation, cleaning of premises and environmental control, sampling and inspection). Certain SOPs may be used to supplement product-specific master and batch production documentation.

Technology transfer report

A documented summary of a specific technology transfer project listing procedures, acceptance criteria, results achieved and conclusions. Any deviation should be discussed and justified.

Validation

Action of proving and documenting that any process, procedure or method actually and consistently leads to the expected results.

Validation master plan (VMP)

A high-level document that establishes an umbrella validation plan for the entire project and summarizes the manufacturer's overall philosophy and approach, to be used for establishing performance adequacy. It provides information on the manufacturer's validation work programme and defines details of and time scales for the validation work to be performed, including a statement of the responsibilities of those implementing the plan.

Validation protocol (or plan) (VP)

A document describing the activities to be performed in a validation, including the acceptance criteria for the approval of a manufacturing process or a part thereof for routine use.

Validation report (VR)

A document in which the records, results and evaluation of a completed validation programme are assembled and summarized. It may also contain proposals for the improvement of processes and or equipment.

14.2 SCOPE

This guidance provides for transfer of QC methods to RU. QC laboratory where technical agreement exists between SU & RU. Such technical agreements may not exist, e.g., testing by national laboratories or testing for procurement agencies:

This guidance provides:

- Principles for transfers.
- General recommendations on the activities necessary to conduct a successful intra- or inter-site transfer.
- Basic considerations needed for a successful transfer in order to satisfy the regulatory authority.

The guidelines will be applied to:

- Manufacturing active pharmaceutical ingredients (APIs).
- Manufacturing and packaging of bulk materials.
- Manufacturing and packaging of finished pharmaceutical products (FPPs).
- Performing analytical testing.

The recommendations provided in these guidelines apply to all dosage forms. However, they need to be adjusted on a case-by-case basis, e.g., by using risk management principles.

Particularly close control of certain aspects will be required for certain formulations such as sterile products, and metered dose aerosols. As each transfer project is unique these guidelines cannot cover all possible situations. These guidelines do not provide guidance on any legal, financial or commercial considerations associated with technology transfer projects.

14.3 ORGANIZATION & MANAGEMENT

Transfer comprises an SU and an RU. In some circumstances there may be an additional unit. This unit may be responsible for directing, managing and approving the transfer. There is a formal agreement between the parties. This specifies the responsibilities before, during and after transfer. A successful technology transfer needs to ensure that the main steps have been executed and documented.

There should be a project management plan. This should identify and control all the necessary activities identified at the start of the undertaking.

The transfer protocol should list the intended sequential stages of the transfer.

The protocol should include:

- Objective
- Scope
- Key personnel and their responsibilities.
- A parallel comparison of materials, methods and equipment.
- The transfer stages with documented evidence that each critical stage has been satisfactorily accomplished before the next commences.
- Identification of critical control points.

The protocol should include:

- Experimental design and acceptance criteria for analytical methods.
- Information on trial production batches, qualification batches and process validation.
- Change control for any process deviations encountered.
- Assessment of end-product.
- Arrangements for keeping retention samples of active ingredients, intermediates and finished products, and information on reference substances where applicable.
- Conclusion, including signed-off approval by project manager..
- The SU should provide the necessary validation documentation for the process and its support functions.

- Usually, an established process is transferred, and such documentation is already available.
- The SU should provide criteria and information on hazards and critical steps associated with the product, process or method to be transferred. This should serve as a basis for a quality risk management (QRM) exercise at the RU.
- The SU and the RU should jointly verify that the following, satisfactorily completed, validation protocols are available: Installation qualification (IQ) and operational qualification (OQ) data for manufacturing equipment, packaging equipment, analytical equipment and qualification of the rooms for both manufacture and packaging.
- The SU and the RU should jointly implement any training programmes that may be required specific to the product, process or method to be transferred, e.g., on analytical methods or equipment usage, and assess training outcomes.
- The SU and the RU should jointly execute the transfer protocol according to a checklist.
- A flow diagram may also be used showing the sequence of steps to be carried out to affect an efficient transfer.
- Any changes and adaptations made during the course of the technology transfer should be fully documented.
- The SU and the RU should jointly document the execution of the transfer protocol in a transfer of technology summary in a report.

14.4 PROJECT TEAM

Any transfer project will be managed by a team comprising members with clearly defined key responsibilities.

The team should be drawn from members of relevant disciplines from both the SU and RU sites.

The team members should have the necessary qualifications and experience to manage their particular aspect of the transfer.

14.5 PRODUCTION: TRANSFER

14.5.1 Processing, Packaging and Cleaning

The RU should be able to accommodate the intended production capacity. Establish if single-batch manufacture, continuous production or campaigns is required. Consideration should be given to the level and depth of detail to be transferred to support production and any further process development and optimization at the RU as intended under the transfer project plan.

Consideration should be given to the:

- Technical expertise
- Site technology
- Site capabilities for the RU.

The SU and the RU should jointly develop a protocol for the transfer of relevant information related to the process under consideration from the SU to the RU, as well as the development of a comparable process at the RU.

14.5.2 Starting Materials

The specifications and relevant functional characteristics of the starting materials: APIs and excipients to be used at the RU should be consistent with materials used at the SU.

Any properties, which are likely to influence the process or product, should be identified and characterized.

14.6 ACTIVE PHARMACEUTICAL INGREDIENT (API)

The SU should provide the RU with the open part of the API master file (APIMF or drug master file (DMF) or active substance master file (ASMF)), or equivalent information.

Any relevant additional information on the API of importance for the manufacture of the pharmaceutical product.

The following are examples of the information which may typically be provided; however, the information needed in each specific case should be assessed using the principles of QRM:

- Manufacturer and associated supply chain
- Step of the API to be transferred
- Flowchart of synthesis pathway, outlining the process, including entry points for raw materials, critical steps, process controls and intermediate
- Where relevant, definitive physical form of the API (including photomicrographs and other relevant data) and any polymorphic and solvate forms
- Solubility profile
- If relevant, pH in solution
- Partition coefficient, including the method of determination
- Intrinsic dissolution rate, including the method of determination
- Particle size and distribution, including the method of determination
- Bulk physical properties, including data on bulk and tap density, surface
- Area and porosity as appropriate
- Water content and determination of hygroscopicity, including water activity data and special handling requirements
- Microbiological considerations in accordance with national, regional or international pharmacopoeial requirements
- Specifications and justification for release and end-of-life limits
- Summary of stability studies conducted in conformity with current guidelines, including conclusions and recommendations on retest date
- List of potential and observed synthetic impurities, with data to support proposed specifications and typically observed levels
- Information on degradants, with a list of potential and observed degradation products and data to support proposed specifications and typically observed levels

- Potency factor, indicating observed purity and justification for any recommended adjustment to the input quantity of API for product manufacturing, providing examples calculations
- Special considerations with implications for storage and or handling, including but not limited to safety and environmental factors (e.g., as specified in material safety data sheets) and sensitivity to heat, light or moisture.

14.7 EXCIPIENTS

- The excipients to be used have a potential impact on the final product.
- Their specifications and relevant functional characteristics should, therefore, be made available by the SU for transfer to the RU site.

The following are examples of the information, which may typically be provided; however, the information needed in each specific case should be assessed using the principles of QRM:

- Manufacturer and associated supply chain
- Description of functionality, with justification for inclusion of any antioxidant, preservative or any excipient
- Definitive form (particularly for solid and inhaled dosage forms)
- Solubility profile (particularly for inhaled and transdermal dosage forms)
- Partition coefficient, including the method of determination (for transdermal dosage forms)
- Intrinsic dissolution rate, including the method of determination (for transdermal dosage forms)
- Particle size and distribution, including the method of determination (for solid, inhaled and transdermal dosage forms)
- Bulk physical properties, including data on bulk and tap density, surface area and porosity as appropriate (for solid and inhaled dosage forms)
- Compaction properties (for solid dosage forms)
- Melting point range (for semi-solid or topical dosage forms)
- pH range (for parenteral, semi-solid or topical, liquid and transdermal dosage forms)
- Ionic strength (for parenteral dosage forms)
- Specific density or gravity (for parenteral, semi-solid or topical, liquid and transdermal dosage forms)
- Viscosity and or viscoelasticity (for parenteral, semi-solid or topical, liquid and transdermal dosage forms)
- Osmolality (for parenteral dosage forms)
- Water content and determination of hygroscopicity, including water activity data and special handling requirements (for solid and inhaled dosage forms)
- Moisture content range (for parenteral, semi-solid or topical, liquid and transdermal dosage forms); microbiological considerations (including sterility, bacterial endotoxins

- Bio burden levels where the excipient supports microbiological growth in accordance with national, regional or international pharmacopeial requirements, as applicable (for general and specific monographs)
- Specifications and justification for release and end-of-life limits
- Information on adhesives supporting compliance with peel, sheer and adhesion design criteria (for transdermal dosage forms)
- Special considerations with implications for storage and or handling, including but not limited to safety and environmental factors
- Regulatory considerations, e.g., documentation to support compliance with transmissible animal spongiform encephalopathy certification requirements (where applicable)
- Information on processed and finished pharmaceutical products information
- The SU should provide a detailed characterization of the product, including its qualitative and quantitative composition:
  - Physical description
  - Method of manufacture
  - In-process controls
  - Control method and specifications
  - Packaging components and configurations, and any safety and handling considerations.

The SU should provide all information on the history of process development; such information may include the following:

- Information on clinical development, e.g., information on the rationale for the synthesis, route and form selection, technology selection, equipment, clinical tests, and product composition;
- Information on scale-up activities
- Process optimization
- Statistical optimization of critical process parameters
- Critical quality attributes
- Pilot report and or information on pilot-scale development activities indicating the number and disposition of batches manufactured
- Information or report on full-scale development activities, indicating
  - the number and disposition of batches manufactured, and
  - deviation and change control (sometimes referred to as change management) reports which led to the current manufacturing process. The change history and reasons, e.g., a change control log, indicating any changes to the **process or primary packaging or analytical methods as a part of process optimization or improvement; and information on investigations of problems and the outcomes of the investigations.**
- The SU should provide to the RU information on any health, safety and environmental issues associated with the manufacturing processes to be transferred, and the implications, e.g., need for gowning or protective clothing.

- The SU should provide to the RU information on current processing and testing, including but not limited to:
- A detailed description of facility requirements and equipment
- Information on starting materials, applicable MSDS and storage requirements for raw materials and finished products
- Description of manufacturing steps (narrative and process maps or flowcharts, and or master batch records)
- Qualification of in processing hold times and conditions
- Order and method of raw material addition and bulk transfers between processing steps
- Description of analytical methods
- Identification and justification of control strategy
- Identification of critical performance aspects for specific dosage forms
- Identification of process control points
- Product quality attributes
- Qualification of critical processing parameter ranges, statistical process control (SPC) charts.
- Design space, in cases where this has been defined
- Validation information, e.g., validation plans and reports
- Annual product quality reviews
- Stability information
- An authorized set of protocols and work instructions for manufacturing
- Environmental conditions or any special requirement needed for the facility or equipment depending on the nature of the product to be transferred
- During the transfer process, the RU should identify any differences in facilities, systems and capabilities
- Communicate the same with the SU about these differences
- Understand the potential impact on ability to run the process to deliver good product quality
- Differences should be understood and satisfactorily addressed to assure equivalent product quality. Based on the information received from the SU, the RU should consider its own capability to manufacture and pack the product to the required standards.
- SU should develop relevant plant operating procedures and documentation before the start of production.
- Process development at the RU should address the following tasks:
  - Comparison and assessment of suitability and qualification of facility and equipment
  - Description of manufacturing process and flow of personnel and of materials at the RU (narrative and or process maps or flowcharts)

- Determination of critical steps in manufacture, including hold times, endpoints, sampling points and sampling techniques
- Writing and approval of SOPs for all production operations
- Dispensing
- Granulation or blending or solution preparation
- Tablet compression
- Tablet coating, encapsulation, liquid filling, primary and secondary packaging, in-process quality control, packaging, cleaning, testing and storage
- Evaluation of stability information, with generation of site-specific stability data if required
- Compliance with regulatory requirements for any changes made, e.g., in terms of batch size.

14.8 PACKAGING

- The transfer of packaging operations should follow the same procedural patterns as those of the production transfer.
- Information on packaging to be transferred from the SU to the RU includes:
  - Specifications for a suitable container or closure system
  - Any relevant additional information on design, packing, processing or labelling requirements
  - Tamper-evident and anti-counterfeiting measures needed for qualification of packaging components at the RU.
- For QC testing of packaging components, specifications should be provided for drawings, artwork and material (for example, glass, card or fibre board)
- Based on the information provided, the RU should perform a suitability study for initial qualification of the packaging components.
- Packaging is considered suitable if it provides
- Adequate protection (preventing degradation of the medicine due to environmental influences)
- Safety (absence of undesirable substances released into the product), compatibility (absence of interaction possibly affecting medicine quality)
- Performance (functionality in terms of drug delivery)

14.9 CLEANING

- During the manufacturing process, pharmaceutical products and APIs can be contaminated by other pharmaceutical products or APIs if the plant is processing different products.
- To minimize the risk of contamination and cross-contamination, operator exposure and environmental effects, adequate cleaning procedures are essential.
- Cleaning procedures and their validation are site specific.

In order for the RU to define its cleaning strategy the SU should provide information on cleaning at the SU to minimize cross-contamination due to:

- Residues from previous manufacturing steps
- Operator exposure
- Environmental impact, including:
- Information on solubility of active ingredients, excipients and vehicles
- Minimum therapeutic doses of active ingredients
- Therapeutic category and toxicological assessment
- Existing cleaning procedures.
- Additional information should be provided, as appropriate and where available, e.g., cleaning validation reports (chemical and microbiological)
- Information on cleaning agents used (efficacy, evidence that they do not interfere with analytical testing for residues of APIs, removal of residual cleaning agents)
- Recovery studies to validate the sampling methodology
- Before the transfer, the SU should provide information on limits for product residues, and the rationale for limit selection
- Based on the information provided by the SU, cleaning procedures should be designed at the RU, taking into account:
- Relevant characteristics of the starting materials (e.g., potency, toxicity, solubility, corrosiveness and temperature sensitivity)
- Manufacturing equipment design and configuration
- Cleaning agent and products residue
- Implementation of processing, packaging and cleaning systems
- Trial batches ("demonstration batches") are normally produced to confirm process capability before initiating formal validation
- Where trial batches are produced, at a minimum, all critical processing parameters and finished product specifications should be assessed
- Once process capability has been established at the RU, assuring that the product, process or method at the RU meets predefined and justified specifications, process validation and cleaning validation can be carried out.

14.10 QUALITY CONTROL: ANALYTICAL METHOD TRANSFER

- Transfer of analytical methods should accommodate all the analytical testing
- This should demonstrate compliance of the product to be transferred with the registered specification
- Analytical methods used to test pharmaceutical products, starting materials, packaging components and cleaning (residue) samples, if applicable, should be implemented at the testing laboratory before testing of samples for process validation studies is performed by the RU
- Process validation samples may be tested at the RU, the SU or a third laboratory
- A protocol defining the steps should be prepared for transfer of analytical methods

- The analytical methods transfer protocol should include a description of the objective, scope and responsibilities of the SU and the RU
- A specification of materials and methods; the experimental design and acceptance criteria; documentation (including information to be supplied with the results, and report forms to be used, if any); procedure for the handling of deviations; references; signed approval; and details of reference samples (starting materials, intermediates and finished products)

The SU's responsibilities for the transfer of analytical methods are to:

- Provide method-specific training for analysts and other quality control staff, if required.
- Assist in analysis of QC testing results
- Define all methods to be transferred for testing a given product, starting material or cleaning sample
- Define experimental design, sampling methods and acceptance criteria
- Provide any validation reports for methods under transfer and demonstrate their robustness
- Provide details of the equipment used, as necessary (part of validation report, if available)

The RU's responsibilities are to:

- Review analytical methods provided by the SU, and formally agree on acceptance criteria before execution of the transfer protocol
- Ensure that the necessary equipment for QC are available and qualified at the RU site
- The equipment used by the RU during the analytical transfer should meet appropriate specifications to ensure the requirements of the method or specification are met
- Ensure that adequately trained and experienced personnel are in place for analytical testing
- Provide a documentation system capable of recording receipt and testing of samples to the required specification using approved test methods, and of reporting, recording and collating data and designation of status (approved, rejected, quarantine)
- Execute the transfer protocol
- Perform the appropriate level of validation to support the implementation of the methods
- Generate and obtain approval of transfer reports.
- Appropriate training should be provided and all training activities and outcomes should be documented
- Reference to compendia monographs (e.g., The International Pharmacopoeia, European Pharmacopoeia, British Pharmacopoeia and United States Pharmacopeia), where available, is expected.

- Possible experimental designs and acceptance criteria for the main analytical testing methods.

14.11 PREMISES AND EQUIPMENT

14.11.1 Premises

The SU should provide information to the RU on the layout, construction and finish of buildings and services, which have an impact on the product, process or method to be transferred.

- HVAC
- Temperature
- Relative humidity
- Water
- Power
- Compressed air

The SU should provide information on relevant health, safety and environmental issues, including:

- Inherent risks of the manufacturing processes (e.g., reactive chemical hazards, exposure limits, fire and explosion risks)
- Health and safety requirements to minimize operator exposure (e.g., atmospheric containment of pharmaceutical dust)
- Emergency planning considerations (e.g., in case of gas or dust release, spillage, fire and fire water run-off)
- Identification of waste streams and provisions for reuse, recycling and/ or disposal

14.11.2 Equipment

The SU should provide a list of equipment, makes and models involved in the manufacture, filling, packing and or control of the product, process or method to be transferred

Should also provide existing qualification and validation documentation. Relevant documentation may include:

- Drawings
- Manuals
- Maintenance logs
- Calibration logs
- Procedures (e.g., regarding equipment setup, operation, cleaning, maintenance, calibration and storage).
- The RU should review the information provided by the SU together with its own inventory list including the qualification status (IQ, OQ, PQ) of all equipment and systems

- Perform a side-by-side comparison of equipment at the two sites in terms of their functionality, makes, models and qualification status.
- The RU should perform a gap analysis to identify requirements for adaptatingthe existing equipment, or acquisition of new equipment, or a change in the process, to enable the RU to reproduce the process being transferred.
- GMP requirements should be satisfied and intended production volumes and batch sizes (e.g., same, scaled-up or campaign) should be considered. Factors to be compared include:
    - Minimum and maximum capacity
    - Material of construction
    - Critical operating parameters
    - Critical equipment components (e.g., filters, screens, and temperature/ pressure sensors)
    - Critical quality attribute
    - Range of intended use
- The facility- and building-specific location of all equipment at the RU should be considered at the time of drawing up process maps or flowcharts of the manufacturing process to be transferred, including flows of personnel and material.
- The impact of manufacturing new products on products currently manufactured with the same equipment should be determined.
- Any modification of existing equipment that needs to be adapted to become capable of reproducing the process being transferred should be documented in the transfer project plan.

14.12 DOCUMENTATION

- The documentation required for the transfer project itself is wide ranging.
- The documented evidence that the transfer of technology has been considered successful should be formalized and stated in a technology transfer summary report.
- That report should summarize the scope of the transfer, the critical parameters as obtained in the SU and RU (preferably in a tabulated format) and the final conclusions of the transfer.
- Possible discrepancies should be listed and appropriate actions, where needed, taken to resolve them.

14.13 QUALIFICATION AND VALIDATION

- The extent of qualification and/or validation to be performed should be determined on the basis of risk management principles.
- Qualification and validation should be documented as prepared by "Drug Regulations: A Not for Profit Organization".

14.14 APPROVED REGULATORY BODIES AND AGENCIES

14.14.1 TIFAC (Technology Information Forecasting and Assessment Council)

As per the recommendations of Technology Policy Implementation Committee (TPIC) in 1985, Cabinet approved the formation of TIFAC in mid-1986 and TIFAC (Technology Information Forecasting and Assessment Council) was formed as a registered society in February, 1988 under the Department of Science and Technology as an autonomous body.

It was mandated to assess the state-of-the-art of technology and set directions for future technological development in India in important socio-economic sectors.

The main objectives of TIFAC:

(a) Ensuring timely availability of requisite technologies relevant to the needs of the country on futuristic basis and minimizing the time gap between the development of new technologies and their utilization.

(b) Establishing a purposeful linkage between technology development and technology import policies, to identify priority areas of research in relation to the socio-economic, environmental and security needs of the country; to evolve and suggest strategies for technological developments based on such priorities; and to draw up programmes of purposeful research in various sectors.

14.14.2 National Research Development Corporation (NRDC)

- NRDC was established in 1953 by the Government of India.

The main objectives of NRDC:

- Develop and commercialise the technologies/know-how/inventions/patents/processes emanating from various national R&D institutions/universities and is presently working under the administrative control of the Dept. of Scientific & Industrial Research, Ministry of Science & Technology.
- NRDC has forged strong links with the scientific and industrial community in India and abroad and developed a wide network of research institutions, academia and industry and made formal arrangements with them for the commercialisation of know-how developed in their laboratories. It has licensed the indigenous technology to more than 4800 entrepreneurs and helped to establish a large number of small and medium scale industries.
- Besides being the torch bearer in the field of technology transfer, NRDC also undertakes a number of activities under its structured promotional programme for encouragement and advancement of research, promotion of inventions and innovations such as meritorious inventions awards, techno-commercial support, technical and financial assistance for IPR protection, value addition services and support for further development of technologies and much more.
- NRDC has also successfully exported technologies and services to both developed as well as the developing countries. NRDC is recognised, particularly in the developing countries, as the source of reliable appropriate technology, machines and services, which are typically suitable for these countries.

14.14.3 BCIL (Biotech Consortium India Limited)

- BCIL was inaugurated in 1990 by the then Prime Minister of India, Hon'ble Shri Chandra Shekhar, in the presence of the Finance Minister, Yashwant Sinha and Dr. Manju Sharma, Secretary, Department of Biotechnology.
- Biotech Consortium India Limited (BCIL) is a public limited company, promoted by the Department of Biotechnology (DBT), Ministry of Science and Technology, Government of India and All India Financial Institutions for providing the necessary linkages among stakeholders and business support for facilitating accelerated commercialization of biotechnology.
- BCIL was incorporated under the Indian Companies Act, 1956. The Board of Directors of BCIL consists of senior representatives of DBT, Council of Scientific and Industrial Research (CSIR), Indian Council of Agricultural Research (ICAR), leading all India financial institutions and the biotechnology industry.

Functions of BCIL

- BCIL has been actively involved in technology transfer, project consultancy, fund syndication, information dissemination, and manpower training and placement related to biotechnology.
- It has assisted hundreds of clients including scientists, technologies, research institutions, universities, first entrepreneurs, the corporate sector, national and international organizations, central government, various state governments, banks and financial institutions.

14.14.4 SIDBI (Small Industries Development Bank of India)

- SIDBI is an integrated approach to development of MSEs. Since its formation, SIDBI has been impacting the lives of citizens across the various strata of society through its integrated, innovative and inclusive approach.
- Be it traditional domestic industry, small, bottom-of-the-pyramid entrepreneurs, medium enterprises to high-end knowledge based industries and export promotions, SIDBI has directly or indirectly touched the lives of more than 360 lakh people in the MSE sector, through various credit and developmental measures.
- SIDBI Vision 2.0 is a strategic initiative by SIDBI aimed at further accelerating this effort by transforming its current role to that of an All India Financial Institution that can create an integrated credit and development support ecosystem for Indian MSEs, thus promoting their inclusive growth.
- The initiative is dedicated to meet both, credit and non-credit needs of MSEs, enabling them to be globally competitive businesses. SIDBI 2.0 is designed for sustainable development of MSE sector in India, based on the three Ps front, namely, profit (economic), people (social) and planet (environment).

14.14.5 APCTT (Asian and Pacific Centre for Transfer of Technology)

- APCTT is a United Nations Regional Institution under the Economic and Social Commission for Asia and the Pacific (ESCAP).

- The Centre was established in 1977 in Bangalore, India. In 1993, the Centre moved to New Delhi, India.
- APCTT promotes transfer of technology to and from small- and medium-scale enterprises (SMEs) in Asia and the Pacific.
- APCTT implements development projects funded by international donors aimed at strengthening the environment for technology transfer among SMEs in Asia and the Pacific; in this respect the Centre makes special efforts to encourage more participation of women in the field of technology.
- APCTT undertakes consultancy assignments in various technology transfer related areas (institution building, human resources development, studies, business partnership development).
- The objective of APCTT is to strengthen the technology transfer capabilities in the region and to facilitate import/export of environmentally sound technologies to/from the member countries.
- All member states and associate members of UNESCAP are the members of APCTT.

14.14.6 TBSE (Technology Bureau for Small Enterprises)

TBSE provides a platform where small enterprises can tap opportunities at the global level for acquisition of technology or establish business collaboration.

Resulting from the joint initiative of the United Nations' Asian and Pacific Centre for Transfer of Technology (APCTT) and Small Industries Development Bank of India (SIDBI) it represents, under one roof, synergy of technology and finance.

TBSE also receives partial funding from the Office of DC (SSI), Government of India. Important features of TBSE services are:

- Offers a professionally managed system for technology and collaboration search.
- Helps in building up confidence between prospective partners.
- Lends a friendly hand in the intricate task of negotiations and matching of perceptions.
- Provides a gateway to global technology market through networking.
- Unique mechanism for arranging technology and finance.
- Takes up project appraisal and preparation of business plan.

Range of Services Technology Information: The Bureau has a large computerised data base on technology options available from different countries. It gives the user updated information on sources of technologies and means of accessing them. Also background information on technology seeking enterprises is maintained and made available to interested technology suppliers and collaborators.

Match Making: It identifies business partners willing to collaborate, brings them face to face and extends support to tie up financial assistance and other requirements for transfer of technology and joint ventures. Collaborating partners are further assisted in drafting agreements, obtaining various approvals and preparation of business plans.

Finance Syndication: Depending on the cost of project, nature and quantum of assistance required, the Bureau undertakes financial syndication through SIDBI covering term loans, foreign currency, venture capital, lines of credit, equity assistance and on selective basis interest-free loan to meet initial expenditure in the pre-technology absorption stage.

Business Collaboration: The Bureau offers support to small enterprises for the export of technologies and the products manufactured by them through business tie-ups as a part of the package. To promote international cooperation amongst SMEs the Bureau organises overseas visits of business delegations.

Support Services: It arranges consultancy services, visits of overseas experts for in-plant counselling: coordinates buyer-seller meets for specific product process technologies and represents the business interests of small enterprises in international events.

14.15 TECHNOLOGY OF TRANSFER (ToT)

Related Documentation- Confidentiality Agreements, Licensing, MoUs, Legal Issues

14.15.1 Introduction - Why Licence?

Ideas, innovations and other expressions of human creativity are converted into private property and protected by law through the intellectual property system. As property, they are tradable assets. Licensing, the right granted by an owner of such an asset to another to use that asset while continuing to retain ownership of that asset, is an important way of creating value with these assets. Licensing creates an income source, disseminates the technology to a wider group of users and potential developers and acts as a catalyst for further development and commercialization.

The legal system of intellectual property rights converts this innovative and creative output into property and thus into valuable tradable assets. Human ingenuity and insight manifest in the form of new and/or original ideas, inventions, information, creative expressions, knowledge and other such intangibles that may be embedded in or relate to the products and services that we so depend on in our daily lives.

Thus, new and improved technology, know-how, confidential information, software and databases, creative expression in the making of instruction manuals, books, plays, movies, videotapes, television productions, music, multimedia, the image, reputation and goodwill linked to trustworthy names of goods and services, business identifiers, etc., can be protected by a range of intellectual property and certain aspects of unfair competition laws.

The intellectual property laws include laws on patents, utility models, trade secrets, trademarks, geographical indications, industrial designs, topographies of integrated circuits, non-original databases, new varieties of plants, and copyright and related rights.

14.15.2 Is Licensing the Right Strategy?

Before embarking on either "licensing-in" technology, which is to acquire rights to technology developed by another, or "licensing-out" technology, which is to grant to another the right to use technology to which one has proprietary rights, through a licensing agreement, it is important to consider the preliminary question as to whether licensing is the right strategy to adopt. It may good for an owner of intellectual property, the best strategy is to manufacture and market the product. If not, however, other options include entering into an outright sale of the intellectual property rights over a given technology. Sale of intellectual property rights through assignment may not be practical because often the buying of intellectual property alone is not attractive without human capital, a product, a developed market and/or an established business or revenue stream. Still, sale or assignment may be an option in some cases.

14.15.3 Patent Information

An agreement to licence technology is often part of a larger business transaction, which may include agreements on a multitude of other issues that are generally linked to, but may be separate from, the agreement to licence technology. The technology sought to be licensed may be protected by one or more patents, subject to copyright and/or may have been kept as a trade secret. There may be other intellectual property rights surrounding the technology, such as trademarks protecting the brand or name of the company, copyright protecting documentation, trade secrets protecting a whole host of confidential information including know-how and so on. Further, there may be a variety of other concerns relevant to the particular business relationship being formalized between the parties. All of these issues may merit different agreements or perhaps constitute different parts of a single agreement.

14.15.4 What is Patent Information?

Since the patent system requires patent applicants to make public disclosure of their inventions, all inventions for which patent protection has been sought are documented, catalogued and made freely available for public consultation either 18 months after the filing of the patent application and/or immediately after the grant of the patent.

Consisting of some 42 million documents published by patent offices all over the world and growing by about a million every year, patent information is the largest repository of technical information in the world.

14.15.5 Content of Patent Documents

A patent document is usually called a patent specification. It is divided in a number of sections.

In most countries, a consistent approach has been adopted to the layout and contents of the sections of a patent specification. The first page (or front page) of a patent document generally displays bibliographic information.

The bibliographic data gives information concerning the patent application, i.e., who filed the application, when and where it was filed, and the technical fields to which the invention relates. The first page usually also includes a title, an abstract and a representative drawing.

Bibliographic information is an essential means of identifying, locating and retrieving patent documents. If the name(s) of inventor(s) and/or of the owner(s) of the invention are known, all past patent applications under their names can be found. If the technical field in terms of the IPC is known, all documents in that technical field can be retrieved.

14.15.6 Memorandum of Understanding (MoU) or Letter of Intent

If both parties have reason to believe that they are adequately prepared for the negotiation then the need for a preliminary understanding in the form of an MoU or Letter of Intent should normally not arise. However, despite the best efforts of the parties, there are situations in which it becomes necessary to enter into such an MoU or Letter of Intent prior to the signing of a licensing agreement. This may happen prior to the commencement of formal negotiations or sometimes during protracted negotiations when, for example, there is a need to publicly announce the launching of a new product or apply for funding. Before entering into an MoU or Letter of Intent it is important not to agree to anything proposed by the other side without understanding its implications for the final licensing agreement. This is particularly true in a country where an MoU or Letter of Intent is treated as legally binding. As with a confidentiality agreement discussed above, any such MoU or Letter of Intent would has to be customized based on the facts and circumstances of a given situation and should be reviewed by an appropriate legal professional.

14.15.7 Subject Matter

The subject matter of a licence agreement may include creations such as inventions, confidential information, the creativity expressed in novels, plays, movies, music, the names of goods and services, business identifiers, etc. These can be owned and protected under intellectual property laws, which, to reiterate, include patents, utility models, trade secrets, trademarks, geographical indications, industrial designs, topographies of integrated circuits and copyright, as well as those that protect against certain types of unfair competition.

As the subject matter of a licence agreement often includes confidential information as well as inventions, as much attention as is devoted to the licensing of patents should also be devoted to such confidential information, including know-how and licensed trade secrets.

In this connection, it is important to include in the agreement one or more clauses superseding the confidentiality agreement entered into prior to the negotiations. Such clause{s) would, inter alia, take into account the following:

(a) Define what is meant by confidential information. Such a definition should, preferably, includes not only that which is disclosed to the recipient but other information which it may receive or be made aware of as a consequence to the agreement.

(b) Ensure that the licensee has or undertaken to put in place procedures for restricting the use of the information for the purposes as specified in the agreement and safeguarding it against disclosure. This may also include the possibility of verifying or auditing such procedures by the licensor or his authorized representative.

(c) Provide for liability in the case of accidental or negligent disclosure of the information to third parties who are not subject to the provisions of the licence agreement and who are not otherwise informed of the confidentiality of such information.

(d) Spell out the exceptions to the obligation, such as if the information is publicly available, that is, it is already known or has become known to the recipient in a legitimate manner or if it had been independently developed by the recipient.

(e) Clarify as to how long these provisions will continue after the termination of the agreement and specify when the information should either be returned or destroyed.

REVIEW QUESTIONS

1. What is technology transfer? Give its importance in pharmaceutical industry.
2. Discuss the WHO guidelines for technology transfer.
3. Briefly explain the technology transfer documentation.
4. Explain the types of equipment qualifications.
5. Explain the technology transfer process for API and finished products.
6. Explain the transfer of technology and documentation for quality control.
7. Explain the practical aspects and problems of technology transfer department.
8. Define validation and explain its scope.
9. Elaborate upon validation master plan (VMP).
10. Discuss the roles of APCTT and TIFAC technology transfer agencies.
11. Write about NRDC licensing process in India.
12. Discuss about SIDBI agency approval process.
13. Write about the BCIL approval process.
14. Write a note on memorandum of understanding (MoUs).

15

REGULATORY AFFAIRS

Learning Objectives

After going through this chapter, you would be able to:

1. Understand the need and roles of regulatory affairs profession.
2. Understand the different regulatory authorities of different countries.
3. Explain the concept of different regulatory submissions.
4. Describe the process of INDA submission.
5. Explain the documentation requirements for NDA submission.

15.1 INTRODUCTION

Regulatory affairs (RA) is one of the challenging professions within the regulated industries, such as pharmaceuticals, food products, cosmetics, agricultural products, banking and energy. With regards, to pharmaceuticals, regulatory affairs is a bridge or interface between the pharmaceutical company and the regulatory authorities of different countries.

The prime objective of RA profession is protecting public health by controlling and constant monitoring of safety, efficacy and quality of medicinal drug products. Regulatory affairs compose a variety of disciplines and job responsibilities, which start during the product development, its manufacture and continue till the product is available for use.

Nowadays, almost every company either domestic or MNC has RA department to keep track on the legislations of countries where the company wishes to market their pharmaceutical products. This process includes collection and analysis of legal as well as scientific requirements of a particular country to get and maintain the regulatory approval of healthcare products.

A drug regulatory authority/agency is a competent government agency which is responsible for ensuring quality, safety and efficacy of drug products. There are many regulatory agencies across the world representing the particular countries. The regulatory authorities should assess the technical data obtained during development of product and proposed procedures of manufacturing and quality control reports.

15.2 BASIC NEED OF RA DEPARTMENT

Any drug product either a new drug or generic drug manufactured by a pharmaceutical company just cannot be commercialized for human use unless it gets regulatory approval. RA department of a pharma company files all the data regarding drug development, manufacture, control, stability studies, labelling, packing, safety and clinical studies of drug products within the standard formats of regulatory documents such as NDA, ANDA, DMF, SNDA, MAA, etc. After filing the particular document is submitted to concerned regulatory authority. Once the regulatory submission made, the concerned agency critically reviews all the information provided whether it is in compliance with the regulations and guidelines, if satisfied regulatory approval is granted for the marketing of the drug for human use.

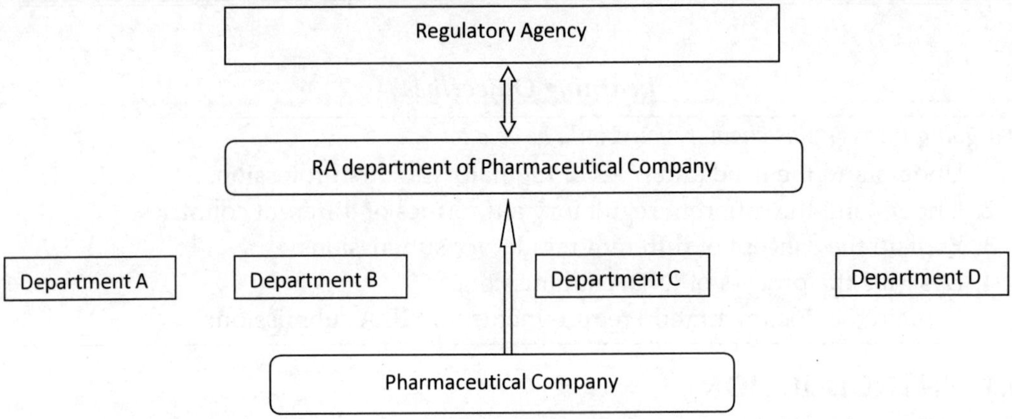

Fig. 15.1: Overview of RA department in pharmaceutical industry

15.3 OBJECTIVES OF RA DEPARTMENT

- To protect human health.
- To ensure the safety, quality and efficacy of drugs.
- To ensure appropriateness and accuracy of product information.

Regulatory affairs of any pharmaceutical industry plays a vital role in the overall development process starting from design and clinical studies compilation, submission of regulatory documents followed by mutual communication with concerned regulatory agencies until the final approval. The main job of RA profession is to provide technical advice on the scientific requirements, and collect, collate and evaluate the scientific data generated by the research and development department.

The RA responsibility just never stops after drug approval. Most of the regulatory submissions, involve maintenance of existing marketing authorization, compiling and submitting so called variation applications to update the approvals as a result of modifications and amendments to manufacturing process, extending product indications by conducting additional clinical studies, updating the data, labelling aspects and renewing the approvals.

The requisites of good RA professional include certain qualities like effective communication skills, writing skills, presentation skills, updating the knowledge of currently available regulations.

15.4 HISTORICAL OVERVIEW OF REGULATORY AFFAIRS

The evolution of pharmaceutical regulations started and implemented after some tragic incidents happened in a few parts of the world. Some of the notable disasters were described as follows.

15.4.1 Sulphanilamide Tragedy

In the year 1937, in US the consumption of sulphanilamide elixir caused death of more than 100 people. Elixir of sulphanilamide was prepared using solvent called DEG (diethylene glycol) which was known to be poisonous to humans. The pharmaceutical company manufacturing the sulphanilamide elixir was not aware of the information and also did not perform any pre-clinical studies on animals. During those days, there were no stringent regulations for assuring the safety and quality of drug products. Because of the lack of information, DEG composed sulphanilamide elixir induced more than 100 deaths and the cause of death was suspected use of poisonous substance DEG. This incident led to the introduction of The Federal Food, Drug and Cosmetic Act with the premarket notification requirement for new drugs in 1938. After implementing the Act, US government mandated all the pharmaceutical companies to perform pre-clinical studies for confirming the safety of drug products and to submit the data to the authority, FDA, before commercializing the drug products to market.

15.4.2 Thalidomide Disaster

The second horrible tragic incident was Thalidomide Disaster. During 1950-60s thalidomide was used as sedative and hypnotic. In Western Germany, this drug was marketed for the first time in 1956. During the period of 1960 the drug spread to 46 countries worldwide. In Europe, Canada and US the pregnant woman who were treated with Thalidomide found that drug caused teratogenic effects with serious birth deformities in the newborn babies. Unfortunately, around 12, 0000 babies were born with severe birth defects worldwide. This incident led to the Drug Amendments Act of 1962 by FDA in US to approve all new drugs by NDA submission for the first time, stating that any new drug developed must be demonstrated for safety on humans. In addition to this FDA also framed cGMP guidelines for manufacturing of drug products.

Similarly, in Europe, the EEC (European Economic Community) Directive 65/65/ EEC laid down regulations related to medicinal/drug products safety, quality and efficacy aspects. Further, after 10 years, in 1975 the European Community (EC) introduced 2 directives related to analytical, pharmacological, clinical studies, administrative principles and regulations for drug products. Further all the regulations were harmonized together and a single regulatory authority was framed for the entire European Union named European Medicines Evaluation Agency (EMEA) in the year 1993.

15.4.3 Tuskegee Syphilis Study (1932-1972)

In 1932, the Public Health Service of US started syphilis study in collaboration with Tuskegee University, which was traditionally known as Black University in Alabama. In the study, investigators enrolled 600 low income African-American males, among which 400 were infected with syphilis, the men were initially informed that study duration will be of 6 months but it was extended for 40 years. Free medical examinations were given; however, participants were not told about their disease. Even though a proven cure (penicillin) became available in the 1950s, the study continued until

1972 with participants being denied treatment. Later, 28 patients died directly from syphilis, 100 died with complications related to syphilis and 40 wives of patients were infected with the disease and 19 children were born with congenital syphilis. Then the study was stopped in 1972 by the US Department of Health, Education and Welfare when the horrifying story was published in many newspapers of US and it was also cited "arguably the most infamous biomedical research study in U.S. history". The incident led to formation of Belmont Report—a set of ethical principles for conducting human studies in 1979 and also office for Human Research Protection (OHRP) was established. In addition to these regulations, institutional review boards were set up for the protection of human subjects in studies involving them.

15.4.4 Nazi Experiments

In Nazi Germany, the German physicians planned and enacted the Euthanasia programme, the systemic killing of people who were found to be unworthy of life. The victims included were mentally retarded, physically challenged and mentally impaired. In addition, during world war II, the German physicians conducted many unethical studies on more than 1000 prisoners without their consent. Many died and some became permanently disabled. Most of the victims were treated worse than animals. The experiments included testing people in seawater, high altitude, bone transplantation, keeping the prisoners in extreme cold condition, torturing with poison bullets, etc.

In 1946, December 9 the American military tribunal made criminal proceedings against 23 leading doctors and administrators for their participation in these inhuman experiments. The accused physicians were charged with murder, torture and other crimes committed in the name of research. Among 23 defendants, 7 were sentenced to death by hanging, 9 were given lifetime prison term and 7 were found not guilty. The judgement by the war crimes tribunal laid down 10 basic principles to which physicians must confirm when carrying out experiments on human subjects in a new code referred as Nuremberg Code. The Nuremberg Code is a set of research ethics/ principles for human experimentation set as a result of the subsequent Nuremberg trials at the end of the World War-II.

15.5 REGULATORY AUTHORITIES

The key role of regulatory authorities is protecting public health by assuring the safety, quality and efficacy of drug products. Each country has its own regulatory authority composed of certain guidelines, regulations and document submission procedures which vary from country to country. After a certain period of time the regulations can be revised and changed accordingly.

Some of the well known and well implanted regulatory authorities of countries are discussed below.

15.5.1 World Health Organization (WHO)

It was framed in the year 1948 on 7th April. It is a specialized, non-political health agency of United Nations located in Geneva, Switzerland as head office.

WHO is responsible for providing leadership in global health related matters. The main objective of WHO is to enhance the knowledge about attaining and maintaining good health. WHO has its regional offices at different parts of world that include India, Egypt, America, Africa and Europe.

Functions of WHO

- Providing worldwide guidance in the field of health.
- Setting up of global standards for health.
- Coordinate with government bodies to strengthen national health programmes.
- Develop and transfer appropriate health technology information.

15.5.2 United States Food and Drug Administration (USFDA)

The USFDA is an agency of US Department of Health and Human Services responsible for the safety regulations of healthcare products such as, drugs, vaccines, medical devices, dietary supplements, veterinary products, biologicals and cosmetics.

Role of FDA

The job of FDA is to make sure that:

- Food products and dietary supplements are found to be safe and clean.
- The drug products and medical devices are safe and effective.
- Cosmetics are safe and animal food and drugs are safe.
- The medicinal products and food products have proper labels.

Functions of FDA

- To promote and protect the public health by helping safe and effective products reach the market in timely manner.
- To monitor the products for continued safety after their commercialization for public use.
- To help public to receive the accurate, science based information required to enhance health.

15.5.3 Central Drugs Standards Control Organization (CDSCO)

CDSCO is the Drug regulatory authority in India responsible for regulating pharmaceuticals, medical devices, vaccines and for permitting to conduct clinical trials. The headquarters of CDSCO is located at New Delhi and it performs the functions under the supervision of Directorate General of Health Services, Ministry of Health and Family Welfare of India. The chairperson of CDSCO is Drugs Controller General of India (DCGI), who is responsible for approval of new drugs, medical devices and clinical trials to be conducted in India.

The DCGI is advised by Drugs Technical Advisory Board (DTAB) and the Drugs Consultative Committee (DCC). There are 6 zonal offices of CDSCO located at Mumbai, Kolkata, Chennai, Hyderabad, Ghaziabad and Ahmadabad. These zonal offices are involved in GMP audits and inspection of manufacturing units of large volume parentrals, vaccines, sera and blood products. In addition to zonal offices, CDSCO also has 3 sub-zonal offices at Jammu, Chandigarh and Bengaluru. These co-ordinate with state drug control authorities under their jurisdiction for uniform standard of inspection and enforcement.

Functions of CDSCO

- Giving approval for new drugs and permission for conducting clinical trials in India.
- Providing licences for blood banks, vaccines, medical devices, r-DNA products and diagnostic agents.
- Amendment to Drugs & Cosmetics Act and Rules.
- Participating in WHO-GMP certification programmes.

15.5.4 European Medicines Agency (EMA)

EMA is the regulatory agency for the European countries. It was officially framed in the year 1995 works across the European Union (EU) and globally to protect public and animal health by monitoring medicines with strict scientific guidelines. The management board is the EMA's integral governance body. The Agency is responsible for the scientific evaluation, supervision and safety monitoring of medicines developed by pharmaceutical companies for use in the EU. EMA serves a market for more than 500 million people living in Europe.

EMA is composed of sevenscientific committees

1. Committee for Medicinal Products for Human Use (CHMP)
2. Pharmacovigilance Risk Assessment Committee (PRAC)
3. Committee for Medicinal Products for Veterinary Use (CVMP)
4. Committee for Orphan Medicinal Products (COMP)
5. Committee for Herbal Medicinal Products (HMPC)
6. Committee for Advanced Therapies (CAT)
7. Pediatric Committee (PDCO)

Functions of EMA

- To promote and protect public and animal health by evaluation and supervision of medicines for human and veterinary use.
- To monitor and supervise the safety of drug products via pharmacovigilance network and take appropriate actions.
- To publish clear and impartial information about medicines and their approved uses. This includes public versions of scientific assessment reports and summaries written in local language.
- To provide scientific advice and assist pharmaceutical industries for developing new medicines.

15.5.5 Medicines and Healthcare Products Regulatory Agency (MHRA)

The MHRA is the agency/authority responsible for ensuring that medicines and medical devices are acceptable/safe for public use in UK. The MHRA also regulates wide range of healthcare products such as vaccines, biological drug products, blood related products and tissue engineered drug products.

The agency was framed on 1 April 2003 with the merger of the Medicines Control Agency (MCA) and the Medical Devices Agency (MDA). It is an Executive Agency of the Department of Health.

Functions of MHRA

- Regulation of clinical trials for drug products and medical devices.
- Monitoring the safety and efficacy of drug products by post-marketing surveillance reporting system.
- Assessment and authorization of medicinal products for sale and supply in UK.
- Monitoring and assuring compliance with MHRA regulations relating to medicines and medical devices.
- Providing technical and scientific information to healthcare professionals.
- Oversee the notified bodies that ensure medical devices manufactureres to comply with regulatory requirements prior to the marketing approval.

15.5.6 Health Canada

In Canada, the drug products and medical devices are regulated by Health Canada. Before giving marketing approval for a product, the Therapeutic Products Directorate (TPD) of Health, Canada evaluates the scientific data of the product's safety, efficacy and quality as directed by Food and Drugs Act and Regulations. The head office of TPD is located at Ottawa, the capital of Canada.

In Canada, about 70% of newer drug product submissions were made over 3 months and 40% in a year. The review process of regulatory submissions to Health Canada takes a time period of 540 days. The drug regulatory approval process is completed by various applications submitted to the authority and the drug product registration in Canada is a challenging task.

Functions of Health Canada

- Scrutinizes the scientific data related to quality, safety and efficacy of drug products and medical devices.
- Assess the potential uses and possible risks of drug products and medical devices.
- Reviews the clinical trial applications and investigational testing applications for drug products and medical devices to assure the studies and methodologies are well designed and scientifically sound that participants are not to be exposed to undue risks.
- Provides Canadian people with science based information that they need to make informed choices.
- Monitors the evolving safety of drugs in development through a review system of adverse events reports that are submitted as requirements of Food and Drug regulations.

15.5.7 Therapeutic Goods Administration (TGA)

Therapeutic Goods Administration (TGA) is the regulatory authority of Australia for regulating the healthcare products including medicines, medical devices, blood products and cosmetics. TGA is a division of the Australian Health Department established under the Therapeutic Goods Act of 1989. The main goal of TGA is to assess and monitor the activities to ensure that therapeutic goods available in Australia are of acceptable standards of quality and safety.

Functions of TGA

- Evaluation of quality, safety and efficacy of prescription drugs, OTC healthcare products, medical devices and biological products.
- To control the export of drugs and medical devices from Australia to other countries.
- To control the advertisements related to drug products and medical devices.
- To monitor the adverse drug reactions of medicinal drug products manufactured in Australia.
- To review and approve the regulatory submissions for the drug products and medical devices.

Table 15.1: List of important regulatory authorities

Name of the Country	Regulatory Authority Name
USA	Food and Drug Administration (FDA)
India	Central Drugs Standard Control Organization (CDSCO)
Europe	European Medicines Agency (EMA)
Canada	Health Canada
Brazil	Agencia Nacional de Vigiloncia Sanitaria (ANVISA)
UK	Medicines and Healthcare Products Regulatory Agency (MHRA)
Australia	Therapeutic Goods Administration
New Zealand	Medicines and Medical Devices Safety Authority (Medsafe)
South Africa	South African Health Products Regulatory Authority (SAHPRA)
Sweden	Medical Products Agency (MPA)
Denmark	Danish Medicines Agency (DMA)
Russia	Ministry of Health of the Russian Federation
Italy	Italian Pharmaceutical Agency (IPA)
Thailand	Ministry of Public Health
Ireland	Irish Medicines Board
Nigeria	National Agency for Food and Drug Administration and Control (NAFDAC)
Germany	Germany's Federal Institute for Drugs and Medical Devices
Sri Lanka	National Medicines Regulatory Authority
Switzerland	Swiss Agency for Therapeutic Products (Swissmedic)
China	National Medical Products Administration (NMPA)
Japan	Pharmaceuticals and Medical Devices Agency (PMDA)
South Korea	Ministry of Food and Drugs Safety (MFDS)

15.6 ROLE OF REGULATORY AFFAIRS DEPARTMENT

- RA department acts as a bridge between the pharmaceutical company and the regulatory authorities across the world.
- Preparation and submission of well organized and scientifically valid regulatory documents such as NDA, ANDA, MAA, DMF.
- Ensure the pharmaceutical companies adhere to the applicable cGMP, ICH, GCP, GLP guidelines, regulations and laws.
- Providing expertise and regulatory knowledge in translating regulatory requirements into practical approaches.
- Providing technical advice to the companies on regulatory matters and climate that would affect their activities.
- As a team member, RA department also contributes in drug development procedures.

15.7 JOB RESPONSIBILITIES OF RA DEPARTMENT

- Filing and documenting the DMF with concerned regulatory agencies in support of NDA/ANDA/INDA/MAA submitted by manufacturer.
- Filing of API dossier in accordance with European Directorate for the Quality of Medicines (EDQM).
- Assessing and filing the amendments to the information in DMF/Dossier of API with regulatory agencies. The major regulations are reported before their final implementation.
- Getting prior approval from customers of API before making major changes related to information given in DMF/dossier. The revised DMF/dossier can be submitted to the customers along with changes filed with the agency.
- Documenting, compiling and submitting the applicant's DMF to the API customers by customer filing with the regulatory agency.
- Preparing and submitting the authorization letter to API customers and regulatory authorities.
- Preparing the technical specifications required for the packaging of API.
- Filing annual, biannual, quarterly reports (changes made in DMF, ASMF and Dossier) with the regulatory agencies.
- Documenting and maintenance of complete profile of all the API's manufactured.

15.8 JOB PROFILE OF RA PROFESSIONALS IN DRUG PRODUCT/ FINISHED PRODUCT MANUFACTURING COMPANY

- Preparing and submitting the regulatory documents, NDA, ANDA, SNDA, BLA and MAA of drug products to the concerned regulatory authorities to get marketing approval.
- Verifying and filing amendments, supplements, and variations related to manufacture, control, labelling, stability studies, and evaluations in NDA, ANDA and MAA with regulatory agencies for prior approval.

- Filing annual/biannual reports with changes made in NDA, ANDA, MAA with the regulatory authorities.
- Collecting the information about the adverse events reported from drug products used by patients and reporting that to higher authorities.
- Documenting and maintaining the complete profile of individual drug dosage forms manufactured in the company.
- Getting involved in drug development process to advice the R & D department about the guidelines, regulations and different procedures.

15.9 REGULATORY REQUIREMENTS FOR DRUG APPROVAL

15.9.1 Drug Development Teams

In the recent years, the drug development and drug discovery process has become essential part of pharmaceutical industries. The drug development and discovery nearly takes an average time line of about 10-15 which requires an investment of approximately US $ 1 bn.

The pharmaceutical and biotechnological industries majorly involved in drug development usually frame different teams/departments to carry out the different processes involved in the drug discovery stages to formulate a suitable drug candidate into pharmaceutical product.

The responsibilities of the drug discovery teams include:

- To prepare and compile the drug development protocols and objectives of drug discovery.
- To frame the timelines for different stages of drug discovery process.
- To review the data of results of methods adopted in the research process.
- To define and monitor the various stages of drug development programme.
- To compare research results and development status and timelines with drug candidates under development by competitors.
- To provide technical guidance and make necessary recommendations on the continuous development of the drug candidate.

The different drug development teams involved in drug research are discussed below.

1. Drug Discovery Project Team

This team is usually composed of small number of research scientists of different scientific disciplines such as chemistry, pharmacology, toxicology, biopharmaceutics, etc. The first objective of this team is to find out a lead drug candidate by initial screening methods such as structural elucidation, molecular structure relationships and combinatorial chemistry. The study then proceeds for pharmacological methods and results obtained were shared with chemists, to prepare the derivatives of active compounds to carry out SAR studies. After recognizing the lead molecule, other team players need to carry out the further studies. The analytical chemistry department performs physical and chemical characterization of the molecule to establish the stability profile. The drug metabolism and pharmacokinetics are assessed by bioanalytical chemistry team. Toxicology team evaluates the potential adverse effects of drug molecule and biopharmaceutics team is involved in formulating the dosage form with proposed route of drug administration.

2. Pre-clinical drug development team

This team is assigned the responsibility of carrying out the pharmacological screening of lead drug molecule, using the animal models. The pre-clinical evaluation studies include:

(a) Toxicological studies
(b) Pharmacodynamic studies
(c) Pharmacokinetic studies

The final job of this team is to prepare, compile an IND and submits it to the respective regulatory authority. As the development of the drug candidate transferred to next stage, clinical study then the preclinical project team becomes as clinical project team.

3. Clinical drug development team

After the submission of IND and its approval the next step is the initiation of clinical trial studies on human subjects. The clinical drug development team further includes new members to expand the roles. The trained clinical investigators will perform Phase 1. 2 and 3 studies. The clinical research associates coordinate and monitor the Phase 1, 2 and 3 studies to ensure that study documents such as protocols, case reports are properly prepared and documented. The quality control department performs the assay, validation procedures to support the manufacturing process. Biostatisticians guide in designing the study groups and help in evaluating the results from both non-clinical and clinical studies.

The 4 phases of clinical trials are described below.

Phase I: The study is conducted on small number of 20-100 healthy human volunteers and the study can be finished within 6-9 months of time period. The main objective of phase I studies is to assess the pharmacokinetic study variations between humans and animals to determine the safe and tolerable drug dose for humans and to document any predicted toxicity.

Phase II: Here, the studies are performed to evaluate the safety and efficacy of drug molecule in patients with target disease. Depending on the type of drug and disease to be treated the study can take time period of 6 months to 3 years. It has 2 phases:

Early phase: The study can be conducted on 20-200 human subjects.

Late Phase: Here, the study is done on 50-300 human subjects.

Phase III: This study is carried out in large patient pool of 200-1000 to further verify the safety and efficacy of the drug. It is also referred as confirmatory phase. The study duration period is 1-4 years. The main aim of the study is to reduce the data errors obtained in phase II studies. After the completion of phase III studies, the New Drug Application (NDA) is prepared, filed and submitted to the concerned regulatory agency. Once the NDA submission is received by the regulatory agency, they review and if accepted regulatory approval is be granted for the drug product to enter the market.

Phase IV: It is called post-marketing-surveillance phase and there is no specific time period for this study. The aim of this phase is to find out and record any possible rare, unknown and serious adverse reactions of drug reported from patients. The reported information has to be communicated to the respective regulatory authority by the manufacturer.

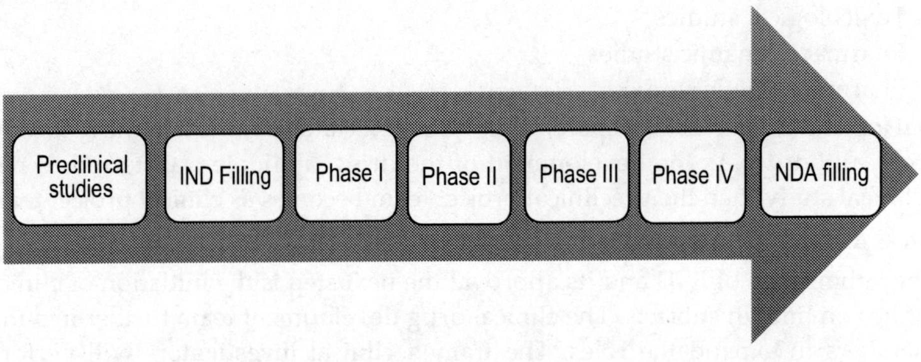

Fig. 15.2: Process of drug development and final approval

4. Drug Development logic plan team

This team is dedicated to coordinate the various studies required for the successful development of research drug molecule and to ensure that the timelines for development is as per the schedule. The required studies and the extent of the development plan depends on 4 criteria of the proposed drug candidate, those are:

(i) The type of drug molecule (macromolecule such as a protein, polypeptide or oligonucleotide or small organic molecule).

(ii) Type of disease to be treated with the drug molecule (life threatening diseases like AIDS, cancers, CVS and CNS disorders and non- life threatening diseases, hypertension, diabetes, inflammation and infectious syndromes).

(iii) The duration of drug therapy (acute with one or a few doses being sufficient for treatment or chronic with prolonged administration necessary to mediate the disease process).

(iv) Route of administration (such as IV bolus injection, infusion or oral, pulmonary, subcutaneous, intramuscular, topical, etc.).

15.10 NON-CLINICAL DRUG DEVELOPMENT

Before performing non-clinical studies, an adequate amount of the active pharmaceutical ngredient (API) must be produced. Non-clinical studies generally require less amount of APIs in milligrams or grams, further for the commercial scale up batches to produce bulk quantity.

For the studies to meet standard regulations, like good laboratory practices (GLP), the production batches of APIs must be qualified and formulated according to good manufacturing practices (GMP) guidelines. The key aspects to be checked during non-clinical drug development are chemistry, manufacturing and control (CMC) systems. The CMC studies include:

- Determination of therapeutic drug dose and method of application of the active ingredients based on product properties and type of animal model used.
- Assessing the detailed physicochemical characterization studies of active drug.
- Carrying out stability studies and impurity analysis.
- Development and validation of methods to estimate the active drug content in body fluids (e.g., blood, plasma, urine) by using pharmacokinetic and pharmacodynamic approaches.

The non-clinical drug development studies and activities are performed throughout the life cycle of the product. The non-clinical studies of drug product are complex in design and are regulatory driven.

The main aims of these studies include:

- To identify the drug candidate that has the higher probability of therapeutic efficiency.
- To evaluate the safety and efficacy.
- To establish solid scientific study results before transmission to the clinical development stage.

The information obtained in non-clinical studies is needed in specific situations for decisions:

- For clinical trials
- For marketing authorization applications
- For post-marketing or monitoring studies

15.10.1 Types of Non-clinical Studies

***In vitro* studies**

These are performed in a well controlled environment outside of a living organism, such as using hepatocyte cultures for metabolism studies.

***In vivo* studies**

These include experiments performed on laboratory testing animals using animal tissues, organs and cells.

The following types of studies are performed:

- Pharmacodynamics (effects of medicines on organism)
- Pharmacokinetics (effects of organism on medicine)
- Toxicity
- Drug effects on pregnancy and fertility

In *silico* studies

In silico refers to an expression meaning performing the experiments using computer software or via computer simulation, for example, predicting the toxicity profile of a product using its chemical structure with data based approaches.

The types of studies include:

- Pharmacogenomics
- Biomarkers effects
- Development of the compound

15.11 PHARMACOLOGY

The pharmacological screening for the research drug products can be performed adopting various *in vitro* methods, for activation and dependency on dosing, schedule and route of administration, calculating the inhibitory concentrations, such as IC_{50} and IC_{90}, for each system evaluated; evaluate the potential resistance for lead candidate, determine the additive, synergistic or antagonistic drug-drug interactions during combination therapy, if appropriate; evaluate possible cytotoxic concentrations of lead drug compound on various types of cells like stem cells, bone marrow and immune system cells.

Pharmacological studies can also be extended to define and characterize the animal models that mimic the human disease to be evaluated and determine appropriate end points for the assessment of biological activity. To evaluate *in vivo* dose-response comparison of lead candidates, calculation of therapeutic doses, e.g., ED_{50} or ED_{10} and therapeutic ratio when combined with no effect or minimum toxic effect dose levels. In addition, other *in vivo* evaluations can also be conducted, but not limited to dosing regimen dependency; administration route; formulation type, disease status, cross-resistance profile, combination therapy for synergism, antagonism, and special models.

15.12 DRUG METABOLISM

The drug metabolism is the process of enzymatic conversion from one form of chemical substance to another form. There are generally 2 major phases of drug metabolism which include different types of reactions. Phase I includes hydrolytic reactions in esters, amides, epoxides. Oxidation of aromatic moieties, alcohols, aldehydes, benzylic and allicyclic carbon atoms. Reduction reactions occur with aldehydes, ketones, nitro and azo compounds. Phase II reactions include conjugations of glucuronic acid, glycine and other amino acids, acetylation and methylation reactions. The enzymes responsible for oxidation, reduction and conjugation include hepatic microsomal enzymes and the major organs influenced with these reactions include brain, heart, lungs, and intestines. The reactions, such as acetylation, sulphation, hydrolysis of alcohols and aldehydes are mediated by hepatic non-microsomal enzymes and the major site of metabolism includes liver and kidneys. In general, the drug metabolism studies are conducted to assess the rate and extent of metabolism of drug candidate in human body. Many *in vitro* experiments can be carried out to determine the metabolic stability of active drug and to compare the fate of drug in animals and humans.

15.13 TOXICOLOGY

Toxicity may exert from the extension of the therapeutic effect of the drug, e.g., use of barbiturates can induce coma, bleeding due to heparin, etc.

The organs that are most likely to be affected by drug toxicity include brain, heart, kidneys, liver, lings, intestine and pancreas

15.13.1 Types of Toxicity

1. Cytotoxicity

It is the most common type of drug toxicity, where the drug or an active metabolite causes severe damage to the body cells. The cells of particular organ are affected, resulting into a potentially fatal loss of function of the liver or kidney, damage to eyes, ears or abnormal clotting of the blood.

2. Carcinogenicity

Any substance, drug, radioactive compound or radiation agent which induces cancer is called carcinogen and the toxicity induced by such agent is referred to as carcinogenicity. Many radioactive substances are considered to be carcinogens, a few examples are tobacco smoke and inhaled asbestos.

3. Mutagenecity

Some drugs can cause permanent changes to the DNA of germ cells -- egg cells and sperm cells – leading to mutations which are inherited by a patient's children, e.g., nitrogen mustard.

4. Teratogenicity

Some drugs can cause birth defects in the development of the foetus, resulting in birth deformities in the newborn babies. The extent and severity of teratogenic effects depends on the different stages of organs to develop at different times during pregnancy. Thalidomide consumption in pregnant women caused birth deformities in more than 12,000 children worldwide during 1950-60 period.

15.14 INVESTIGATIONAL NEW DRUG APPLICATION (INDA)

IND is a regulatory submission made to FDA or to any respective regulatory authority to get permission for conducting the clinical studies for a new/innovator drug product. The Federal Food, Drug and Cosmetics Act states that drugs should have an approved marketing authorization (MAA) before they can be commercialized. The IND application allows a company to initiate, plan and conduct the clinical trials for their new drug products.

IND is required for a:

- new/innovator drug candidate,
- drug not being approved for the intended purpose under investigation,
- new dosage form, and
- new combination drug therapy.

IND is not required for:

- a drug that doesn't require human studies, but is intended for *in vitro* and *in vivo* animal studies,
- non-clinical studies, and
- studying an approved drug for approved indication.

Essentials of IND

- The IND must provide adequate data and information to FDA for evaluating the drug suitability for use in proposed clinical study.
- The objective of the initial IND should be the general investigational plan and the protocol for the first proposed human study.
- To assure that the human subjects who participate in the proposed study will not be exposed to unreasonable and significant risk.

15.14.1 Types of IND

IND is of two types:

1. **Commercial IND:** It is required to get marketing authorization approval for a new drug product.
2. **Non-commercial IND:** It is of following types.
   - 2.1 **Investigator IND:** In this type, the physician acts as both sponsor and investigator.
   - 2.2 **Emergency IND:** It allows FDA to authorize the use of an experimental drug in an emergency condition.
   - 2.3 **Treatment IND:** It is required for getting approval of investigational drug to be used to treat a serious or life threatening disease or if there is no alternative therapy available.

15.14.2 INDA Content and Format

1. Cover sheet (FORM FDA 1571)
2. Table of contents
3. Introductory statement and a general investigational plan
4. Investigators brochure
5. Clinical study protocols
6. Chemistry, manufacturing and control information
7. Pharmacology and toxicology information
8. Previous human experience with the investigational drug
9. Other relevant information
10. Protocol amendments, any changes in the protocol

1. Cover sheet: Form FDA 1571

- **Sponsor:** Sponsor is the person who takes the responsibility to initiate the clinical investigation for the new drug. The sponsor can be a pharmaceutical company, a private or academic organization or an individual. The IND sponsors are required to get a signed FDA form 1572 from the clinical investigator with the following information:
  - Date of submission
  - Name and contact address of investigator(s)
  - Contents of application
  - Name of investigational drug product and its IND number

- Name and address of the person responsible for monitoring of clinical investigations
- Name of sponsor's authorized representative

2. Table of contents

It is an index page including all the contents as headings and subheadings with proper assigned page numbers and description.

3. Introductory statement and investigational plan

The introductory statement includes the following information:

- The description of investigational drug.
- Pharmacological classification or category of drug.
- Structural formula, dosage form of drug, and route of administration of drug.
- Summary of previous human experience to assess the drug safety studies.
- Aims, objectives and timelines for the proposed clinical investigation.

The investigation plan includes description of clinical studies planned for the investigational drug, purpose of the study, indications to be used, types of trials to be conducted, number of human subjects for the study, risks associated and potential benefits of the study.

4. Investigator's brochure

The investigator's brochure (IB) should include the following information:

- Structural formula of the drug.
- Summary of pharmacological, toxicological, pharmacokinetic effects in animals.
- Safety and efficacy study profiles.
- Purpose of the study.
- Dose/dose frequency, dosage form and storage indications of drug product.
- Monitoring procedures.

5. Clinical study protocols

A clinical protocol is a study document that should briefly describe the information about the conduction and proposed clinical investigation including the study objectives, trial design, selection of human subjects, and procedure of clinical studies. The clinical protocols must also contain the following information:

- Name, address and qualification of each investigator involved in the study.
- Name and address of the clinical site.
- Study subjects inclusion and exclusion criteria.
- Estimate of the number of subjects to be enrolled in the clinical investigation.
- The study duration of clinical investigation.
- Methods to minimize the study errors.

6. Chemistry, Manufacturing and Controls (CMC)

This section outlines the adequacy of methods used to manufacture and evaluation procedures like impurity analysis, stability studies, quality control checks and assay for the investigational drug. It also includes safety concerns, method of preparation of drug formulation, reagents and solvents used for study and acceptable limits of analytical studies to ensure the purity and quality of the drug.

7. Pharmacology and toxicology information

This section of IND describes the information about the pharmacological effects, mechanism of action of and pharmacokinetic profile of the drug. If the information is not known then clinical acceptance of the drug will be hold. In addition, an integrated summary of toxicological effects of drug reported in animal studies can be included to support the safety of the proposed human investigation.

8. Previous human experience with the investigational drug

In this section, if the drug is already studied on humans or if the clinical investigations have been done in any other country then the obtained data can be used as supporting document as previous human experience. But if the drug is to be tested on human subjects for the first time, then this information is not required.

The required information is pharmacokinetic, pharmacodynamic study reports and reported adverse reactions. In addition to this, if any information regarding the safety of drug is available in any publications that can be used as reference source.

9. Other relevant information

This section includes any additional information required for the special topics as required if by the FDA such as drug dependence, drug abuse potential, radioactive substance dose, studies conducted in paediatric patients, etc. In addition to the above said information, some other essential aspects of investigational new drug also should be included such as:

- The financial disclosure statement of each investigator and sub-investigator.
- Informed consent form copies.
- Drug master files.
- Previous study reports or supporting study literatures.

10. Protocol amendments

This refers to the revised or changes made in the protocol such as addition of clinical investigators, changes in the study design, procedures and the document is submitted to conduct new clinical studies that are not described in the existing investigational drug product. The protocol amendments include a copy of new protocol and a detailed summary of differences between the old and revised protocol. A method of data collection in amendment can be asked by FDA to ensure the specifications like new/revised protocol, new investigator.

After the compilation and submission of IND to FDA, the sponsor should wait for 30 days. During this period, the FDA will review the IND to ensure that research studies are safe and within the compliance of standard regulatory guidelines.

15.15 FDA REVIEW PROCESS OF IND

Once FDA receives the IND it is forwarded to review team called Center for Drug Evaluation and Research (CDER). On arrival at the review division, it is critically evaluated by different experts of chemistry, medical, biopharmaceutics, microbiology, statistics, pharmacology and toxicology departments to ensure the safety of study subjects enrolled for clinical investigation. Once the IND is submitted, the sponsor should not initiate the clinical study until a period of 30 days. If there are any major issues found regarding the safety of human subjects in the proposed study, the FDA can hold or reject the proposal. If FDA is satisfied with the information provided in IND, it can approve the IND and also permits to conduct clinical trials for the investigational drug by sending the acceptance notification to the sponsor.

15.16 INVESTIGATOR'S BROCHURE

The investigator's brochure (IB) is a document of compilation of the non-clinical and clinical study data on the investigational product that are relevant to the study of products in humans. The purpose of IB is to provide the information to clinical investigators and others involved in the clinical studies to facilitate the understanding of rationale for the trial design and its compliance, other key concepts of protocol like dose, dose frequency, interval, route of drug administration and safety monitoring procedures.

The information provided in IB should in a simple, understanding, concise, objective oriented that enables a physician or other investigators to understand and make their own unbiased risk-benefit assessment of the appropriateness of the proposed trial. For this purpose, a medically well qualified person should generally participate in the editing of an IB, but the contents of the IB should be approved by the disciplines that generated the described data. The IB should be reviewed at least once yearly and must be accordingly revised in compliance with sponsor's written procedures. In general, sponsor is responsible for updating of IB to make it available to the investigator and investigator is responsible for providing the updated IB to the respective institutional review boards (IRBs).

The general considerations of IB include:

1. Title page

It should include the information about the name of sponsor, details of each investigational product including its chemical, generic and brand name, and release rate. It is also suggested to provide the edition number, reference to the number and supersede edition date of the document. The format of IB title page is shown below:

Title Page of Investigator's Brochure

Sponsor's Name: ____________________

Name of the product: ____________________

Research Number: ____________________

Names: Chemical/generic name (if approved):____________

Trade name (If approved): ____________

Edition number: ____________

Release date: ____________

Replaces previous edition number: ____________

Date: ____________

2. Confidentiality Statement

The sponsor may wish to include statement informing the investigator/recipient to consider the IB as confidential document for the sole information and use of the investigator's team and the IRB/IEC.

3. Contents of Investigator's Brochure

3.1 Table of contents

An example of table of contents is described in the following table.

Table 15.2: IB table of contents

SI. No.	Name of the content
1	Table of contents
2	Summary
3	Introduction
4	Physical, chemical and pharmaceutical properties of formulation
5	Non-clinical studies
5.1	Non-clinical pharmacology
5.2	Pharmacokinetics and product metabolism in animals
5.3	Toxicology
6	Effects in humans
6.1	Pharmacokinetics and product metabolism in humans
6.2	Safety and efficacy
6.3	Marketing experience
7	Summary of data and guidance for the investigator

3.2 Summary

A brief summary should be given specifying the potential physical, chemical, pharmaceutical, pharmacological, toxicological, pharmacokinetic, metabolic and clinical aspects that are related to the clinical development stage of the investigational drug product. The summary report should not exceed two pages.

3.3 Introduction

This section includes the information of chemical name, generic name or trade name of the investigational products, all active ingredients, the pharmacological category and advantages of investigational products, the need of research and the anticipated diagnostic or therapeutic indications.

3.4 Physical, chemical and pharmaceutical properties of formulation

This section should describe the information of investigational product(s) regarding the chemical, structural formula, physical, chemical and pharmaceutical properties.

To permit appropriate safety measures to be taken in the course of study, a description of formulation used, excipients used should be provided with proper justification. The storage instructions and handling of the product should also be included.

3.5 Non-clinical studies

This section should include a brief summary of data of all the relevant non-clinical pharmacology, toxicology, pharmacokinetic and metabolism studies of investigational product. The summary should address the methods used, results and discussions with potential findings to the evaluated therapeutic, unfavourable and unintended effects on humans.

The following information should be documented in this section:

(a) Number and sex of animals tested
(b) Number of species of animals used
(c) Unit dose (mg/kg)
(d) Dose interval
(e) Dosing duration
(f) Route of drug administration
(g) Information about systemic distribution
(h) Results of the following aspects:
- Nature and frequency of pharmacological or toxic effects
- Severity of toxic effects
- Reversibility of effects
- Duration of effects
- Dose response

3.5.1 Non-clinical pharmacology

In this section, a brief summary of the pharmacological studies of the investigational drug and its significant metabolites found in animal studies should be provided. The summary should also include some studies adopted to evaluate the therapeutic activity and studies used to assess the safety and other pharmacological actions.

3.5.2 Pharmacokinetics and product metabolism in animals

This section should include the summary of studies of pharmacokinetics and biological transformation and disposition of the investigational product conducted in all the animal species used for the studies. The results of findings should address the absorption, local and systemic bioavailability of investigational product, its metabolites and their relationship to the pharmacological and toxicological outputs in animal species.

3.5.3 Toxicology

In this section a brief report of the toxicological effects found in the relevant studies conducted in different animal species should be included with the details of single dose, repeated dose, carcinogenicity, reproductive toxicity and mutagenicity findings.

3.6 Effects in humans

This section provides information of pharmacokinetics, metabolism, pharmacodynamics, dose response, safety, efficacy and other pharmacological studies conducted on humans. If possible, a brief summary of each trial completed can also be provided. Information should also be provided regarding results of any use of the investigational product(s) other than from in clinical trials, such as from experience during marketing.

3.6.1 Pharmacokinetics and product metabolism in humans

This section includes the information of investigational products with reference to following studies:

- Pharmacokinetic studies: Absorption, metabolism, plasma protein binding, distribution and elimination.
- Bioavailability of the investigational product using reference dosage form.
- Population subgroups: Age, sex and impaired organ function.
- Drug:Drug and drug-food interaction studies.
- Other relevant pharmacokinetic data.

3.6.2 Safety and Efficacy

In this section, a summary of information related to safety, efficacy, pharmacodynamics, dose response studies of investigational product performed in human subjects should be included.

3.6.3 Marketing experience

This section of IB should include the information of investigational product that has been approved in any other countries and the also the countries where the same product has not been approved or withdrawn from market can also be provided. This is followed by significant information such as dosage form, route of administration and adverse reactions reported.

3.7 Summary of data and guidance for the investigator

This section should provide an overall summary of the non-clinical and clinical data with reference to possible risks and adverse reactions, pharmacological and toxicological studies conducted for the investigational drug product.

15.17 NEW DRUG APPLICATION (NDA)

The new drug application (NDA) is regulatory approval granted by FDA to the innovator products and for new drug dosage forms. In US, NDA is the driving force through which sponsors formally propose the FDA for getting the approval of new/innovator drug products.

15.17.1 Goals of NDA

- Assessment of safety and efficacy of new drug product in its proposed uses and its potential benefits and possible risks.
- Verifying the labelling aspects of the new drug product is in compliance with standard regulations.

- Assessing the methods used for quality, identity and purity of new drug product are following the GMP guidelines or not.

The NDA submitted to FDA can be prepared in following three formats:

I. **Archival copy:** It contains NDA covering letter, FDA-356h form, administrative information of company, index and case report forms.

II. **Review copy:** It includes the technical sections of NDA with cover letter, index, form FDA-356h, table of contents, labelling section and summary report.

III. **Field copy:** It is needed for FDA inspections during pre-approval of facilities. In addition to that, it also includes the CMC and validation aspects.

The NDA document consists of 20 different sections in addition to the FDA-356h itself. The content of every NDA may be variable based upon nature of drug and volume of information available at the submission time.

The NDA has total of 12 important sections with particular specification for each.

15.17.2 NDA Document Contents

Section 1: Index

It is the first section of NDA placed on the first page. It includes the details of all the sections included with the headings and page numbers. Each section may further have subsections included in the index page.

Section 2: Labelling aspects

This section includes the sample labelling draft for the use on the container, cartons and packages of the product.

Section 3: Summary format and content

In this section a brief summary should be provided. The data obtained must be represented in tables of graphical pictures and the overall summary report should be within 50-200 pages.

A. Annotated package insert

It includes proposed text of labelling requirements for the drug product. The proposed information of package labelling must be mentioned with reference to volume and page number to the provided information in the summary and in the technical sections of the applications.

B. Pharmacological class, scientific rationale, intended use and potential uses

This section should include a brief summary about the pharmacological category of drug, the scientific rationale of the drug, the intended uses and the potential benefits of the drug.

Section 4: Chemistry, manufacturing and controls (CMC)

This section must include a summary of overview for the drug substance and for the finished drug product.

A. Drug substance

A description of drug substance referring to its physical, chemical characteristic properties and stability aspects can be included.

B. Finished drug product

For the finished drug product(s) the following information should be provided.

- Composition and type of dosage form.
- Name and contact address of the manufacturer.
- Type of container and closure system used.
- Stability studies.
- Specifications for the drug product and evaluation methods to assure the standards.

Section 5: Nonclinical Pharmacology and Toxicology Summary

This section includes the information about the following types of studies:

- Pharmacological studies
- Acute toxicity studies
- Multidose toxicity studies
- Carcinogenicity studies
- Mutagenicity studies
- Special toxicity studies
- ADME studies

Section 6: Human Pharmacokinetics and Bioavailability section

This section should provide a brief summary of bioavailability study, bioequivalence studies conducted for new chemical entities to demonstrate that the formulation proposed for NDA approval is significantly bioequivalent to the standard reference drug used in early clinical trials. In addition, a brief summary of pharmacokinetic parameters such as C_{max}, T_{max}, V_d, plasma and renal clearance of drug product should also be included in this section.

Section 7: Microbiology

This section should include the major important features of anti-infective drug with following details:

- The biochemical basis of drug's action.
- Antimicrobial spectrum of the drug.
- Any known resistance mechanism to the drug.
- Clinical microbiological methods

Section 8: Clinical Data Section

This is an important and most complicated section of NDA which provides the data regarding the safety and efficacy of the drug for its intended use with the following details:

- Overview of clinical investigations
- Clinical pharmacology study reports
- Controlled and uncontrolled clinical study reports
- Integrated summary of drug safety and efficacy
- Drug abuse and overuse information
- Integrated summary of benefits and risks associated with drugs.

Section 9: Safety updates report

This includes the data that could affect the statement of draft label, warnings, contraindications, precautions and adverse events.

Section 10: Statistics

This section includes a brief description and documents of statistical approaches used to evaluate the clinical studies and other safety information.

Section 11: Case Report Tabulations

This section provides information about the completed data of each patient from Phase 1 clinical pharmacology study, Phase II, Phase III and safety data from all clinical studies.

Section 12: Case Report Forms

It includes the information about the patients who have died during the course of clinical studies and also patients dropped from the study.

15.18 REVIEW AND APPROVAL OF NDA

Once NDA is submitted to FDA, it conducts a review process for the received NDA to confirm the compliance with the regulations. FDA will either accept the filing or may send refusal letter to the applicant within 60 days of time period. The possible reasons for the rejection of proposal may include incomplete information provided in Form FDA 356h, incorrect formatting, no inspection of manufacturing facilities, translations of all sections of the document not being in English language, no availability of GLP compliance procedures.

CDER is responsible for assessing the NDA submitted by means of different expert groups such as pharmacology, chemistry, microbiology, biopharmaceutics, statistics and pharmacology. All the expert members review the critical aspects of NDA contents and if any additional information required, the sponsor will be informed for the same by FDA and the applicant would be notified to submit the report within 4 months of notification received. After verifying the received information, the FDA may either accept if all the provided information is in compliance with the regulations and if it is not acceptable, the submitted NDA proposal will be rejected.

15.19 BIOEQUIVALENCE STUDIES

Bioequivalence (BE) refers to the bioavailability comparison of two or more drug products, in which the formulation containing the same API are said to be bioequivalent, if the rate and extent of both drug formulations is same. BE has gained increased attention, because of increased availability and importance of generic drugs in the present pharmaceutical market.

BE studies are basically required to compare two products so as to compare their biological equivalence. Bioequivalence is finding the significant variations in the rate and extent to which the APU in formulations becomes available at the site of action when administered at same dose under same conditions. It is determined by comparing the biological study parameters like plasma concentration of drug, urinary excretion rate, and pharmacodynamic effects.

Objectives of BE studies

- To justify the equivalence of a new drug product as an alternative for an approved drug product to be pharmaceutically same or equivalent as that of approved drug.
- To ensure the clinical effectiveness of drug products by measuring the bioequivalence study parameters.
- To assess the risk of bioinequivalence and risk of pharmaco-therapeutic failure or diminished clinical safety.

15.20 TYPES OF BE STUDIES

Bioequivalence studies are performed by different in vitro and in vivo methods which are briefly discussed as follows:

15.20.1 Pharmacokinetic Studies

The rate and extent of absorption of active drug at the site of action can be well described by using the pharmacokinetic measures to find out the drug release from the formulation into blood stream. In order to assess the rate and extent of systemic exposure and systemic absorption some pharmacokinetic parameters such as AUC, C_{max} and T_{max} can be studied.

These approaches are needed to understand the predetermined relationship that exists in between the concentration of drug at the site of action and at systemic circulation. The pharmacokinetic studies are more prominent to assess bioequivalence for the drug products by determining the drug amounts in biological fluids such as blood, plasma and urine. There are two major types of pharmacokinetic methods for measurement of BE of drugs and they are:

1. Plasma level-time studies
2. Urinary excretion studies

15.20.2 Pharmacodynamic Studies

The pharmacokinetic studies provide more accurate, sensitive and reproducible results, however, if these approaches cannot give the good end points, then pharmacodynamic studies are helpful to demonstrate the bioequivalence of drug products. The essential component of BE study by pharmacodynamic response is the dose-response relationship study. Pharmacodynamic evaluation measures the effect on a pathophysiological process after administration of two different products to serve as a basis for BE assessment. Pharmacodynamic studies are necessary for the following situations:

- For the drug or its metabolite that cannot be analyzed quantitatively in plasma or urine.
- If the drug concentration measurement cannot be used as alternative endpoint for the demonstration of efficacy and safety of a pharmaceutical product.

The two most commonly used pharmacodynamic methods are:

1. Acute pharmacological response
2. Therapeutic response

15.20.3 Comparative Clinical Studies

These are required, if there are no proper pharmacokinetic and pharmacodynamic approaches available to establish the BE of certain drug products. For example, for the orally administered drug products to assess the active moieties in biological fluids cannot be determined by any of the pharmacokinetic and pharmacodynamic studies.

15.20.4 *In vitro* Dissolution Studies

Under certain circumstances, the bioequivalence of drug products can be determined by *in vitro* methods. *In vitro* dissolution studies are mostly recommended for the BE measurement of drugs having high permeability and high solubility. The *in vitro* dissolution studies are also required to reduce the number of *in vivo* methods and to support batch-to-batch product quality.

15.21 CLINICAL RESEARCH PROTOCOL (CRP)

Every clinical study begins with the development of a clinical research protocol. CRP is the document that describes the conduction of clinical trials with study design, objectives, method, statistical considerations and ensures the safety of human subjects involved in the study.

Need of clinical research protocols

- To clarify the research question
- To compile existing knowledge
- To formulate a hypothesis and objectives
- To decide about a study design
- To clarify ethical considerations
- To apply for funding
- To have a guideline and tool for the research team

15.21.1 Components of Clinical Research Protocols

1. Title page

The title page of clinical research protocol includes the following:

- Protocol title, protocol identifying number, date, and any amendment(s).
- Details of the sponsor, investigator(s), and sponsor's medical expert.
- Details of the person(s) authorized to sign the protocol.
- Details of the qualified physician who is responsible for trial-site related medical decisions (if other than investigator).
- Details of the clinical laboratory and other medical and/or technical department(s) and/or institutions involved in the trial.

2. Introduction

Study subject/hypothesis should be clearly identified and briefly described in introduction.

3. Abstract

Abstract is a summary of the information in a document. Abstract must be:

Accurate, which correctly reflects the purpose and content of manuscript.

Concise and specific ,to make sentence informative and as possible as brief.

Non-evaluative , to report information objectively.

4. Objectives of study

The study objectives should be clearly stated as hypotheses to be tested. It should have a corresponding discussion in the statistical section. A detailed description of primary, secondary and exploratory objectives can be included in this section.

5. Study Rationale

Every clinical research protocol must have a section of scientific rationale, with a brief explanation of necessary study of the product in the patient population or in the event of an observational study, to know the importance of the study design. The risk and benefit ratio of the study also should be clearly stated by the investigators.

6. Study Design

The scientific integrity and the data resulted from the proposed study largely depends on the study design adopted. This section should critically describe the following aspects:

- The methods of measurement of primary and secondary endpoints.
- A schematic diagram with study design, procedures, study types and stages.
- Possible measures to be taken to minimize the bias.
- Details of dosage form, dose, labelling and packaging of investigational product(s).
- The approximate time duration of participant exposure in the study, time line of different studies to be conducted.
- Criteria for the discontinuation of the clinical study during unavoidable circumstances.
- Accountability procedures for the investigational product, including the placebo and comparator.
- Maintenance of study treatment randomization codes and procedures for breaking codes.

7. Selection, inclusion, exclusion and withdrawal of subjects

- The important criteria for selecting the human subjects for the clinical study include age, gender, type of disease, patient treatment history, and other medical conditions. The other possible reasons for eligibility criteria include rationale of the study, safety concerns, regulatory issues and practical considerations.
- The inclusion and exclusion criteria are the conditions that must be met in order to participate in the trial.
- The procedures for withdrawal of the participants include:
    - When and how participants can be withdrawn from the study.
    - How or whether the participants can be replaced into the study.
    - Follow up for the participants withdrawn from the clinical study.

8. Statistical methods and considerations

The data that may be subjected to the statistical approach may be specified with certain studies, parameters, formula and which may be adopted for analysis of data, may be proposed in blue prints in advance. The sample size and sampling procedure should be described properly for selecting the number of subjects for the study designed.

9. Ethical and regulatory considerations

The proposed clinical investigation/study should be carried out according to following ethical guidelines:

- Declaration of Helsinki
- Belmonte Report
- Protection of Human Subjects
- Institutional Review Board Regulations
- Good Clinical Practice

10. Data management

This section describes the method of data gathered, documented, submitted, verified and archived. The protocol should provide general information of data management activities associated with the protocol. The data management plan describes the procedures to ensure the integrity regarding:

- Details of data system design and development.
- Data collection methods.
- Data entry and editing methods.
- Data monitoring, reporting and documenting methods.

11. Financing and Insurance

This section describes how the study will be financed and insured. In some research networks, these issues are addressed in a separate agreement and need not be included in the protocol.

12. Publication policy

It describes the procedures and policies regarding the publication of output of the study. In a few research studies, the guidelines and policies were made for investigators for the publication process. Researchers must be familiar with and to adhere with institutional and sponsor policies and publication requirements.

15.22 BIOSTATISTICS IN PHARMACEUTICAL PRODUCT DEVELOPMENT

Statistics is the scientific study of the numerical data based on the natural phenomena. It deals with collection, organizing, interpreting and reporting of data. Biostatistics is the application of statistics to a wide range of topics in biology. The approach of biostatics is also widely used in pharmaceutical industry for research and development.

Biostatics in pharmaceuticals is required:

- For evaluating the therapeutic response of drugs. For example, attention effect of caffeine, comparing the analgesic effect of plant extract and NSAID.
- To explore the changes produced by the drug either due to the action of drug or by chance.
- Comparing the action of two or more drugs of different dosages of same drug using statistical methods.
- Finding the association between disease and risk factors such as coronary artery disease and risk factors like smoking.
- In public health, including epidemiology, environmental health and healthcare management.
- In the design and analysis of clinical trials in medicine.

15.22.1 Basic Biostatistics Approach

A. **Descriptive Statistics;** It includes the collection, organization, summarization and presentation of data.

B. **Inferential Statistics:** It consists of generalizing from samples to populations, performing hypothesis tests, determination of relationship or influence of variables/factors and making predictions.

15.22.2 Commonly used Terms in Biostatistics

Data: It is the value or representation of a measurement. Dataset is a collection of data values that forms a dataset and each value in dataset is referred to as datum or data value.

Variable: A variable is a characteristic or an attribute that can take different values. It is of 2 types: dependent and independent variables.

Dependent variable includes the factors that is dependent on or influenced by the independent variables, i.e, variable to be affected by changes in the independent factors. Dependent variables can be termed outcome.

Independent variables are those required for the purposes of the studies to be investigated and are independent of the effects to be studied.

Population: It consists of all subjects that are being studied. Sample population is a part of population or a group of subjects selected from a population.

15.22.3 Types of Measurement Scales

Nominal scale: It divides the data mutually into exclusive categories in which no order can be imposed on the data. No ranking order can be placed on the data.

E.g: Gender: male or female, religion—roman, catholic.

Ordinal scale: It classifies that data into grades that can be ranked, however precise variations between the rankings do not exist.

E.g: Level of pain: None, mild, moderate and severe.

Interval scale: It grades the rank data and small differences between units of measures do exist but there is no meaningful zero.

E.g: Temperature in °C in 4 different days

Day	:	1	2	3	4
Temperature (°C)	:	35	40	43	46

Ratio scale: It includes all the characteristics of interval measurement, and there exists a true zero.

E.g: Weight in pounds of 6 individuals: 126, 132, 116, 152, 144.

IV. Sampling Techniques

Random sampling: In this type, the subjects are selected by random numbers.

Systematic sampling: Here, the subjects are selected by using the nth number after the first subject is selected randomly from 1 through n^{th}.

Stratified sampling: In this, subjects are selected by dividing the population into groups and the subjects within the groups are randomly selected.

Cluster sampling: Here, the subjects are selected by using an intact group called cluster, that is, representative of the population.

15.23 DATA PRESENTATION FOR FDA SUBMISSIONS

The regulatory submissions such as NDA, ANDA, BLA and marketing authorization to FDA includes a set of data which includes non-clinical and clinical studies. The presentation of the data to FDA should be made in the standard format as recommended by authorities. The NDA regulatory submission to FDA can be presented in the following format:

15.23.1 Format of Text

(a) Content

In general, the NDA submission contains large number of data, which cannot be included completely within the body of document. The data collected for individual subject or patient that may be important, then only critical aspects must be included in the discussion section. The specific data can be presented within the body of the document instead of separate appendix that will be easy to assess the data. The data that is of less importance can be precisely described and placed in the appropriate appendices.

(b) Tone of text

The subject matter or information can be generally conveyed through writing skills, knowledge about the subject matter in the viewpoint of writer on a particular subject. It is advised to avoid legal language on one hand and colloquial or informal language on the other.

(c) Conciseness

FDA review of regulatory documents is a complex process, since the reviewers have to go through bulk content of the document. Hence, the following points should be followed in order to speed up the review and make easy for the reviewers to assess the submitted data.

- It is recommended to keep the language in simple and understanding.
- To speed up the process, some acronyms and abbreviations can be used.
- Editing the content and peer review before final submission to FDA helps to avoid unwanted words, phrases and grammatical errors.
- Sentences can often be combined by the deletion of redundant phrases, thus improving the flow of the text.

(d) Correctness

For the scientific merit of submission, it is advised that the text content should be in agreement with the data represented in tables and similarly, the tabular data should be in agreement with data source. If there is difference between the text data and source documents, the submission may be suspect and the reviewer may require more time to scrutinize the raw data to get the conclusion and report it.

(e) Consistency

All the abbreviations, punctuation, writing format and other text formats should be consistent and must be uniform in all the documents.

(f) Outline of sections and subsections

The critical review of document depends on the relationship of one section to another. In general, the decimal system is followed for outlining the system in most word processing software applications. One more popular approach is alphanumeric system which includes combination of words and numbers as section headers.

(g) Indenting

FDA advises that large sections indenting in the text must be avoided for the easy review. The text content should be presented at the left side margin with proper headings to identify the sections. Multiple indenting will waste the space of document and also will be quite confusing. Short titles are highly recommended and presenting the indent with bullets, arrows and points are useful to avoid enormous information.

15.23.2 Tabular Presentation

Inclusion of tables in the text is recommended wherever necessary for the substantial reduction of content. Multiple tables with large content should be avoided unless they are not important. If they are required, they can be included in the same volume in the appendix. Information from the tables should not be repeated in the text except as part of a concluding statement about the tabular data or trends seen in the data.

(a) Title

All the tables included in the text should be serially numbered and tables should have descriptive titles.

(b) Data source

Each table in the text should identify the source of data present in it. It is usually done in footnote of the table. The volume and page numbers of the tables are inserted at the end of page.

(c) Footnotes

Footnotes can be represented as superscripted letters but not as symbols or numbers which confuses the data. For statistical data symbols like asterisks (*) can be used. For multiple tables, footnotes are assigned as letters in the same order as they appear in the specific pages.

(d) Orientation

Tables as portrait are more preferred rather than landscape format. Suppose if the data doesn't fit in portrait format, axes of tables can be changed and rearranged with descriptions. Tables can be further revised as separate sections under the same column headings with description.

(e) Order of presentation

The data can be usually presented in the same order when similar data is present in multiple tables. Suppose the first column has the data of active drug and the second column is about the placebo, then the same order has to be followed in all the tables.

15.24 MANAGEMENT OF CLINICAL TRIALS

The key aspects for management of clinical trials are discussed as follows.

(a) **Investigator selection:** The first step of the clinical investigation is the selection of clinical investigator. As per the US federal regulations of GCP and ICH-GCP regulations, sponsor has to select well qualified, scientifically sound and experienced clinical investigator to carry out the clinical studies for the investigational drug products.

(b) **Pre-investigational site visit:** After the selection of potential investigator, pre-investigational site inspection is conducted at the investigation site by the identified investigator and with their staff in order to check the site facilities and requirements for initiating the clinical trials. In general, the pre-investigational site visit is done by the authorized person usually appointed by the sponsor company.

(c) **Study initiation visits:** After the completion of pre-investigational site visit the next process is the study initiation visit. The initiation visit is a training programme. It is the last training programme as protocol for the investigators and their staff before selecting the trial subjects and initiating the trails. During the clinical trial study, the investigator should critically review the following:
- Study protocols
- Adverse event report and document
- Case report forms
- Product dispensation and accountability
- Review of regulatory documents and source documentation

(d) **Trial conduct and execution:** There are many other key components to trail execution that include: informed consent form, IRB review, adverse reaction reporting, financial disclosure and document maintenance. For the overall success of clinical trial, each component is important.

(e) **Periodic monitoring visits:** As per the CFR and ICH-GCP regulations, the sponsor should regularly monitor the progress of clinical study at the site where the trial is being conducted. The purpose of the periodic visit by the sponsor is to ensure that the clinical investigator and the staff adheres to GCP guidelines as per the protocol to assure that rights of clinical trial subjects protected and the data obtained is accurate, original and scientifically sound.

(f) **Subject recruitment:** The recruitment of trail subjects should be done in short time as far as possible. The challenging part is the availability of subjects meeting the trial criteria especially when competing trials are made at site. There should be proper planning for the selection of trial subjects that meet the protocol criteria. No one has to force the subjects without their consent to participate in the clinical trials.

(g) **Product accountability:** Since clinical trials are conducted to evaluate new investigational drug to get regulatory approval from the regulatory agencies, it is mandatory that there must be strict control on the investigational product. The responsibility for the accountability of the product resides on the clinical investigator. The verification of all the used/unused disposition of product is done by the sponsor. Throughout the processing of clinical study, the records of product accountability should be maintained with details of date, quantity used batch number of product and subject number.

(h) **Adverse events and adverse drug reactions reporting:** The drug safety is inversely proportional to adverse drug reactions. In US, for drug safety FDA has mandated strict regulations. As per US federal regulations, sponsor has to report any adverse events and reactions occurred from the investigation drug during investigational stage and also at the post-marketing stage.

(i) **Study closeout visits:** After the completion of trial study at the investigational site, the study must be closed. The study is only closed, when all the trial subjects have finished the clinical studies or withdrawn and all data issues have been rectified and resolved in the final process. After this process only the investigator can proceed to close-out the visit from the site.

(j) **Records retention and inspections:** Record retention is critical to the ongoing viability of the study data. The FDA or other healthcare authorities may conduct an on-site inspection to verify the data from a given site at some time after submission of the New Drug Application (NDA). This information must be readily available at the site. Both the CFR and the ICH require that the records be retained for two years after the date of a marketing application is approved.

REVIEW QUESTIONS

1. What is a drug regulatory affairs? Give its importance in pharmaceutical industry.
2. Discuss the historical perspectives of drug regulatory affairs.
3. Define drug regulatory authority. Enlist the important drug regulatory authorities of different countries.

4. Discuss the drug regulatory authorities of Europe, US and India.
5. Discuss the role of regulatory affairs professionals in pharmaceutical industry.
6. Describe the job responsibilities of RA professionals in API and finished drug manufacturing units.
7. Explain the role of different drug development teams involved in research and development of new drugs.
8. Describe the INDA process for getting the clinical trials approval.
9. Explain the documentation contents of NDA in brief.
10. Describe the investigator's brochure contents.
11. Enumerate the different non-clinical studies for the drug development process.
12. Define bioequivalence and explain the different methods of bioequivalence studies.
13. Discuss the clinical research protocol with briefing the contents of documentation.
14. How the biostatistics play vital role in the pharmaceutical drug development?
15. Describe the different biostatistics approaches used in the drug development process.
16. Describe the different aspects of data presentation formats for FDA regulatory submissions.
17. Explain the management of clinical trials with special emphasis on the key components.

16

QUALITY MANAGEMENT SYSTEMS (QMSs)

Learning Objectives

After going through this chapter, you would be able to:

1. Understand the basic concept of quality and need of total quality management in an organization.
2. Explain the approach of QbD and principles of six sigma concept.
3. Understand the concept, procedure, types and guidelines of out-of-specification and change control.
4. Describe the quality standards of ISO 9000 and ISO 14000 series.
5. Explain the NABL certification process and GLP regulation.

16.1 INTRODUCTION

Quality management system (QMS) is a quality approach, which includes compilation of documents, processes, procedures, regulations and responsibilities to achieve the objectives and policies of quality. It is helpful for the organization as a guiding approach to meet the needs of customers and the regulatory authorities. In addition, the QMS also improves the company sales and enhances the growth of company in the competitive market in a cost-efficient manner. The global standards for QMS have been regulated by ISO 9001 series.

Quality is an essential aspect to retain the potential market of pharmaceutical industry. In pharmaceutical sector, the QMS approach has emerged as mandatory requirement to retain the identity, purity and safety of pharmaceutical products. The quality standards for the pharmaceuticals for human use are governed by the ICH Q10.

16.2 IMPORTANT ELEMENTS IN QMS

1. **Quality planning:** It is a process that converts the quality policy into processes and instructions to meet the objectives and statements.
2. **Quality assurance:** It is a vital department and part of QMS which assures that the process or the requirements for the quality of product are fulfilled.
3. **Quality control:** It is the department which evaluates and monitors the processes to ensure that the requirements for the product quality are in compliance with the regulatory standards.
4. **Quality improvement:** This process includes the methods and other appropriate actions that are to be taken to improve the quality of products.

16.3 CONCEPT OF QUALITY

Quality means excellence in services, especially to the degree they confirm to standard requirements and to satisfy the needs of customers. Quality is conformance to standards and requirements. It is the degree to which performance meets the expectations.

The American National Standards Institute (ANSI) and the American Society for Quality (ASQ) define quality as: "The totality of features and characteristics of a product or service that bears on its ability to satisfy given needs."

In healthcare sector, quality is defined as providing the right services in right way from the first time and every time for every patient regardless to his/her ability to pay 24 hours/7 days a week/365 days/year.

16.4 NEED OF QUALITY

- Today's competitive market is demanding availability of good quality products at cheaper cost. So having just high quality standards is not enough, internal cost of reputation maintenance should be less.
- There is a shift in customer demanding more about quality aspects instead of priority based approach.
- There is a need to reduce the internal cost of products with poor quality because of change over from low volume, high price to high volume.
- As systems have become more complex, the reliability requirements for suppliers of components have become more stringent.
- Higher customer expectations are getting spawned by increased competition.

16.5 QUALITY ASPECTS

1. **Measurable quality:** It can be defined with certain objectives, policies saying in compliance with or adherence to the standards. Clinically, these standards may take the form of practice parameters or protocols or may establish acceptable expectations for patients and organizational outcomes. These quality standards serve as guidelines for excellence.
2. **Perceptive quality:** It is the degree of excellence that is perceived by the recipient or observer of care rather than by the provider of care. It is generally based on the degree of caring expressed by physicians, nurses and other staff than on the physical environment and technical competence.
3. **Appreciative quality:** It is based on the appraisal of excellence beyond the minimal standards and criteria. It requires the judgments of skilled, experienced practitioners and caring people.

16.6 CONCEPT OF QUALITY MANAGEMENT TRIOLOGY

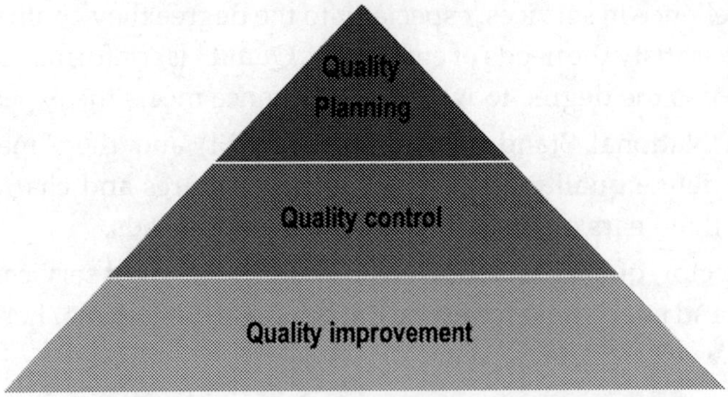

Fig 16.1: Quality management triangle

The quality management trilogy includes the following three aspects.

16.6.1 Quality Planning

It basically includes identifying and tracking the customers' requirements and expectations. Once the needs of customers are identified, then new systems will be designed by planning strategy. The quality planning also includes identifying function and process issues critical to effective outcomes; and developing new processes capable of achieving the desired outcome.

16.6.2 Quality Control

It includes developing process and measures the outcome performance. Quality control system monitors the actual performance and detects the variance from the expected results. It also summarizes the data and performs the initial assessment and analysis.

16.6.3 Quality Improvement

It involves analyzing the causes of process failure, dysfunction and insufficiency to systematically develop the solutions to solve or overcome chronic problems. Quality improvement also includes collaboratively studying and improving selected existing processes and outcomes in governance, management, clinical and support activities.

16.7 TOTAL QUALITY MANAGEMENT (TQM)

Total quality management (TQM) is referred to as an integrated organizational network system required enhancing the quality at every level. It involves all the processes to produce a perfect product by a series of measures requiring team effort of an organization to reduce the quality defects at every stage in the production.

According to international organization for standards, TQM is defined as "a management approach for an organization, centred on quality, based on the participation of all its members and aiming at long-term success through customer satisfaction and benefits to all the members of the organization and to the society."

16.7.1 Key Elements of TQM

(a) Focus on the customer

The basic approach to improve the quality is to identify the customers of the organization. External customers are those who receive products or services of the organisation. Internal customers refer to the employees who receive the output of other employees.

(b) Employee involvement

Since the prime objective of any organization is to improve the quality, all the employees should be actively involved in quality improvement approaches and initiatives. The front line employees have close contact with the external customers and thus make the most contribution to quality. All the employees of the organization must have the authority to innovate and improve the quality.

(c) Continuous improvement

For any organization to sustain and retain its position the quality should be improved continuously and quality is a never ending process, where all the employees work together to improve the performance, speed and number of features of the product or service. Continuous improvement means small, incremental improvement that occurs on a regular basis. It eventually adds up to vast improvement in quality. The foundation of total quality is a management philosophy that supports meeting customer requirements through continuous improvement.

16.7.2 TQM Tools for Quality Problem Solving

There are many statistical tools which can be used to monitor the quality checks, defects and to reduce or eliminate the quality errors of products.

1. **Cause and effect diagrams:** It is also called "fish-bone" diagram which identifies various causes for the quality problems. This diagram reflects the relationship between the causes and effects for the quality error.

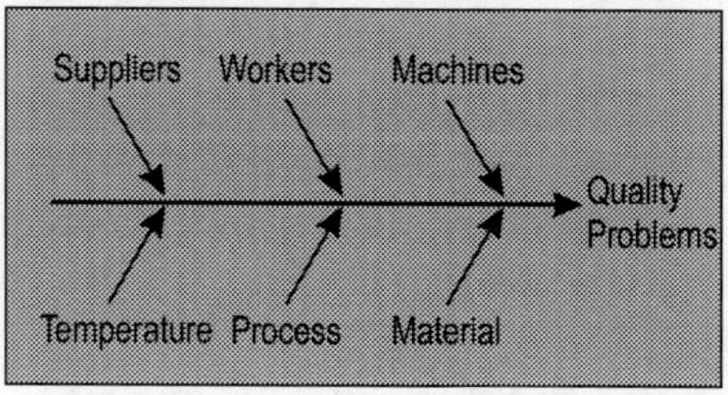

2. **Flowcharts:** It includes a series of events as individual steps as connecting lines to show some changes in the process when improvements were made. Flowcharts are required to document the steps of process.

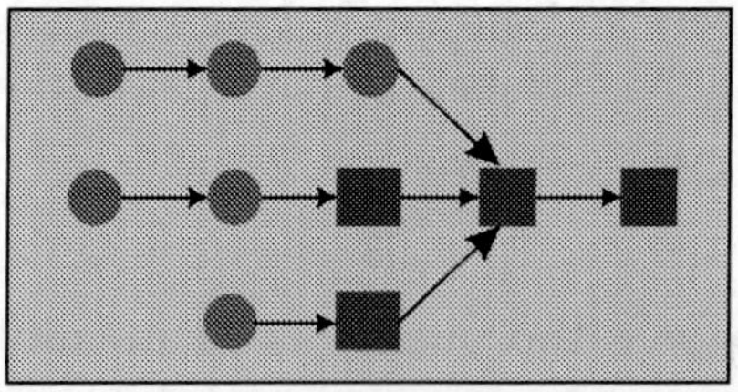

3. **Checklists:** Checklists are the simple data check-off sheets designed to identify the types of quality errors at each work station, such as per machine, per batch, per operator.

Defect Type	No of Defects	Total
Broken zipper	✓✓✓	3
Ripped material	✓✓✓✓✓✓✓	7
Missing buttons	✓✓✓	3
Faded colour	✓✓	2

4. **Control charts:** These are important tools used in the statistical process control. These charts identify when the data is consistent or when there are upper control and lower control limits to show whether the process is in or out of control.

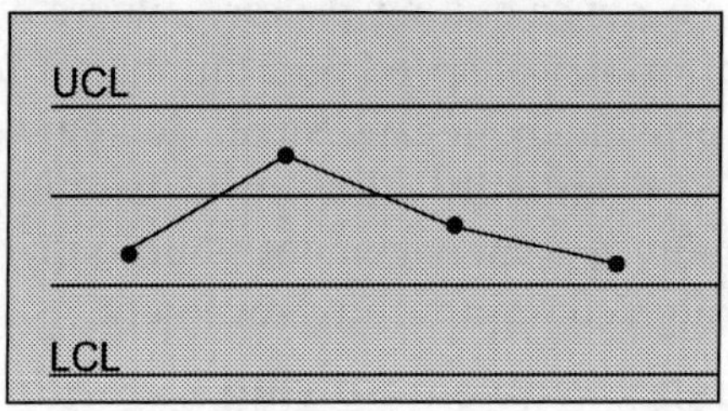

5. **Scatter plots:** These are the graphs that show how the two variables are related to one another. In these plots, the data can be used as regression analysis to establish the equation for the relationship.

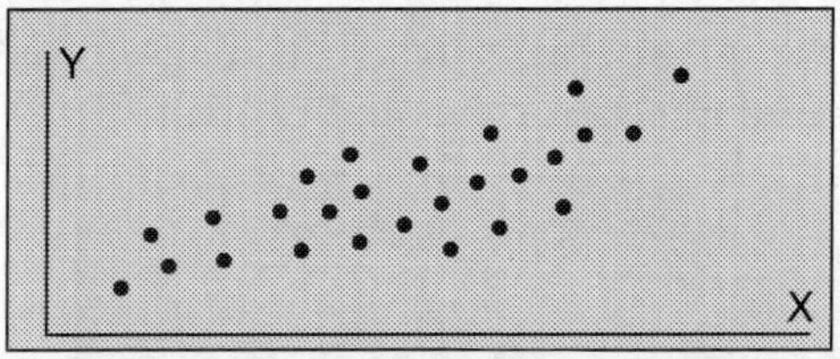

6. **Histograms:** These are bar charts that show the frequency distribution of observed values of a variable like service time at a bank drive-up window.

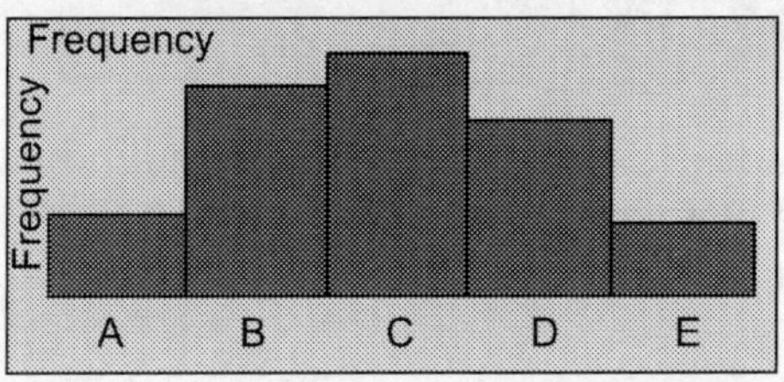

7. **Pareto analysis charts:** It was named with an Italian economist, Velfredo Pareto who discovered a method that displays the degree of importance for each element. Pareto analysis is also called 80-20 rule, since it was analyzed as 80% of the quality issues result from the 20% of the causes.

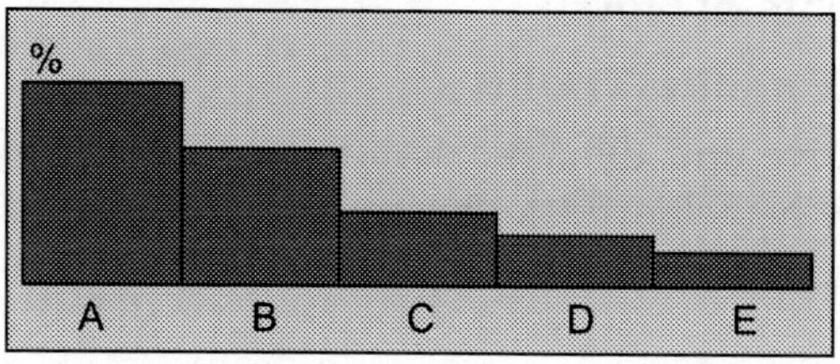

Advantages of TQM

- Improved reputation by detecting the quality faults and problems and implementing the approaches to reduce the quality defects.
- The employees are motivated by leadership qualities, teamwork and active involvement.
- TQM reduces quality defective products.
- Improves the quality products or service continuously.
- Financial benefits include lower costs, higher returns on sales, investment, and the ability to charge higher rather than competitive prices.

Disadvantages of TQM

- Initial introduction cost.
- Benefits may not be expected for many years.
- Employees and workers may be resistant to change.

16.8 QUALITY BY DESIGN (QBD)

The quality by design (QbD) is a systematic approach to development that begins with predefined objectives and emphasizes product and process understanding based on the sound science and quality risk management.

The concept of QbD was first introduced by Joseph M Juran who proposed that concept of quality can be planned. QbD approach is also mentioned in ICH Q8 guidelines, which states that, to identify quality cannot be tested in products, i.e., quality should be built into product by design.

The main objective of QbD is to ensure the quality products, for that product and process characteristics important to desired performance must result from combination of prior knowledge and new estimation during knowledge.

Benefits of QbD

- It is required for designing and developing formulations and manufacturing processes to ensure predefined quality.
- It is helpful to understand how the formulation and manufacturing process variables influence the quality of a product.
- It ensures the product quality with effective control strategy.
- It is beneficial for more effective and efficient control of change.

- It includes cost savings and less batch failures.
- It is a good business approach to minimize deviations, costly investigations and to avoid regulatory compliance issues.

16.8.1 The Key Elements of QbD

1. Target product quality profile (TPQP)

It is defined as prospective and dynamic summary of the quality characteristics of a drug product that can be achieved to ensure that the desired quality, safety and efficacy of the drug product is realized. The TPQP forms the basis for product design in the following way.

- Dosage form of drug product
- Route of administration
- Dose/strength of drug product
- Therapeutic category of drug product
- Drug product quality criteria

2. Critical quality attributes (CQA)

Once the TPQP is identified, the next step is to identify the relevant critical quality attributes. A CQA is a physical, chemical, biological or microbiological property or characteristic that should be within an appropriate limit, range or distribution to ensure the desired product quality. Prior product knowledge, such as accumulated laboratory, non-clinical and clinical experience with a specific product quality attribute is the key in making these risk assessments.

The CQAs are basically associated with

- Drug substance/ API
- Excipients
- Intermediates
- Drug product

3. Critical process parameter (CPP)

A CPP is defined as a parameter whose variability has an impact on a critical quality attribute and should be monitored or controlled to ensure the process produces desired quality product. CPPs have direct impact on CQAs.

Process robustness is defined as the ability of process to demonstrate acceptable quality, performance and tolerate variability in inputs at the same time.

The example, CPPs include temperature, pH, feed rate, mixing speed, cooling rate, etc.

4. Quality risk assessment

Risk is defined as the combination of the probability of occurrence of harm and the severity of that harm. Quality risk management is a systematic approach for the assessment, control, communication and review of risks to the quality of drug product across the product life cycle. The initial list of potential parameters that can affect CQAs can be extensive but can be reduced by quality risk assessment (QRA).

According to the ICH Q9 guidelines, the QRA provides a basis to initiate and follow a risk management process.

5. Design space

According to ICH Q8 guidelines, design space is a multidimensional combination and interaction of input variables and process parameters that have been demonstrated to provide assurance of product quality. The design space is implemented by the applicant and it is subjected to regulatory assessment and approval.

Working within the design space is not considered a change. Movement out of the design space is considered to be a change and would normally initiate a regulatory post approval change process.

6. Control strategy

Control strategy is defined as a planned set of controls that are derived from the current product and process understanding that assures process performance and product quality. The ability to evaluate and ensure the quality of in-process and final product based on process data which typically include a combination of measured material attributes and process controls. The control strategy can include the following aspects:

- Procedural controls
- In-process controls
- Lot- release testing
- Process monitoring
- Characterization testing
- Comparability testing
- Stability testing

16.9 SIX SIGMA CONCEPT

Six sigma is a set of techniques and tools for the process improvement. It was developed for the first time by the firm Motorola in 1986. Bill Smith, the father of six-sigma, introduced this quality improvement concept to Motorola. Six sigma is now an enormous brand in the world of corporate development.

Six-sigma concept is believed to improve the quality of process outputs by identifying and removing the causes of defects. Six-sigma includes collection of managerial, statistical and methods that focuses on reducing variations in processes and preventing deficiencies in product.

16.9.1 Six Sigma Methods

1. Six sigma: DMAIC

DMAIC principle is used for the projects that are aimed to improve the existing business process.

Define the system, the voice of the customer and their requirements and the project objectives specifically.

Measure the key aspects of the current process and collect the relevant data.

Analyze the data to investigate and verify the cause and effect relationships. Determine what the relationships are and attempt to ensure that all the factors have been considered. Find the root cause of the defect by proper investigation.

Improve the current process based upon data analysis using methods such as design of experiments (DoE), and standard work to create a new, future state process. Carry out pilot runs to establish process capability.

Control the future state process to ensure that any deviations from target are corrected before they result in defects. Implement control systems such as statistical process control, production boards, and visual workplaces and continuously monitor the process.

2. Six sigma: DMADV

DMADV principle is used for the projects designed to create new products or process designs.

Define design goals that are consistent with customer demands and the enterprise strategy.

Measure and identify the CTQs (characteristics that are critical to quality), product capabilities, production process capabilities and risks.

Analyze to develop and design alternatives, create a high level design and evaluate design capability to select the best design.

Design an improved alternative, best suited per analysis in the previous step.

Verify the design, setup pilot runs, implement the production process and hand it over to the process owner.

Six-Sigma Implementation Roles

Executive leadership: This group comprises top level management people like CEOs who are responsible for setting up a vision.

Champions: They take the responsibilities for implementation of six-sigma across the organization in an integrated manner.

Master black belts: These people act as in-house coaches on six-sigma. They dedicate themselves 100% for six-sigma implementation in the organization. They assist champions, guide black belt and green belt members.

Black belts: They work under master black belts to apply six-sigma concepts to specific projects.

Green belts: They are the employees guided by black belts and they are responsible to take up the six-sigma implementation.

16.9.2 Out of Specifications (OoS)

If any of the analytical results of a batch or product are falling outside the standard limits or specifications, such incident is referred to as "out of specification". The OoS test results includes all the suspected results that fall outside the predetermined specifications.

The OoS results can be observed during the analysis of:

- Raw materials
- Intermediates
- In-process parameters
- Finished API
- Packaging materials
- Stability studies

The OoS can occur due to the following types of errors:

1. Laboratory errors

These include the following reasons:

- Using methods that are not validated
- Using laboratory equipment that are not calibrated
- Not following the SOPs
- Not following standard procedures

2. Process related errors

These errors are due to:

- Operator errors
- Equipment failure
- Deviation from the validated procedure
- Quality of raw material and intermediates used
- In-process quality checks during manufacturing

3. Sample homogeneity errors

These errors are are due to:

- Sampling errors
- Handling of samples
- Pooling of samples

There are different guidelines available for handling the OoS investigations for products/batches and they are:

- MHRA guidelines
- USFDA (CDER) guidelines

A. MHRA guidelines

It includes the following types of investigations.

Phase I: Laboratory investigation

It is related to the quality control checks/parameters along with rechecking of the documents with same analyst and re-testing with different analyst with original same sample.

The phase I is subdivided again into two sections.

Phase 1a: primary lab investigation

Phase 1b: extended lab investigation

Phase II: Manufacturing investigation

In manufacturing investigation, the production department person should investigate

- Process parameters
- Drying parameters
- Input raw materials quality
- Training of persons
- Cleaning of equipment
- Environmental factors

Phase III: Extended manufacturing investigation

In phase III investigation, the production, quality control and quality assurance department investigate the following:

- Sampling error by person
- Authorized for re-sampling
- Re-analysis of re-sampled material with different analyst

If with the 3 investigations, the root cause is not found, define the corrective and preventive action (CAPA) or if not divert the matter to R & D/ ADL or QA. Conclusions should be drawn from all the team members and the fate of batch will be decided by the head of QA department.

B. USFDA (CDER) guidelines

It includes the following types of investigation:

Phase I: Laboratory investigation

It includes checking of quality control parameters with addition of rechecking of documents with same analyst and retesting with different analyst with original sample. If the analyst observed same result with re-analysis, report the same to QC head then log the OoS, review the documents with reports. If there is no abnormality found during primary investigation, then report the same results and considered valid OoS and report to quality head who then recommends re-testing of sample. Then repeat the test thrice with different analysts and report the average result, if the result complies the report release the batch and if it doesn't complie report to QA head and continue the OoS investigation with phase II.

Phase II: Manufacturing investigation

In manufacturing investigation, the production person should investigate the following:

- Input quality of raw materials
- Process parameters and critical process parameters
- Reconciliation of raw materials
- Output of raw materials
- In-process parameters results
- Cleaning of equipment
- Training of persons
- Contamination verification

If there is no assignable cause observed during manufacturing investigations, same is reported to QA head. Then QA, QC and production department will evaluate the investigations and after that QA head may recommend for re-sampling. The QC analyst shall analyze the sample as per SOP and report result either passes or fails. If pass defines the CAPA release the batch and if fails, reject the batch and divert the report to R&D/ADL lab. Then QA head shall decide the fate of batch for re-process, rework or for destruction.

All these activities for investigation, corrective actions and preventive actions should be recorded and reviewed and archived.

If OoS batch is to be reprocessed then the below given steps are to be followed:

- Follow the written, approved BMR for re-processing of the batch.
- Sample as per the SOP for sampling of material.
- Analyze the material according to the SOP and STP.
- Evaluate the quality of the batch.
- Keep the batch for stability studies and evaluate their results.
- Communicate the OOS results to the customers.

16.10 CHANGE CONTROL

Change refers to any modification in equipment, manufacturing process, utilities, facilities, designs, formulations, packaging materials, software and all associated documents such as SOP, BMR, BPR, MFR, etc.

Change control is a formal system to document, evaluate, approve and implement changes that might affect the validated status of facilities, equipment and processes. Change is permanent planned alteration to any approved process or procedure that may affect safety, quality and efficacy of drug and blood products. Change control, the key element of quality management system, is a regulatory requirement and is inspected by authorities like FDA, MHRA and CPA.

16.10.1 Scope of Change Control

- Change control reduces the risk that changes made impact the quality and process characteristics.
- Any change made to previously approved requirements need review and also authorization to keep the system in the state of proven suitability.
- Formal change control ensures that all changes are evaluated for their effect on product quality or validation status.

16.10.2 Change Control Principles

- As the change control is considered to be one of the essential aspects of quality management systems, logically the person responsible to implement and approve the changes is QA head.
- Change control process is not department specific; it is the task of whole company.
- Change control monitors all types of changes that can influence the process or product quality and states the measures necessary for implementing the changes or not to make the changes.

- All the changes should be made according to approved written company policies and objectives.

Elements of change control

Initiator: In general, any changes can be proposed or introduced by initiator. Initiating changes involves filling out a change request form which then moves through a process or system of review and approval.

Change control committee: It comprises members from different departments such as production, quality control, regulatory affairs and engineering. Depending on the type of changes made the committee can include legal, sales and marketing department members also.

Change administrator: In pharmaceutical companies, cGMP requires that all changes must be received and approved by QA department. In such companies, there must be a change administrator; generally the head of QA will be assigned for that purpose.

16.10.3 Steps of Change Control

1. **Record/classify:** Initiator proposes a change by filling change request form. The change control team records then and categorizes it.
2. **Asses:** Assessors then make their risk analysis by answering to series of questions regarding risk, business and process and follow this by making judgment on who should carryout change and then it is sent for planning.
3. **Plan:** The planning team plans the change in detail as well as construct regression plan in case if the change is backed out.
4. **Build:** The team then makes solutions which will be then tested. They will then seek approval and request a time and date to carry out the implementation phase.
5. **Implement:** In this phase, the finalized changes are implemented.
6. **Evaluation:** Once the changes are implemented, they will be evaluated.
7. **Close:** Once the implanted changes are evaluated and accepted the change control document will be closed.

16.10.4 Classification of Changes

A classification procedure may help to determine the level of testing, validation and documentation required to justify the changes of validated process. Changes can be classified as minor and major depending on the nature and extent of changes or the effect of these changes on process and products.

16.10.5 Minor Changes

These changes influence a unit requiring control. Minor changes will have low risk and low impact. Some of the minor changes include:

- Change of cleaning agents
- Change in cleaning process parameters
- Change in purchase procedure
- Change in batch size of product
- Change in manufacturing site address

16.10.6 Major Changes

These changes influence the product quality of process reliability. Major changes are found to have high risk and high impact. Some of the major changes include:

- Changes in process parameters
- Change in product composition
- Change of processes to other manufacturing site
- Replacement of equipment parts or accessories
- Changes to HVAC system.

16.11 ISO 9000

ISO, International Standards Organization, was framed for the first time in year 1947. It is a federation of 143 countries national standard bodies. The headquarters of ISO is located at Geneva, Switzerland. ISO is standard to indicate the quality awareness.

ISO is the process that typically shifts an organization's culture to allow successful TQM implementation. Organizations with ISO certification are known to have well established global industrial standards and are well recognized.

ISO 9000 is a series of standards that are developed and published by the ISO, that define, establish and maintain an effective QA system for manufacturing and service industries. The ISO 9000 series of standards are related to quality management systems and formed to help the organizations to ensure that they meet the needs of customers and other stakeholders in accordance with statutory and regulatory requirements.

ISO 9000 is a set of five guideline standards that define the requirements for an effective quality management system. Among the five, only three are certification standards (ISO 9001, 9002 and 9003) and both ISO 9000 and 9004 are guidelines for the other three. ISO 9000 standards basically deal with the fundamentals of quality management systems, including the eight management principles on which the quality of standards is based.

The eight quality management principles are:

1. Customer focus
2. Leadership
3. Involvement of people
4. Process approach
5. System approach to management
6. Continual improvement
7. Decision making approach
8. Mutual beneficial relationship

16.11.1 Objectives of ISO 9000 Standards

- To facilitate the international trade of goods and services.
- To enhance the competency by improving the quality of products and services in cost effective manner.
- To promote and implement TQM approach in the organization.

16.11.2 ISO 9000 Series

1. **ISO 9000:** It describes the basic fundamental quality principles and provides guidelines for the selection and application of each standard.
2. **ISO 9001:** It serves as model for assuring the quality in design, development, production, installation and servicing.
3. **ISO 9002:** It serves as model for quality assurance in the production and installation of manufacturing systems.
4. **ISO 9003:** It includes the guidelines for quality assurance for final testing and inspection.
5. **ISO 9004:** It includes the guidelines for the applications of standards in quality management and quality systems.

ISO 9000 and ISO 9004 are guidance standards. They describe what is necessary to accomplish the requirements outlined in standards 9001, 9002 or 9003.

16.11.3 Benefits of ISO 9000 Series Standards

- ISO registration and certification has a significant bearing on market credibility.
- ISO standards provide opportunity to compete with higher companies.
- ISO certification can increase customer confidence and satisfaction.
- ISO certification gives confirmation that the organization is committed to have quality products.
- ISO standards may facilitate trade and increased market opportunities.

16.11.4 ISO 9000 Series Clauses

The requirements of the standard are specified in following clauses of the standard:

- Quality management system
- Management responsibility
- Resource management
- Product realization
- Measurement, analysis and improvement

16.11.5 ISO 14000

ISO 14000 standards were implemented in 1972 in United Nations organized international forum in which United Nations Environment Program (UNEP) was launched. Later, in the year 1996 different ISO 14000 series standards were framed by International Organization for Standardization.

ISO 140000 includes the standards for the organizations that are committed to protect environment while taking care of their customers. The ISO 14000 is similar to the quality standards of IS0 9000 series. ISO 14000 is both product and process oriented which determines the environmental impacts of product and services to establish, maintain and evaluate environmental management system (EMS).

ISO 14000 standards are required for:

- Small, medium, large and multi-national industries and business sectors.
- Different service sectors such as hospitals, hotels, etc.

- Different government organizations.
- All types of organizations of all sizes, anywhere in the world.

16.11.6 ISO 14000 Policy

- Improvement of chemical management system software.
- Improvement of management of industrial water waste.
- Improve the chemical hazard waste management via solvent recovery system.
- To include methods of evaluating the environmental impacts and systems.
- To establish framework for the setting and reviewing the objectives and goals.
- To implement, maintain and document the ISO 14000 standards regulations.

16.11.7 ISO 14000 Series Standards

1. ISO 14001: Environmental management systems (EMS)

An environmental management system (EMS) is a framework that helps a company achieve its environmental goals through consistent control of its operations. The assumption is that this increased control will improve the environmental performance of the company.

EMS has the following aspects

- It is a systemic approach of handling the environmental issues of organizations.
- It is based on Plan-Do-Check-Act (PDCA) model.
- It focuses on continual improvement of system.
- It addresses immediate and long-term impact of an organization's products, services and processes on the environment.
- It serves as a tool to improve environmental performance.

2. ISO 14004: General guidelines of EMS

The ISO 14004: 2016 provides a basis for an organization to establish, implement, maintain and improve a robust, credible and reliable environmental management system. The ISO standards help the organization to achieve the intended objectives of its environmental management system.

3. ISO 14010: Environmental auditing

These standards generally include the guidelines of environmental auditing and they are:

ISO 14010: It includes the general principles of environmental auditing.

ISO 14011/1: It includes the auditing procedures of environmental management systems.

ISO 14012: It includes the qualification criteria for the auditors to conduct auditing of environmental management systems.

4. ISO 14020: Environmental labelling

The objectives of ISO 14020 are stated to be harmonized with the self-environmental declared claims with following aspects:

- Accurate and verifiable environmental claims that are not misleading.
- Prevention of unwarranted claims.

- Reduction in confusion of marketplace.
- Adaptation of international trading system.
- Increased potential for market to stimulate environmental improvements.

5. ISO 14030: Environmental performance evaluation (EPE)

EPE process provides information to facilitate management decisions about the environmental performance of an organization. This series of standard is a companion to ISO 14001: 2015 that requires organizations to demonstrate an improvement in environmental performance. These standards provide powerful tools for organizations providing a system to track their progress towards more sustainable economy.

6. ISO 14040: Life cycle assessment (LCA)

The life cycle assessment of ISO 14040 is required for:

- Finding out the opportunities to enhance the environmental performance of products at various stages in their life cycle.
- Informing decision-makers in industry, government and non-government organizations.
- Selecting relevant measures of environmental performance.
- Implementing an eco-friendly labelling scheme and making an environmental claim.

16.11.8 Benefits of ISO 14000 Standards

- They held organizations to meet and maintain the regulatory and legislative requirements.
- It minimizes and eliminates the environmental impact of products, activities and resources.
- It helps in maintaining an efficient quality system in an organization.
- It builds the confidence in customer on the quality of product supplied.
- It promotes environmental awareness and also acts as competitive barrier.

16.12 NATIONAL ACCREDITATION BOARD FOR TESTING AND CALIBRATION LABORATORIES (NABL)

NABL is an autonomous agency that gives accreditation of technical competence of testing, calibration, and medical laboratory testing and reference material producer. NABL is established under the Department of Science and Technology (DST), Government of India and is registered under the Societies Act. NABL was established with the objective to provide government, industries, society in general with third-party assessment scheme of the quality and technical competence of testing and calibration laboratories.

In order to achieve this objective, NABL provides laboratory accreditation services to laboratories that are performing tests/calibrations in accordance with NABL criteria based on internationally accepted standard for laboratory accreditation ISO/IEC 17025.

These services are offered in a non-discriminatory manner and are accessible to all testing and calibration laboratories in India and abroad, regardless of their ownership, legal status, size and degree of independence. The headquarters of NABL in India are located at New Delhi.

NABL Accreditation is currently given in the following fields. See Table below.

Testing Laboratories	Medical Laboratories	Calibration Laboratories
♦ Biological	• Clinical biochemistry	♦ Electro-technical
♦ Chemical	• Clinical pathology	♦ Mechanical
♦ Electronics/Electrical	• Histopathology	♦ Thermal and optical
♦ Fluid flow	• Microbiology	♦ Radiological
♦ Mechanical	• Cytopathology	♦ Fluid flow
♦ Photometry	• Genetics	
♦ Radiological	• Haematology	
♦ Thermal/Forensic	• Immunohaematology	

16.12.1 Benefits of NABL Accreditation

- Improvement in business because of increased customer satisfaction and confidence.
- Saves time and money due to reduction or elimination of the re-testing needs.
- Better control of laboratory operations and feedback system to know whether good quality control and assurance system are technically competent enough.
- Customers can search and identify the laboratories accredited by NABL for their specific requirements from the directory of Accredited Laboratories.
- Comparison of facility's performance with that of other peer facilities.
- Enhancement in the performance of tests/calibrations following with investigation and identification of causes of unsatisfactory incidents and implementing suitable corrective actions to preventing the re-occurrence of certain problems.
- Providing awareness, training and education about NABL system to the employees and workers of an organization.
- Evaluation of methods, including the establishment of method precision and accuracy and estimation of measurement uncertainty.

16.12.2 NABL Accreditation/Certification Process

The process of NABL accreditation includes the following stages.

Stage 1: Application filling

The applicant has to fill all the required information with enlisting the tests/calibration procedures along with range and measurement of uncertainty for which the laboratory is competent to perform. Laboratory can be apply for NABL accreditation either for all or part of few testing and calibration purpose in the different forms of NABL 151, NABL 152 and NABL 153. The laboratory must be specific to the scope of NABL accreditation for applying. The laboratory should submit 5 copies of duly filled application form for each field of testing/calibration along with the five sets of quality manual and should pay the prescribed application fees. Once the application is received at NABL head office, the secretary will send acknowledgement to the laboratory. The application will be screened initially and then a unique customer registration number will be assigned to the laboratory for further processing. Then the NABL secretary nominates a lead assessor to give adequate report on the application submitted by the laboratory. One copy of adequacy report will be sent to laboratory for taking any necessary corrective action to be taken if required. After that, the laboratory is requested to submit the corrective action report to NABL secretary office. After receiving the corrective action report, a pre-assessment audit will be done for the laboratory. The laboratory must be well prepared by conducting internal audit before the pre-assessment.

Stage 2: Pre-assessment audit

The NABL secretary will direct the lead assessor to carry out the pre-assessment audit at the laboratory premises. The pre-assessment helps the laboratory to be well prepared for the final assessment. One copy of the pre-assessment report will be provided to laboratory for taking any necessary corrective action questioned during the audit. Then the laboratory must submit the report of corrective action to the NABL secretary. Once the laboratory confirms the completion of corrective actions, the final assessment of the laboratory will be scheduled by the NABL.

Stage 3: Final assessment

The NABL secretary shall plan the final assessment at the laboratory site for its compliance to NABL criteria and for that purpose an assessment team shall be appointed. The team should consist of lead assessor and other technical staff in the relevant field depending upon the scope to be addressed. The team experts can raise non-compliance issues if found and the same can be written and informed to the laboratory so that an opportunity will be given to address the non-conformance before closing the assessment meeting. The lead assessor will provide a copy of consolidated report to the laboratory and send the original report copy to the NABL secretary's office. Laboratory should take necessary measures on the remaining non-conformance and other issues and should submit a report to NABL within a period of two months.

Stage 4: Corrective re-assessment

Once the satisfactory corrective action from the laboratory is received, the NABL accreditation team checks the findings of the assessment team and may recommend any additional corrective action, if any by the laboratory. Then the team verifies whether the recommendations in the assessment report are in compliance with NABL regulations as well as within the claims made by the laboratory in its application. Then the NABL committee shall make appropriate recommendations regarding the accreditation of laboratory to NABL secretary. The laboratory will be given an opportunity to appeal against the findings of assessment or decision on accreditation by writing to NABL Director. If possible, NABL will depute its technical personnel during the assessment time as coordinator and NABL observer. Sometimes, NABL may at its own cost depute a newly trained technical assessor as observer subject to convenience of the laboratory to be accessed.

Stage 5: Grating of accreditation

If the NABL accreditation committee is satisfied with final assessment of the laboratory, then issues accreditation certificate with unique number and QR code to the laboratory. The accreditation certificate will be valid for a period of three years and NABL shall conduct periodical surveillance checks for the laboratory at intervals of each year. The laboratory shall renew the accreditation certificate prior to six months of expiration of its validity.

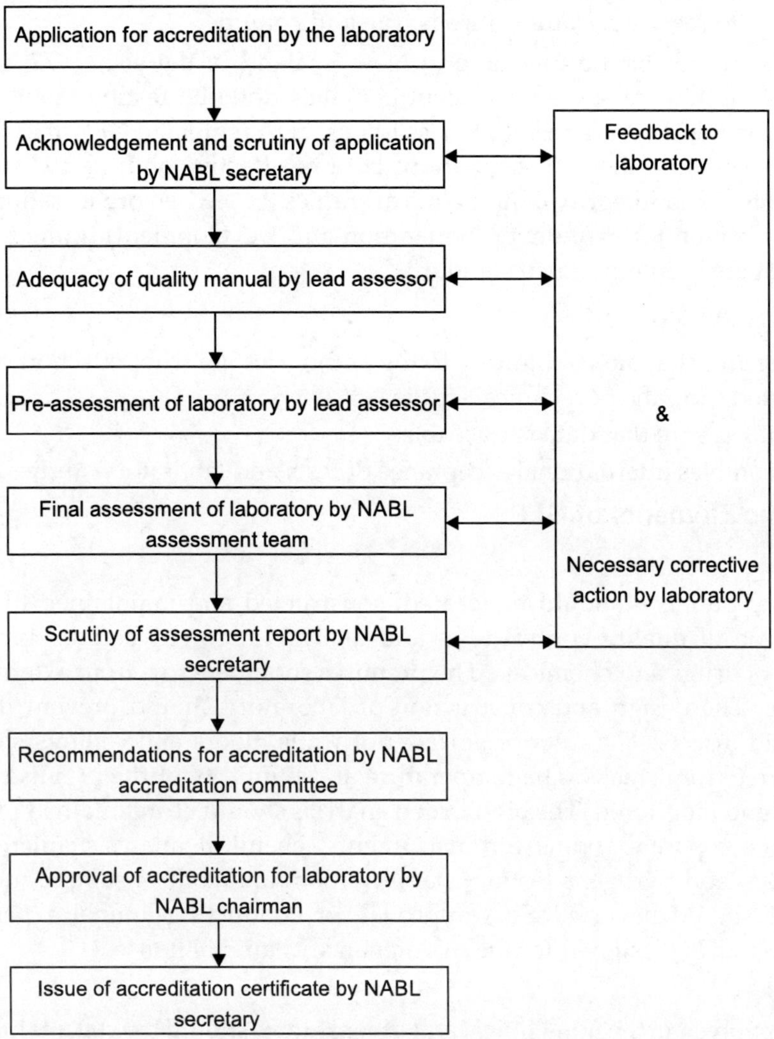

Fig. 16.2: Flow diagram of NABL accreditation process

16.13 GOOD LABORATORY PRACTICES (GLP)

Good laboratory practices (GLP) is a set of principles that provide a framework within which laboratory studies are performed, planned, monitored, recorded, reported, reviewed and documented. GLP specifically refers to quality system management controls for research institutes and organizations to ensure the uniformity, consistency, reliability, reproducibility, quality and integrity of pharmaceuticals and chemicals including non-clinical safety studies from physicochemical properties through acute to chronic toxicity tests.

GLP generally applies to non-clinical studies conducted for the assessment of quality, safety and efficacy of drugs and pharmaceuticals. GLP helps to assure the data submitted to regulatory authorities is true and genuine.

GLP was introduced for the first time in New Zealand in the year 1972. GLP was initiated in US following some fraudulent activities done by testing laboratories in data submission to FDA. As a result of these issues, FDA regulated GLP in 21 CFR Part 58 in the year 1978 and the GLP regulations became effective on June 1979 to assure the quality, safety and integrity of non-clinical studies. In 1981 an organization named OECD (Organization for Economic Cooperation and Development) framed the GLP principles that are of international standard.

16.13.1 Objectives of GLP

- GLP assures that data submitted to the authorities are true reflection of results generated from the non-clinical studies.
- GLP makes sure that data is traceable.
- GLP promotes international acceptance of tests and laboratory studies.

16.13.2 Basic Elements of GLP

(a) Premises

The laboratory premises should be located, constructed and maintained to suit the performance of all quality control tests and analysis required before, during and manufacture of drugs and chemicals. The premises should be free from external noise and pollution. The design and construction of laboratory should prevent the entry of rodents and insects. The interior surfaces of walls, floors and ceilings should be smooth and free from cracks. The temperature and humidity of the premises should be controlled and monitored. The bio-burden analysis should be maintained regularly. There must be separate rooms for instruments, chemical analysis, microbiology studies, sterility and pyrogens testing, stability room and control sample room. The animal house should have CPCSEA approval for conducting animal experiments. Proper SOPs must be designed for the maintenance of animal house.

(b) Personnel

The persons involved in the non-clinical and other studies should be well qualified with adequate experience and knowledge and must be familiar with the GLP principles and regulations. There must be study director as head of the laboratory who is responsible for maintenance of SOPs, protocols and documentation. The study director also has responsibilities of organizing audits, taking up of corrective action and investigating technical complaints.

(c) Equipment

The laboratory instruments and equipment should be serviced and calibrated at suitable intervals according to written procedures by persons or a service agency and validated. (SOP for operation & calibration). Readily available records must be maintained for each one of them. Next servicing or calibration due date should also be mentioned on them. The written operating instructions should be readily available or preferably be displayed for each instrument. The records shall have name of equipment, manufacturer's name, instruction manual, model number, list of spares and accessories, etc. The defective instrument should be withdrawn from use until the fault has been rectified.

(d) Reagents

The testing reagents should be stored in a separate room and they should be properly labelled for their unique identification. The reagents used in laboratory should be prepared by competent persons as per the standard procedures. The labels on the reagent container should display the concentration, standardization factor, manufacturing date, shelf life, storage instructions and signature of chemist who prepared it. The reference standards and working standards should be properly dated and stored in proper conditions. They should be properly handled and carefully used in consultation with senior chemist.

(e) Sampling

Sampling should be done by a trained and authorized person for the analysis. The person should follow sampling procedures, SOPs and safety precautions during sampling process. The sample container should bear label with details of name of material, batch number, manufacturing date, expiry date, name of manufacturer and quantity sampled. The container should be marked as 'sampled' with signature of person who has sampled the product after sampling. The equipment used for sampling must be cleaned after use and should be stored separately from other laboratory equipment.

(f) Documentation

The purpose of documentation is to define specifications for materials, method of manufacturing, control systems and to provide trial to permit investigation of any defective batch of products. The procedures and specifications used for all the raw materials, intermediates and finished products and all the tests and methods of analysis should be properly documented. All the data obtained from the results, analytical reports, various in-process parameters, calibration reports, checklists and draft reports should be properly documented in standard formats and maintained. All the documents must have proper titles and they should be arranged and kept in the racks for easy identification whenever they are required. The documents should be signed, reviewed, approved and dated appropriately by authorized staff.

(g) Records

The records of all the observations were documented properly. Detailed records of test results, analytical reports of all the materials, intermediates, finished products, in-process checks, calibrations and environmental monitoring should be compiled properly. Any changes or corrections made during review should be marked or highlighted. The authorized persons have access to maintain data integrity and confidentiality. The records should have the following details:

- Name of sample
- Date of receipt of sample
- Batch/Lot no.
- Testing protocols
- Analysis signature
- Opinion and sign of approved analyst
- Manufacturing and expiry date
- Date of batch release
- Any other relevant information

(h) Standard operating procedures (SOPs)

The SOPs are required for:

- Analysis of drugs
- Handling and sampling of products
- Clearing, maintenance and calibration of equipment
- Storage and sampling of test and control articles
- Responsibilities of audit team
- Healthy and safety precautions
- Storage and maintenance of microbial cultures
- Training sessions
- Housekeeping
- Retention and disposal of control samples
- Complaints and product recall procedures

(i) Quality system and audits

The quality assurance in-charge person should check the format of study plans, quality policy and their compliance with GLP regulations. Any non-conformity found should be noted by internal audits and should be corrected by taking corrective actions and should be documented. The head of the laboratory should schedule and conduct the audit. Audit should be conducted at least once in a year to cover the training records of staff, complaints and customer feedback received from laboratory employees and other laboratory requirements and future plans.

REVIEW QUESTIONS

1. Define quality management system. Enlist the important elements of QMS.
2. Define the term quality. Explain the concept of quality with reference to different quality aspects.

3. Discuss the concept of quality management trilogy.
4. What is TQM? Discuss the advantages and disadvantages.
5. Discuss the TQM key elements in detail.
6. What are the different TQM tools used for solving quality issues? Explain them.
7. Define quality by design (QbD). Enlist the benefits of QbD approach.
8. Explain the key aspects of QbD in pharmaceutical sector.
9. Define six-sigma concept. Enumerate the DMAIC six sigma principles.
10. Describe the DMADV- six sigma concept. Add a note on the implementation system of six-sigma approach.
11. Define OoS and list the different reasons for OoS.
12. Explain the different types of investigations for handling of OOS.
13. Define change control and give its scope.
14. Discuss the change control elements and steps involved in change control system.
15. Enlist the different types of changes with examples for change control system.
16. Write about ISO 9000 series regulations.
17. Explain the different ISO 9000 series standards with benefits.
18. Describe the ISO 14000 standards.
19. What is NABL? Give its benefits.
20. Enlist the different fields that seek NABL accreditation.
21. Describe the process of getting NABL approval and accreditation.
22. Define GLP. Give its objectives.
23. Discuss the various key elements of GLP system.

17

Indian Regulatory Requirements

Learning Objectives

After going through this chapter, you would be able to:

1. Understand the organization and functions of CDSCO.
2. Know the organizational structure and responsibilities of state licensing authority.
3. Understand the concept and documentation of certificate of pharmaceutical product (COPP).
4. Explain the drug regulatory approval process in India.
5. Understand the regulatory requirements and approval process of new drugs in India.

17.1 INTRODUCTION

Central Drugs Standard and Control Organization (CDSCO) is the main Indian regulatory authority for regulating drugs, pharmaceuticals, vaccines, medical devices and clinical trials. CDSCO serves same functions as that of FDA, EMA, PMDA, TGA, the different regulatory authorities of different countries. The Indian government has decided to put all the medical devices, IVDs, including implants and contraceptives under review of CDSCO for their regulatory approval. CDSCO is the Indian central drug authority for discharging functions assigned to Central Government of India under the provisions of Drugs & Cosmetics Act, 1940. CDSCO performs its functions under the Directorate general of Health Services, Ministry of Health and Family Welfare, Government of India.

17.2 ORGANIZATIONAL STRUCTURE OF CDSCO

17.2.1 Drugs Controller General of India (DCGI)

The DCGI is responsible for regulating and approval of new drugs, medical devices and clinical trials. In general, DCGI will be appointed by the Central Government of India and under the DCGI state drug control organization will carry out the functions. The DCGI is advised by the other authorities Drugs Technical Advisory Board (DTAB) and Drugs Consultative Committee (DCC). The headquarters of CDSCO are located at New Delhi.

The CDSCO has six zonal offices at Mumbai, Kolkata, Chennai, Ghaziabad, Ahmedabad and Hyderabad. These zonal centres are involved in GMP audits and in the inspection of premises of manufacturing plants of parenterals, vaccines, sera and blood products.

In addition to zonal offices CDSCO also has sub-zonal offices at Chandigarh, Jammu and Bengaluru. These centre coordinates with state drug control authorities which come under their jurisdiction for uniform standard inspections and enforcement. The CDSCO has its central testing laboratories at various locations of India as follows:

- Central drug laboratory, Kolkata
- Central drug testing laboratory, Mumbai
- Central drug testing laboratory, Chennai
- Regional drug testing laboratory, Guwahati
- Regional drug testing laboratory, Chandigarh

These testing laboratories perform quality control checks for assuring the quality and efficacy of drugs and cosmetics manufactured in India.

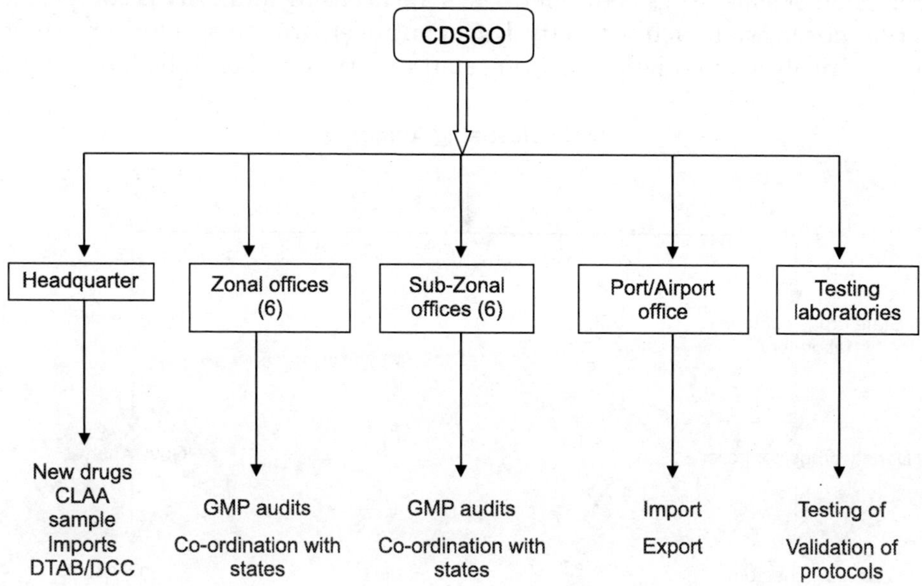

Fig. 17.1: Organizational structure of CDSCO

17.2.2 Responsibilities of CDSCO

- Approval of new drugs, biological drug products and medical devices.
- Granting permission to conduct clinical trials.
- Licensing of blood blanks, large volume parenterals, vaccines, sera, r-DNA medicinal products, medical devices and *in vitro* diagnostic agents.
- Participation in WHO, FDA, GMP certification activities.
- Amendment of provisions pertaining to Drugs & Cosmetics Act.
- Banning of certain medicinal drugs and cosmetics.
- Compilation and publication of Indian Pharmacopoeia.
- Grant to test manufacturing licence, personal licence, NOC for export of drug products.

- Testing and analysis of drugs and cosmetics by central laboratories.
- Monitoring of adverse drug reactions.
- Providing guidance on technical matters related to drugs and cosmetics.
- Co-ordination of the activities of central and state licensing authorities.
- Performing the activities as per the technical guidance of DTAB and DCC.
- Regulation of standards and control the quality of imported drugs in India.

17.3 STATE LICENSING AUTHORITY

The state licensing authority generally performs the functions assigned under the supervision and guidance of CDSCO, which is the central licensing authority. Each state of India has their own state licensing authorities to perform their functions under the supervision of state drugs controller. The state licensing authority is composed of different supporting staff such as deputy drugs controller, drugs inspector, government analyst, chief analyst and other supporting staff to carry out their functions assigned to them.

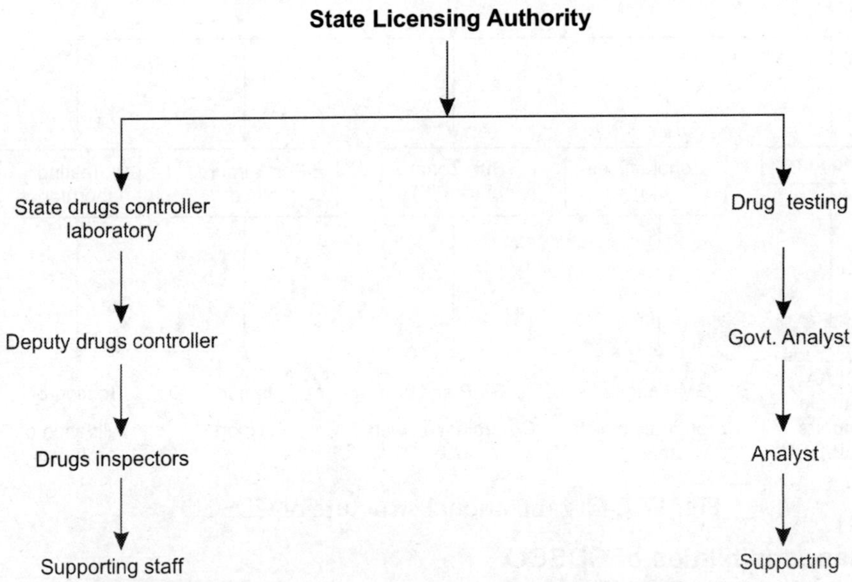

Fig. 17.2: Organizational chart of state licensing authority

17.3.1 Responsibilities of State Licensing Authority

- Issuance of licence for manufacturing, sale, distribution of drugs and drug testing laboratories.
- To carryout pre- and post-licensing inspection for drugs and cosmetics manufacturing units.
- Approval of drug products for manufacturing.
- To oversee the manufacturing process for drugs manufactured by respective state units and those marketed in the state.
- To perform the administrative actions.

- To recall the sub-standard drugs from market after market complaints.
- To conduct testing and analysis of drugs and cosmetics manufactured by respective state manufacturing units.

17.4 CERTIFICATE OF PHARMACEUTICAL PRODUCT (COPP)

17.4.1 Definition

The WHO Certification Scheme for a Certificate of Pharmaceutical Product (COPP) is an international voluntary agreement to provide assurance to countries participating in the scheme, about the quality of pharmaceutical products moving in international commerce.

Certificate of pharmaceutical product is a scheme developed by the WHO in response to the request of WHO member states to facilitate international trade in pharmaceutical products between member states. It was first developed in 1975. Since then it was revised in 1988, 1992 and in 1997.

17.4.2 Purpose

A COPP is in the format recommended by the WHO. It is the importing country who requires the COPP for the pharmaceutical product and a special type of certificate which enables a given pharmaceutical product to be registered and marketed in the exporting country of interest and forms parts of the marketing authorization application.

This certificate describes the characteristics of the medicinal product approved in the exporting country, includes information about the applicant of the certificate and is according to the model recommended by the World Health Organization. This is a certificate issued by the inspectorate establishing the status of the pharmaceutical, biological, radiopharmaceutical or veterinary product listed and the GMP status of the fabricator of the product.

Ideally, a COPP should not be required in countries that have the capabilities to conduct full reviews. The COPP should be used when a pharmaceutical product is under consideration for a product licence/marketing authorisation or when administrative action is required to renew, extend or vary such a licence.

17.4.3 Aim and Scope

The COPP is a legal document that declares a certain manufacturing company is legally allowed to sell their pharmaceutical product in the country they are producing. When registering a pharmaceutical product overseas, the Government body in charge of approving the application will usually require a COPP to ensure that the product is being sold as a commercial finished product in the country that is producing it.

A COPP demonstrates in question that the imported medicine is of the appropriate standard of quality, safety and efficacy to allow marketing in their market, having undergone rigorous testing and examination to regulatory authorities in the exporting country and also demonstrates that it follows the correct guidelines and procedures of good manufacturing practice (GMP), increasing the level of quality and indeed safety of the product. The COPP is needed when the product is intended for registration or its renewal (licensing, authorization or prolongation) by the importing country, with the scope that the product is distributed or commercialized in that country.

Certification has been recommended by WHO to help undersized drug regulatory authorities or drug regulatory authorities without proper quality assurance facilities in importing countries to assess the quality of pharmaceutical products as prerequisite of registration or importation.

17.4.4 Types of COPP

1. WHO 1975 type COPP

The WHO 1975 version is a certificate to be issued by exporting country regulatory authority stating: a) the authorized product has to be placed on the market for its use in the country also, the permit number and issue date, or b) that the non-authorized product has been placed on the market for its use in the country and also add the reasons why it is needed; Also, that; a) As recommended by World Health Organization, the manufacturer of the product conforms to GMP requirements. b) Only within the country of origin the products to be sold or distributed; or c) To be exported to manufacturing plant where the product is produced and at suitable intervals subject to inspections.

2. WHO 1988 type COPP

Unlike the WHO 1975 version, the competent authority of the exporting country should have: all labelled copies and product's detailed information in the country of origin.

3. WHO 1992 type COPP

This is intended for use by the competent authority of an importing country in two situations:

(a) When the question arises related to importation and sale licence.
(b) For licence renew, extend, review or changes.

The following information is required for the certificate:

- Whether a licensed product is required to be placed on the market or not.
- Also if the satisfied information submitted by the applicant that the certifying authority of the manufacture of the product undertaken by another party.
- Inspection has been carried out of the manufacturer of product.
- If the certificate is provisional or permanent.
- Is the dosage forms, packages and/or labels of a finished dosage form manufactured by an independent company or by the applicant?
- State the names of the importing and exporting (certifying) countries.

Here besides three types of COPPs also we have another specific type of the U.S. FDA COPPs. The U.S. FDA issued "Pilot- COPP" for the remaining products which are neither exported nor manufactured in the United States. It is only when no other country has given an approval for the finished medicinal product registration.

17.4.5 Content of the COPP

A CPP has two distinct parts:

(a) Evidence of quality, safety, and efficacy (QSE) Review
(b) Evidence of compliance with GMP.

Content and format

- Importing country
- Exporting country
- Name, form of dosage and its composition of the product (API per unit dose).
- Registration information (licensing)
- Marketing status of the product in the exporting country.
- Licence no. of the product (containing licence holder details; involvement of licence holder in manufacturing if any) and also add date of issue.
- Summary of technical basis on which the product has been licenced (if required by the issuing authority)
- Currently marketed product's information
- Details about the product's applicant
- If lacking is there in the exporting country, need to mention the information about reasons.

Key challenges of the interpretation of the COPP scheme

- Difference in product names between certifying and requesting countries.
- The COPP confirms GMP status, additional GMP certificates should not be necessary.
- The COPP is a legal document, additional apostille and/or legalization should not be requested.
- Requirements for the 'country of origin' or 'source country' have multiple definitions and should be clarified as it could refer to the country of any one of the following: first approval or marketing, manufacture, packaging, final release, or main headquarters of the pharmaceutical company.
- The COPP provides evidence of a positive QSE review in the issuing country. A full dossier should not be requested.
- The scheme refers only to the manufacturer of the dosage form but some importing countries require additional manufacturers to be listed.
- The COPP issued is a snapshot of the market authorization (MA) in the issuing country and may not necessarily reflect the entire situation in the importing country.

Advantages of the scheme

- To grow business in foreign country, necessary to obtain the COPP certificates by pharmaceutical companies.
- The scheme provides the standard format that is expected to be used.
- Enables recipient COPP countries to gain assurance on the QSE of the product in the issuing country.

- Obliges certifying authorities to disclose important information to the importing country.
- By supporting the review and approval process it facilitates patient's access to quality medicines.

The COPP may be required to support a regulatory submission. This can be submitted at the beginning of, or during the health authority review. According to the WHO scheme, COPPs should not be required in countries that require full ICH CTD dossiers and have the capability to conduct full QSE reviews.

The COPP only reflects the approved manufacturing sourcing route of the certifying country.

Most recipient authorities expect that the drug product they will receive mirrors that which has been approved by the authority issuing the COPP. When developing a global submission strategy COPP requirements are considered early during the planning phase. If required HAs should be open to discussion in advance of the regulatory submission to give advice and agree on the content of the submission including the COPP to move forward as quickly possible.

17.5 CERTIFICATE OF A PHARMACEUTICAL PRODUCT

This certificate, which is in the format recommended by WHO establishes the status of the pharmaceutical product and of the applicant for the certificate in the exporting country. It is for a single product only since manufacturing arrangements and approved information for different dosage forms and different strengths can vary.

The COPP provides the information of the following.

1. **Certificate no. of COPP:** The certificate number of COPP should be enclosed in the specified format recommended by WHO.
2. **Name of exporting country** i.e. (certifying country): The name of the country (certified country) to which the product is being exported must be mentioned in the certificate.
3. **Name of importing country,** i.e. (requesting country): The name of the countries (requesting countries) from which the product is being imported from certified country must be mentioned in the certificate.
4. **Name and dosage form of the product:**

Table 17.1: Essentials of product

Active ingredient	International non-proprietary names (INNs) or national non-proprietary names
Amount per unit dose	The formula (complete composition) of the dosage form should be given on the certificate or be appended.
Complete composition including excipients	Details of quantitative composition are preferred but their provision is subject to the agreement of the product licence holder.
Is this product licensed to be placed on the market for use in the exporting country?(yes/no)	When applicable, append details of any restriction applied to the sale, distribution or administration of the product that is specified in the product licence.

5. Status of the product actually on the market in the exporting country

If the product is actually marketed in the exporting country, the COPP should be provided with the following details:

- Number of product licence and date of issue: Indicate, when applicable, if the licence is provisional, or the product has not yet been approved.
- Product licence holder (name and address):
- Status of product licence holder:

Specify whether the person responsible for placing the product on the market:

(a) Manufactures the dosage form.

(b) Packages and/or labels a dosage form manufactured by an independent company.

(c) Involved in none of the above.

- **For categories b and c** the name and address of the manufacturer producing the dosage form, is this information can only be provided with the consent of the product's licence holder or, in the case of non-registered products, the applicant. Non-completion of this section indicates that the party concerned has not agreed to inclusion of this information. It should be noted that information concerning the site of production is part of the product licence. If the production site is changed, the licence has to be updated or it is no longer valid.
- Is a summary basis for approval appended? (yes/no).

This refers to the document, prepared by some national regulatory authorities, that summarizes the technical basis on which the product has been licensed.

- Is the attached, officially approved product information complete and consonant with the license? (yes/no/not provided).

This refers to product information approved by the competent national regulatory authority, such as summary product sharacteristics (SPC).

- Applicant for certificate, if different from licence holder (name and address). In this circumstance, permission for issuing the certificate is required from the product's licence holder. This permission has to be provided to the authority by the applicant.

6. Periodic inspection of the manufacturing plant by the certifying authority

If the certifying authority arranges for periodic inspection of the manufacturing plant in which the dosage form is produced, the following details are to be included in the COPP.

- Periodicity of routine inspections (years)
- Has the manufacture of this type of dosage form been inspected? (yes/no)
- Do the facilities and operations conform to GMP as recommended by the World Health Organization? (yes/no/not applicable)

7. The information submitted by the applicant satisfy the certifying authority on all aspects of the manufacture of the product undertaken by another party

This section is to be completed when the product's licence holder or applicant conforms to status.

(b) or (c) as described in note above. It is of particular importance when foreign contractors are involved in the manufacture of the product. In these circumstances the applicant should supply the certifying authority with information to identify the contracting parties responsible for each stage of manufacture of the finished dosage form, and the extent and nature of any controls exercised over each of these parties.

8. Other details of Manufacturing premises

The following details which is to be enclosed in the COPP are:

- Address of certifying authority
- Telephone and Fax
- Name of authorized person
- Signature
- Stamp and date

17.6 TYPES OF DRUGS FOR WHICH COPP MAY BE ISSUED

- Approved drug products
- Active pharmaceutical ingredients (API)
- Over-the-counter drug (OTC) products
- Unapproved drug products
- Homeopathic drugs

Who can apply for COPP?

A complete application for export certification must be submitted by the person/ company who exports the drug.

The certification is intended for a drug which meets the applicable requirements of the Act or Food Drug and Cosmetic Act 801(e)(1) requirements [21 U.S.C.381(e)(1)].

Process to apply for a COPP:

(A) Submit Form no. 3613b– Located on the FDA internet www.fda.gov/downloads/ AboutFDA/Reports Manuals Forms/Forms/UCM052388

(B) Requirements for COPP application:

- Applicant contact information
- Trade name (the drug product's brand name)
- Bulk substance generic name
- Name of applicant
- Status of product licence holder
- Listing of manufacturing location on COPP
- Complete manufacturing facility address
- Facility registration number
- Importing countries
- Authorization to release information

- Number of certificates requested
- Certification statement
- Billing contact
- Marketing status in the exporting country

Process Time of COPP

- Drugs in compliance are normally issued within twenty government working days of receipt of complete and an accurate COPP application.
- Certificates may not be issued.
- Returned – missing information application with a letter identifying the missing information.
- Rejected – manufacturing facilities are not in compliance with good manufacturing practices (GMPs).
- Denied – drug products are not in compliance as per regulation (e.g., misbranded drug).
- Expiration of COPP.
- Certificate expires on 2 years from the notarization date or as noted.
- After expiry date, a new COPP application has to be submitted.

Format of Certificate of Pharmaceutical Products (COPP) (as per WHO GMP guidelines)

No. of certificate: ....

Exporting (certifying) country: ....

Importing (requesting) country: ....

Name and dosage form of product: ....

Active ingredient(s) and amount(s) per unit dose: ....

1. Is this product licensed to be placed on the market for use in the exporting country? If yes, complete Box A. If No complete Box B.

A.

Product's -licence holder (name and address):

Status of licence holder: a/b/c (key in appropriate category)

Number of product licence and date of issue: ----------------------------

Is an approved technical summary appended? Yes/ No

Is the attached, officially approved product information complete and in consonance with the licence? Yes/no/not provided (key in as appropriate)

Applicant for certificate, if different from licence holder (name and address): ------------
----

B.

Applicant for certificate (name and address): ---

Status of applicant: a/b/c (key in appropriate category) Why is marketing authorization lacking?

Not required/not requested/under consideration/refused (key is as appropriate) Remark:

2. Does the certifying authority arrange for periodic inspection of the manufacturing plant in which the dosage form is produced? Yes/no/not applicable (key in as appropriate)

If no or not applicable proceed to question 3.

2.1 Periodicity of routine inspections (years): ....

2.2 Has the manufacture of this type of dosage form been inspected? Yes/no (key in as appropriate)

2.3 Do the facilities and operations conform to GMP as recommended by the World Health Organization? Yes/no (key in as appropriate)

3. Does the information submitted by the applicant satisfy the certifying authority on all aspects of the manufacture of the product? Yes/no (key in as appropriate)

If no, explain: ....

Address of certifying authority: ....

Telephone number: ....

Fax number: ....

Name of authorized person: ....

Signature: ....

Stamp and date: ....

17.7 APPROVAL OF NEW DRUG IN INDIA

If any company in India wants to manufacture or import a new drug, they need to apply to seek permission from the licensing authority (DCGI) by filling in Form 44 also submitting the data as given in Schedule Y of Drugs and Cosmetics Act, 1940 and Rules 1945.To prove its efficacy and safety in Indian population they need to conduct clinical trials in accordance with the guidelines specified in Schedule Y and submit the report of such clinical trials in specified format.

Demonstration of safety and efficacy of the drug product for use in humans is essential before the drug product can be approved for import or manufacturing of new drug by the applicant by Central Drugs Standard Control Organization (CDSCO). The regulations under Drugs and Cosmetics Act, 1940 and its rules 1945, 122A, 122B and 122D describe the information required for approval of an application to import or manufacture of new drug for marketing. For an investigational new drug, the sponsor needs to provide detailed information to the DCGI about:

1. Generic name
2. Patient status
3. Brief description of physicochemical/biological
4. Technical information like
   - (a) Stability
   - (b) Specifications
   - (c) Manufacturing process
   - (d) Worldwide regulatory status
   - (e) Animal pharmacology and toxicity studies

5. Published clinical trial reports
6. Proposed protocol and pro forma
7. Trial duration
8. Drug master file
9. Undertaking to report serious or life-threatening adverse drug reactions.

The information regarding the prescription, samples and testing protocols, product monographs, labels must also be submitted. It usually takes three months for clinical trial approval in India. The clinical trials can be registered in the Clinical Trials Registry of India (CTRI) giving details of the clinical trials and the subjects involved in the trials. The rules to be followed under the Drugs and Cosmetics Rules, 1945 are:

1. Rule 122 A : Application for permission to import new drug.
2. Rule 122 B: Application for approval to manufacture new drug other than the drugs specified under Schedule C and C (1).
3. Rule 22 D: P Application for permission to import or manufacture fixed dose combination.
4. Rule 122 DA: Application for permission to conduct clinical trials for new drug/ investigational new drug.
5. Rule 122 E: Definition of new drugs

There's a provision in Rule-122A of Drug and Cosmetic Act, 1940 and Rules, 1945, that if the licensing authority finds out that if everything is in the interest of public health then he may allow the import of new drugs, based on the data of the trials done in other countries. Another provision, Rule-122A, is that clinical trial may be allowed in any new drug case, which are approved and already being used for many years in other countries.

Similarly, in Rule 122-B, application for approval to manufacture new drug other than the drugs classifiable under Schedules C and C (1) and permission to import or manufacture fixed dose combination (122-D).

17.7.1 Purpose

The main purpose of regulating all the medicinal products by regulatory agencies is to safeguard public health. Regulatory agencies' work is to make sure that the pharmaceutical companies comply with all the regulations and standards, so that the patient's well-being is protected. Through the International Conference on Harmonization (ICH) process, the common technical document (CTD) guidance has been developed for Japan, European Union, and United States. Most countries have adopted the CTD format. Hence, CDSCO has also decided to adopt CTD format for technical requirements for registration of pharmaceutical products for human use.

It is apparent that this structured application with comprehensive and rational contents will help the CDSCO to review and take necessary actions in a better way and would also ease the preparation of electronic submissions, which may happen in the near future at CDSCO.

17.7.2 New Drug Application (NDA)

New drug application (NDA) is an application submitted to the individual regulatory authority for authorization to market a new drug, i.e., innovative product. To gain this permission a sponsor submits pre-clinical and clinical test data for analyzing the drug information, description of manufacturing procedures.

After NDA receives by the agency, it undergoes a technical screening. This evaluation ensures that sufficient data and information have been submitted in each area to justify "filing" the application that is FDA formal review.

At the conclusion of FDA review of an NDA, there are three possible actions that can send to sponsor:

- Not approvable: In this letter list of deficiencies and explain the reason.
- Approvable : It means that the drug can be approved but minor deficiencies that can be corrected like labelling changes and possible request commitment to do post-approval studies.
- Approval: It state that the drug is approved.

If the action taken is either an approvable or a not approvable, then FDA provides applicant with an opportunity to meet the agency and discuss the deficiencies.

Phases of clinical trials

- Pre-clinical study: Mice, rat, rabbit, monkeys
- Phase I: Human pharmacology trial, estimation of safety and tolerability
- Phase II: Exploratory trial, estimation of effectiveness and short-term side effects
- Phase III: Confirmatory trial, confirmation of therapeutic benefits
- Phase IV: Post-marketing trial, studies done after drug approval

Some of the rules and guidelines that should be followed for regulation of drugs in India are:

- Drugs and Cosmetics Act, 1940 and its Rules, 1945
- Narcotic Drugs and Psychotropic Substances, 1985
- Drugs Price Control Order, 1995
- Consumer Protection Act, 1986
- Factories Act, 1948
- Law of Contracts (Indian Contract Act, 1872)
- Monopolistic & Restrictive Trade Practices Act, 1969
- ICH GCP Guidelines
- Schedule Y Guidelines
- ICMR Guidelines
- Registry of Trial

Stages of approval

1. Submission of clinical trial application for evaluating safety and efficacy.
2. Requirements for permission of new drugs approval.
3. Post-approval changes in biological products: quality, safety and efficacy documents.
4. Preparation of the quality information for drug submission for new drug approval.

1. Submission of Clinical Trial Application for Evaluating Safety and Efficacy

All the data listed below has to be produced.

(a) Phase-I & phase-II clinical trials

I. General information

- Introduction about company: Brief description about company
- Administrative headquarters: Provide address of company headquarters
- Manufacturing facilities: Provide address of company headquarters
- Regulatory and intellectual property status in other countries.
- Patent information status in India and other countries

II. Chemistry manufacturing control

- Product description: A brief description of the drug and the therapeutic class to which it belongs.
- Product development
- Strain details
- Information on drug substance
- Information on drug product

III. Non-clinical data: References: schedule - Y, amendment version 2005, Drugs and Cosmetics Rules, 1945

IV. Proposed phase-I / II studies: protocol for phase-I / II studies

(b) Phase-III clinical trial

All the information is as same as phase-I & phase- II clinical trials

- General information
- Chemistry manufacturing control
- Non-clinical data
- Proposed phase-III studies

2. Requirements for permission of new drugs approval

The manufacturer/sponsor has to submit application on Form 44 for permission of New Drugs Approval under the provisions of Drugs and Cosmetic Act, 1940 and Rules, 1945. The document design is as per the international submission requirements of common technical document (CTD) and has five modules.

Module I: Administrative/Legal Information

This module should contain documents specific to each region; for example, application forms or the proposed label for use in the region. The content and format of this module can be specified by the relevant regulatory authorities.

Module II: Summaries

Module 2 should begin with a general introduction to the pharmaceutical, including its pharmacologic class, mode of action and proposed clinical use. In general, the introduction should not exceed one page. The introduction should include proprietary name, non-proprietary name or common name of the drug substance, company name, dosage form(s), strength(s), route of administration, and proposed indication(s). It contains the CTD summaries for quality, safety, efficacy information. This module is very important, as it provides detailed summaries of the various sections of the CTD. These include: A very short introduction, quality overall summary, non clinical overview, clinical overview, non-clinical written and tabulated summaries for pharmacology, pharmacokinetics, and toxicology.

Module III: Quality information (Chemical, pharmaceutical and biological)

Information on quality should be presented in the structured format described in the guidance M4Q. This document is intended to provide guidance on the format of a registration application for drug substances and their corresponding drug products. It contains all the quality documents for the chemistry, manufacture, and controls of the drug substance and the drug product.

Module IV: Non-clinical information

Information on safety should be presented in the structured format described in the guidance M4S. The purpose of this section is to present a critical analysis of the non-clinical data pertinent to the safety of the medicinal product in the intended population. The analysis should consider all relevant data, whether positive or negative, and should explain why and how the data support the proposed indication and prescribing information. It gives final copy of all of the final non-clinical study reports.

Module V: Clinical information

Information on efficacy should be presented in the structured format described in the guidance M4E. It gives clinical summary including biopharmaceutics, pharmacokinetics and pharmacodynamics, clinical pharmacology studies, clinical efficacy, clinical safety, synopses of the individual studies and final copy of detailed clinical study reports.

3. Preparation of the quality information for drug submission for new drug approval

1. Drug substance (name, manufacturer)
2. Characterization (name, manufacturer)
    - Physicochemical characterization
    - Biological characterization
3. Drug product (name, dosage form)
4. Control of drug product (name, dosage form)
5. Appendices
    - Facilities and equipment (name, manufacturer)
    - Safety evaluation adventitious agents (name, dosage form, manufacturer).

Fees for Clinical Trial/Approval of New Drugs

- Phase I (IND) ₹ 50,000
- Phase II (IND) ₹ 25,000

- Phase III (IND) ₹ 25,000
- Approval of new molecule ₹ 50,000
- Approved new drug: Within 1 year of approval ₹ 50,000
  After 1 year of approval ₹ 15,000
- Approval of new claim, new dosage form, etc., ₹ 15,000.

REVIEW QUESTIONS

1. Discuss the new drug application process for the approval of new drugs.
2. Discuss the Indian regulatory requirements for drug registration.
3. Write the roles and responsibilities of state licensing authorities.
4. Write the CDSCO regulatory requirements for new drugs in India.
5. Discuss the organizational structure and functions of CDSCO.
6. Explain the process of certification of pharmaceutical product (COPP) in India.
7. Write the organizational structure and functions of state licensing authority.
8. Write the regulatory requirements for the new drugs approval in India.
9. Write the requirements of COPP and its purpose.
10. Write the WHO-GMP format of Certificate of Pharmaceutical Products (COPP).

Index

A

Active pharmaceutical ingredient 271
Actuators 185
Additives 68
Aerosol package, components of 179
Aerosols over other dosage forms, advantages of 179
Antimicrobial agents, use of 163
Approved regulatory bodies and agencies 280
Aquasol system 188
Asian and Pacific Centre for Transfer of Technology 281

B

Balling 94
Basic biostatistics approach 316
Bioequivalence studies 311
  types of 312
Biopharmaceutical classification
  significance of 15
  system 14
Biostatistics, commonly used terms in 316
Biotech Consortium India Limited 281

C

Capsule shell, components of 79
  production of 79
Capsules
  quality control tests for 84
  sizes of 80
  special techniques in 83
Central Drugs Standards Control Organization (CDSCO) 291
  organizational structure of 346
  responsibilities of 347
Certificate of Pharmaceutical Product (COPP) 349, 352
  content of 351
  types of 350
Change control 333
  principles of 333
  scope 333
  steps in 334
Changes, classification of 334
Chemical stability 11
Clarity 164
Cleaning 275
Clinical research protocol 313
Clinical trials, management of 319
Closures 110
Coated tablet, quality control test for 60
Coating equipment 52
Coating solution, general formulation of 56
Cold cream 211
  characteristics 211
  formulation of 211
  method of preparation of 211
Cold filling apparatus 191
Colourants 59
Comparative clinical studies 313
Compounding 138
Compressed gas filling apparatus 192
Compression 94
Compression granulation 23
Containers 110, 182
  factors influencing choice of 231–233
  legal and official requirements for 233

D

Damp mass 27
  screening into pellets or granules 28
Direct compression 22
Dispersion system 188
Dissolution parameters 45
Documentation 279
Drug approval regulatory, requirements for 296
Drug content tests 41
Drug content, uniformity of 41
Drug development teams 296
Drug metabolism 300
Drug release tests 42
Drugs Controller General of India (DCGI) 346
Dry powder layering 94
Dry powders 120
Dry screening, sizing the granulation by 28

E

Emulsions 119
Ester hydrolysis 12
European Medicines Agency (EMA) 292
Excipients 272
Extrusion 91
Eye drops, containers for 172
  formulation and preparation of 168
Eye lotions and intraocular solutions, containers for 175
Eye ointments, containers for 175
  formulation and preparation of 170

F

FDA regulations 233
FDA, review process of 304
FDA submissions, data presentation for 317
Film coating, materials used for 55
  methods 50
Film defects 60
Film formers 56
Filtration 139
Foam system 189
Formulation 100

G

Glass 110
Glass containers 226
  evaluation parameters 235-236
  quality control of 235
Globulation 94
GMP considerations 245
Good laboratory practices
  basic elements of 342
  objectives 342

H

Hair dyes 216
  formulations of 216
  method of preparation 220
  requirements of 216
Hard gelatin capsule shells, production of 78
Hard gelatin capsules 77
  formulation of 81
  filling of 81
Health Canada 293
Hot melt extrusion 93
Human eye, anatomy and physiology of 154
Hydrolysis 11
Hypodermic route 98

I

In vitro dissolution studies 313
Indian regulatory requirements 346
Injection, routes of 97
Intradermal route 98
Intramuscular injection 98
Intraocular dosage forms 161
Intravenous route 98
Investigational new drug application 301
  content and format 302
  goals of 308
  types of 302
Investigator's brochure 305
ISO 14000 336
  benefits of 338
  policy 337
  standards 337
ISO 9000 335
  objectives of 335
ISO 9000 series 336
  benefits of 336
  clauses 336

L

Layering techniques 94
Letter of intent 285

Licensing strategy 283
Lipstick 200
    characteristics of 201
    formulation of 201
Liquid and semi-solid manufacturing processes
    scale-up of 254
    manufacture of 204
Liquid manufacturing, critical aspects of 252
Liquid orals, filling and packing of 75

M

Measurement scales, types of 316
Medicines and Healthcare Products Regulatory Agency (MHRA) 292
Memorandum of Understanding 285
Metal containers 229
Moist granulation 26
Multi-station press 32

N

National Accreditation Board for Testing and Calibration Laboratories (NABL) 338
        accreditation/certification process 339
        benefits of 339
National Research Development Corporation 280
Nazi experiments 290
New drug application 308
    document for 309
    review and approval of 311
New drug application 357
New drug in India, approval of 356
Non-clinical drug development 298
Non-clinical studies, types of 299

O

Ocular inserts 160
Opaquant extenders 60
Ophthalmic dosage forms 154
    packaging and labelling of 171
    requirements of 161
    types of 157
Ophthalmic emulsions 158
Ophthalmic forming solutions 157
Ophthalmic gels 159
Ophthalmic ointments 159
    manufacture of 171
Ophthalmic solutions 157
    manufacture of 169
Ophthalmic suspensions 157
Optical isomerisation 13
Out of specifications 330
Oxidation 12

P

Packaging 275
Packaging and labelling 144
Packaging materials, stability aspects of 233
    quality control of 234
Parenteral dosage forms 116
Parenterals, types of 99
Particle size 3, 167
    determination of 4
    shape of 4
Patent documents, content of 284
Patent information 284
Pelletization techniques 91-95
Pellets
    advantages of 90
    desirable properties of 95
    limitations of 91
    technological advantages 90
    therapeutic advantages 91
Pharmaceutical aerosols
    formulation of 186
    manufacture of 190
    quality control for 193
    stability testing of 192
    testing of 195
Pharmaceutical product development, biostatistics in 315
Pharmaceutical products, materials used for packaging of 226
Pharmacodynamic studies 312
Pharmacokinetic studies 312
Pharmacology 300
Pilot plant design 240
Pilot plant, operation 241
    general considerations 243
Pilot plant, scale-up for semi-solid products 253
Plastic 113
Plastic containers 227
    disadvantages of 229
    quality control of 237
Plasticizers 59

Polymerisation 13
Powder flow property 5
Preformulation 99
    applications of 15
Preformulation studies, objectives and goals of 1
Preservatives 163
Pressure filling apparatus 191
Production transfer 270
Project team 270
Propellants 180
Pyrogens, significance in parenteral dosage forms 125
    source of control 125

Q

QMS, important elements in 322
Quality assurance and control 144
Quality by design 327
    key elements of 328
Quality control 145, 324
    analytical method transfer 276
Quality improvement 324
Quality management triology, concept of 324
Quality planning 324
Quality
    aspects 323
    concept of 323
    need of 323
RA department
    basic need of 287
    historical overview of 288
    objectives of 288

R

RA department, job responsibilities of 295
RA professionals, job profile of 295
Racemisation reaction 13
Regulatory affairs department, role of 295
Regulatory authorities 290
Rotary press, features of 32
    advantages of 34
Rotary tablet machine 32
Rubber based components 230
Rubber closures 115
    quality control of 237

S

Scale-up and post-approval changes (SUPAC) 255
Sealing 141
Shampoos
    characteristics of 205
    formulation of 205
    manufacture of 210
Simple liquids 74
Single punch tablet press 31
    advantages of 32
    components/functional parts of 31
Six sigma concept 329
Six sigma methods 329
Small Industries Development Bank of India 281
Soft gelatin capsules
    composition of 86
    formulation of 86
    manufacturing of 87
    packaging and storage stability for 89
    quality control test for 88
Solutes 106
Solution system 187
Solutions 116
Solvents 58
Specialized coating 61
Spheronization 91
Spray drying 95
Stability 165
Starting materials 271
State licensing authority 348
    responsibilities of 348
Sterile solids 120
Sterility 162
Sterilization 143
Subcutaneous route 98
Subdermal implants 124
Sugar coating 47, 49
Sulphanilamide tragedy 289
Sun protection factor 221
    formulation of 221
    levels of packaging 225
    types of 223

Sunscreens 220
Surface area 3
Surfactants, use of 167
Suspension system 188
Suspensions 117
    formulation components of 72
Synthetic polymers 56
Systems, types of 187

T

Tablet compression cycle 33
Tablet compression machines 30
Tablet manufacturing, compression problems in 34
Tablet
    administered by other routes 19
    classification of 18
    defects in 34
    equipment and tooling 28
    excipients and formulation 20
    friability of 40
    general appearance 38
    ideal characteristics of 17
    ingested orally 18
    manufacturing of 22
    organoleptic properties 38
    processing problems 35
    quality control tests 37
    strength tests 39
    used in oral cavity 19
    used to prepare solutions 19
Tablets pilot plant, design for 246
Tamper proof feature 176
Technology Bureau for Small Enterprises 282
Technology Information Forecasting and Assessment Council 280
Technology of transfer 283
Thalidomide disaster 289
Therapeutic goods administration 293
Three-phase system 187
Tonicity 167
Toothpaste 213
    basic requirements of 213
    formulation of 214
    manufacture of 216
Topical ophthalmic dosage forms, site of application for 156
Topical preparations, administration for 156
Total quality management (TQM) 324
    key elements of 325
    tools for quality problem solving 325
Toxicity, types of 301
Toxicology 300
Tuskegee syphilis study 289
Two-layer system 188
Two-phase system 187

U

United States Food and Drug Administration 291
USP dissolution
    test apparatus 44
UV radiation, effects of 220

V

Valves 183
Vanishing cream 212
    characteristics of 212
    formulation of 212
    method of preparation 213
Vehicles 100
Viscosity 164

W

Water based system 187
Wet granulation 26
World Health Organization 290